Values and Visions

Changing Ideas in Services for People with Learning Difficulties

Edited by

Terry Philpot
Editor, *Community Care*

Linda Ward PhD
Senior Research Fellow, Norah Fry Research Centre,
University of Bristol; Programme Adviser (Disability),
Joseph Rowntree Foundation

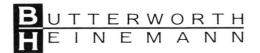

Butterworth-Heinemann Ltd
Linacre House, Jordan Hill, Oxford OX2 8DP

A member of the Reed Elsevier group

OXFORD   LONDON   BOSTON
MUNICH   NEW DELHI   SINGAPORE   SYDNEY
TOKYO   TORONTO   WELLINGTON

First published 1995

British Library Cataloguing in Publication Data
A catalogue record for this book is available from the British Library.

ISBN 0 7506 2248 2

Typeset by Wilmaset Ltd, Birkenhead, Wirral
Printed in England by Biddles Ltd, Guildford and Kings Lynn

Contents

List of Contributors

Peter Allen

Peter Allen is the head of a clinical psychology service in the East End of London, where he has worked since 1984. In this time he has been centrally involved in the return of people with learning difficulties to the community from a hospital in Essex. He is strongly committed to the development of high quality services, and to the inclusion of people with learning disabilities in shaping, commenting on and influencing their services. He is an associate consultant with the National Development Team, and has also worked in the local authority sector and with a voluntary organisation.

Dorothy Atkinson

Dorothy Atkinson is a senior lecturer in the School of Health and Social Welfare at the Open University. Her background is in social work and social work education, and includes several years' experience of working with people with learning difficulties. Her research has included looking at the social networks of people with learning difficulties living in the community. Her OU work has been primarily in the learning field, including editing (with Fiona Williams) the anthology *Know Me As I Am*. Her current interest is in exploring how biographical and oral history approaches can enable people with learning difficulties, especially women, to find out and reclaim their individual and shared pasts.

Carol Baxter

Carol Baxter is senior lecturer in race and health, University of Central Lancashire. She was previously an independent consultant primarily concerned with equal opportunities and service research within the public and voluntary sector. She has written extensively on the subject of equity within health and social welfare agencies and is a leading authority on the development of service access policies. She is co-author (with K. Poonia, Z. Nadirshaw and L. Ward) of *Double Discrimination: Services for People with Learning Difficulties From Black and Ethnic Minority Communities* (1990).

Stephen Beyer

Stephen Beyer has worked as a researcher on services for people with disabilities in the voluntary, social services and university sectors. Now deputy director of the Welsh Centre for Learning Disabilities – Applied Research Unit, he has been associated for many years with research and development in the context of the All-Wales Strategy. Over the last ten years he has been particularly associated with research and development in supported employment, day centres and in other forms of day provision in Wales. Stephen Beyer has also been involved in national initiatives on Quality Action, and the changeover of day centres to new forms of support. He is currently the secretary of the Association of Supported Employment Agencies which promotes good practice in supported employment and campaigns for its wider availability as an important route into employment for people with learning disabilities.

Tim Booth

Tim Booth is professor of social policy in the Department of Sociological Studies at the University of Sheffield. He is the author of several books including *Home Truths: Old People's Homes and the Outcome of Care* (Gower, 1985), *Developing Policy Research* (Gower, 1988), *Outward Bound: Relocation and Community Care for People with Learning Difficulties* (with K. Simons and W. Booth, Open University Press, 1990) and *Parenting Under Pressure: Mothers and Fathers with Learning Difficulties* (with W. Booth, Open University Press, 1994)

Wendy Booth

Wendy Booth is a research associate in the Department of Sociological Studies at Sheffield University. She is the adviser to Huddersfield People First, a member of the Maternity Alliance Disability Working Group and a citizen advocate. She is co-author (with T. Booth and K. Simons) of *Outward Bound: Relocation and Community Care for People with Learning Difficulties* (Open University Press, 1990) and *Parenting Under Pressure: Mothers and Fathers with Learning Difficulties* (with T. Booth, Open University Press, 1994)

Hilary Brown

Hilary Brown has a background in education and residential care in Britain and the USA and has been involved in staff training at a senior level in health, social services and the voluntary sector. She has worked on training materials and training for trainers and has a long-standing interest in sexuality issues for people with learning disabilities. She has also completed a course in organisational consultancy at the Tavistock Institute. She is currently directing research on the sexual abuse of adults with learning disabilities and difficult sexual behaviours. Her publications include: *Lifestyles and the Bringing People Back Home* series of video-assisted training packs; with A. Craft (eds) *Thinking the Unthinkable: Papers on Sexual Abuse and People with Learning Difficulties* (1989, FPA) and *Working with the Unthinkable: A Trainers' Manual on the Sexual Abuse of Adults with Learning Disabilities* (1992, FPA); with H. Smith, 'Whose ordinary life is it anyway? A feminist critique of the normalisation principle'. *Disability, Handicap and Society*, (1989) 4:224 and *Normalisation: A Reader for the 1990s* (1991, Routledge); with V. Turk, Defining sexual abuse as it affects adults with learning disabilities. *Mental Handicap*, (1992) 20(2), 44–55 and The sexual abuse of adults with learning disabilities: Results of a two year incidence survey. *Mental Handicap Research*,

(1993) 6(3), 193–216. Recent papers include: Lost in the system: The filtering of knowledge about the abuse of adults with learning disabilities (In press, *Care in Place*) and 'An ordinary sexual life?: A review of the normalisation principle as it applies to the sexual options of people with learning disabilities. *Disability, Handicap and Society*, 9(2).

Paul Cambridge

Before joining the centre in 1992, Paul Cambridge worked at the Personal Social Services Research Unit (PSSRU) and in local government. His work at the PSSRU included a series of research projects which included the government's 1983 Care in the Community Programme, an evaluation of the long-term outcomes and costs of care in the community for people with learning difficulties and a comparison of the quality and costs of services provided by community support teams for people with learning difficulties and challenging behaviours (with J. Mansell and E. Emerson). His research interests are the organisational processes of community care (commissioning inter-agency working and care management) and HIV and people with learning difficulties (including men with learning difficulties who have sex with men). His publications include *Demonstrating Successful Care in the Community* (with M. Knapp, 1988, University of Kent), *Evaluating the Challenge* (with E. Emerson and P. Harris, 1991, King's Fund Centre), *Care in the Community: Challenge and Demonstration* (with M. Knapp *et al.*, 1992, Ashgate) and papers on case management and HIV in community services.

Jean Collins

Jean Collins worked with people with learning difficulties for ten years before studying social anthropology at the London School of Economics. Awarded a BSc in 1985 she went on to earn a DPhil at the University of Sussex. Her doctoral thesis examined social support systems in England, and she has contributed widely to the debate on community care. She has also taught social anthropology and undertaken detailed research into the social implications of divorce law. She became assistant director of Values Into Action, the national campaign with people who have learning difficulties, in 1991 and director in 1994.

Ann Davis

Ann Davis is director of social work research and development, the Department of Social Policy and Social Work, the University of Birmingham. She has worked with people with learning difficulties as a residential social worker, a local authority field social worker and a welfare rights trainer and advocate. She has a particular interest in issues of poverty, social security and community care and has researched and written on the subject.

Ruth Eley

Ruth Eley is head of adult services in Liverpool social services directorate. She has a particular interest in the involvement of service users in planning and delivering services and in anti-discriminatory practice within services.

Lynne Elwell

Lynne Elwell worked as a photographer until having her children. When Nicola, the second of her five children, became disabled at the age of eight months, she decided to stay at home to support her. Until she was 14, Nicola took part at home in an intensive programme of intellectual and physical stimulation. Through Nicola, Lynne became aware of the traditional response to disabled people from society and services. For the past ten years Lynne Elwell has worked on behalf of her daughter, taking part in and leading training, working with families and recently through citizen advocacy and circles of support. She is also renewing her interest in photography to produce positive images of disabled people.

Pat Fitton

Pat Fitton's experience of profound and multiple disabilities comes from caring for her daughter Kathy, who died in 1991 at the age of 27. She worked in several parents' groups to improve services and has campaigned to increase parental participation in planning procedures in social services and health. She has recently taken early retirement after teaching in inner London secondary schools since 1964. During her last post as deputy headteacher she was involved with the integration into mainstream of children with a range of disabilities. Her book *Listen to Me: Communicating the Needs of People with profound Intellectual and Multiple Disabilities* (Jessica Kingsley Publishers, 1994) details strategies for parents and carers based on Kathy's life. With Jean Willson and Carol O'Brien she has written *Home at Last* (1995), which gives a detailed account of the project set up for her daughter and that of Jean Willson.

Margaret Flynn

Margaret Flynn is an assistant director of the National Development Team. She is interested in policy, legislation, research and planning as it relates to people with learning difficulties.

Peter Flynn

Peter Flynn lives by himself. He does lots of voluntary work which he enjoys. He especially likes doing errands for people such as shopping. He also likes working with older people. He loves going to college where he studies maths and computers. He has quite a few credits for maths and English at college. He keeps an eye on his family by visiting them. He has friends and likes seeing them.

Rob Hancock

Rob Hancock is senior education officer and team leader of the Disability, Advisory, and Resource Team in South Glamorgan. He has worked and taught in a variety of continuing education settings, including the South Glamorgan

Community Education Service, colleges of further education in the voluntary sector, and Henley College. Contributions to other publications include *Widening Horizons* (1981) and *Towards Integration* (1989).

Bob Hudson

Bob Hudson is a visiting fellow in community care studies at the Institute of Health Studies, University of Durham and senior lecturer in social policy at New College Durham. He has spent many years teaching front-line professionals and managers in health and social care, and is now working on a consultancy basis on a variety of projects related to the health and community care reforms. He writes a regular feature for the *Health Service Journal* on policy issues and has published widely in academic quarterlies. His latest book, *Making Sense of Markets in Health and Social Care* was published in 1994.

Michelle McCarthy

Michelle McCarthy originally trained as a social worker and worked in what was then called a community mental handicap team. She later worked for four years with David Thompson on the Sex Education Team (formerly the AIDS Awareness/Sex Education Project). As part of her work on this team she was involved in individual and group work with women with learning difficulties, staff training and consultancy and policy development. In 1993 she was appointed lecturer in learning disability in the Tizard Centre at the University of Kent, where she is involved in teaching, research and consultancy. She is also currently studying for a PhD, researching the sexual experiences and sexual abuse of women with learning difficulties.

Mary Myers

Mary Myers is a consultant psychiatrist for people with learning difficulties, and for 20 years has worked in Sheffield and Rotherham. She has been involved in the King's Fund 'An Ordinary Life' initiative since its origins in 1979, and contributed to the National Development Team's activities during the same period. Following a study tour in 1983 of value-based and individualised community services in the USA, she has continued to visit and learn from transatlantic experiences, including new approaches to the needs of people whose behaviour challenges us to understand them. Mary Myers provides consultancy and training for special needs, and is special adviser in learning disabilities to the North West Regional Health Authority.

Connie Lyle O'Brien and John O'Brien

Connie Lyle O'Brien and John O'Brien learn, along with people with disabilities, their families and friends, and innovative service providers, about how communities become better able to support all their members. Their work involves them in action-learning projects to increase the openness of schools, neighbourhoods, workplaces and associations, and to improve the effectiveness of support services. Their affiliation with the Centre on Human Policy at Syracuse University provides the opportunity for reflection and enables them to write about what they learn with activists and innovators. Connie Lyle O'Brien provided direct services to people moving out of institutions and worked as an organiser of family members wanting to advocate for better schools and community services. Her recent major projects include working with disabled people to redesign personal assistance services (attendant care) policies in order to allow substantially disabled people to live in their own home, and working with parents and teachers to create inclusive school classrooms. She is an associate editor of *Mental Retardation: A Journal of Policy and Perspectives*. John O'Brien provided direct services to people in institutions, lived in a group home, worked in a day service, and worked on a management team responsible for the design, management and evaluation of a regional service system. He is currently studying the organisation of the work of supporting inclusion. He is an associate consultant with the National Development Team in the UK.

Terry Philpot

Terry Philpot is editor of *Community Care*. He had edited several books, including *Social Work* (Lion, 1985) and *Last Things: Social Work with the Dying and Bereaved* (1989). He is co-editor (with C. Hanvey) of *Practising Social Work* (Routledge, 1993) and of *Sweet Charity: The Role and Workings of Voluntary Organisations* (to be published by Routledge). He is author of *Managing to Listen: A Guide to User Involvement for Mental Health Service Managers* (King's Fund Centre, 1994). He is also the author of *Action For Children* (Lion, 1994). He is an honorary member of the council of the NSPCC and was formerly a member of the social work committee of NCH Action for Children and of the advisory council for the Centre for Policy on Ageing. He has won several awards for his journalism. In 1990 he visited Czechoslovakia, as a British Council fellow, to look at services for people with learning difficulties. He has won several awards for journalism.

Helen Platts

Helen Platts has worked in social services and the voluntary sector, managing and developing services for people with learning difficulties. She is currently general manager at the National Development Team for People with a Learning Disability where she is involved in consultancy and policy advice work. Her particular interests include day services and involving service users in the management and development of organisations.

Gillian Rees

Gillian Rees works at the McIntyre Garden Centre in Bromley where she is studying agriculture along with Maths and English. She also works at Oakfield day centre where she does packing work and goes to an English group. Recently she took part in the Jobsearch programme at Oakfield which led to her working at Sainsbury's for work experience. She has also been awarded the English Speaking Board's Levels 1, 2 and 3 for excellence in spoken communication. She lives at Selby Houses, a group home in south London, where she is a member of the management committee.

Diane Richler

Diane Richler is executive vice-president of the Canadian Association for Community Living, which works to assist communities to be inclusive of persons who have a learning difficulty. The association is a federation of ten provincial and two territorial associations with more than 400 local associations and over 40,000 members. Ms Richler was previously director of the Roeher Institute and has worked for over 20 years supporting organisations of persons with intellectual disabilities, their families and their friends to be agents for social change. She has particular interests in deinstitutionalisation and inclusive education. She was one of the major architects of a national deinstitutionalisation strategy which has resulted in partnerships between the federal government and the Canadian Association of Community Living with provincial governments and provincial associations for community living. With Gordon Porter, she edited *Changing Canadian Schools: Perspectives on Disability and Inclusion*, which is the primary Canadian textbook on inclusive education. In addition to numerous speaking engagements in Canada and the United States, Ms Richler has been invited to lecture in England, France, New Zealand, China, Sweden and Mexico. She is currently co-ordinating a project to develop social policy that will be inclusive of children with a disability throughout the Americas in co-operation with the Inter-American Children's Institute and CILPEDIM, the regional federation of the International League of Societies for Persons with Mental Handicap in the Americas.

Gwyneth Roberts

Gwyneth Roberts is a senior lecturer in social policy in the School of Sociology and Social Policy, University of Wales, Bangor. She also works part-time for the National Development Team. Her particular interests are in the areas of legal and social policy and how these affect the lives of people with learning difficulties.

Jackie Rodgers

Jackie Rodgers works at the North Fry Research Centre at the University of Bristol. She began her career as a nurse and midwife, then took a degree in social policy as a mature student. After graduating, she carried out research on childcare needs for a voluntary organisation. In 1992, she joined the Norah Fry Research Centre to continue the centre's work on the health needs of people with learning difficulties. In 1993, she was awarded a South West Regional Health Authority research training fellowship, to allow her to undertake research which emphasises the experience of health and health care from the point of view of people with learning difficulties. Jackie Rodgers has a strong interest in women's issues, and supports a local women's group organised by women with learning difficulties.

Oliver Russell

Oliver Russell is a reader in mental health at the University of Bristol. He has been honorary director of the Norah Fry Research Centre since its inception in 1988. Trained as a child psychiatrist, he has worked for more than 20 years in services for people with learning difficulties. He is a scientific adviser to the Department of Health and to the Welsh Office. He is on the editorial board of the *British Journal of Learning Disabilities* and is currently editing a textbook for psychiatrists in training.

Philippa Russell

Philippa Russell is director, Council for Disabled Children and is seconded on a part-time basis as an associate director, the National Development Team for people with learning difficulties. In 1990 she was awarded the Rose Fitzgerald Kennedy Centenary Award for women who had contributed to the development of services for people with learning difficulties. She is an honorary member of the British Paediatric Association and of the council of the NSPCC, and a member of the Prince of Wales's Advisory Group on Disability and chairperson, Mental Health Foundation committee of inquiry on children with learning disabilities and challenging behaviour. Her interest in family support arises from her own experience of a son with learning difficulties and awareness that families are still an often undervalued, much criticised but committed and caring basis for community living for people with learning difficulties.

Marcia Rioux

Marcia Rioux is executive director of the Roeher Institute, Canada's national institute for the study of public policy affecting people with a learning difficulty and other disabilities. Dr Rioux came to the institute as a visiting scholar in 1986 and was appointed director in 1987. The institute's mandate is to provide insight into the social policy, programmes, laws and other features of Canadian society that affect the capacity of people with disabilities to exercise their rights and fully participate in society. She has a master's degree in sociology from Carleton University in Ottawa and a doctorate in jurisprudence from the School of Law, University of California, Berkeley. Her previous experience includes a range of research, policy analysis and policy development initiatives, including work done as director of research at the Canadian Advisory Council on the Status of Women and as policy analyst and senior researcher for the Law Reform Commission of Canada. In addition to delivering a number of lectures and extensive involvement in community development in Canada, Marcia Rioux has represented the Roeher Institute in England, France, the Caribbean, eastern Europe and Central America. She has published over 50 articles and monographs in Canadian law, public policy and medical journals and government publications. Her forthcoming book, *The Equality–Disability Nexus*, provides a careful examination of the factors and attitudes that have shaped current policy and legislation, which in turn have dictated equality and entitlement in society.

Tony Ryan

Tony Ryan is a research officer in the Health Research Centre, Sheffield Hallam University on a research project, funded by the Joseph Rowntree Foundation, which is evaluating the quality of life for people with learning difficulties living in the community. Previous work has included research which monitored the community placements of ex-residents of long-stay hospitals in the North Western Health Region. He also worked as a research assistant for Solihull Council on a project assessing local service needs for people with learning difficulties.

Helen Sanderson

Helen Sanderson works as a development officer for the Mancunian Community Health NHS Trust where she is involved in quality assurance, person-centred planning, and service development for people with profound and multiple disabilities. She has a background in occupational therapy and a Masters in quality assurance. She is currently researching communication issues and planning for people with profound multiple disabilities for a PhD, and evaluating user involvement in person-centred planning supported by a grant from the Joseph Rowntree Foundation. She also works as a part-time regional tutor for Birmingham University on the distance learning course 'Interdisciplinary work with people with profound multiple learning difficulties'. She has contributed to course material for the Open University, Manchester University and the Royal National Institute for the Blind Certificate in Multiple Disability.

Ken Simons

Ken Simons has been working as a contract researcher in the learning difficulties field for nearly a decade. Previous work includes a project which looked in detail at the relocation of people with learning difficulties from long-stay hospital, a study of the experiences of people involved in self and citizen advocacy, and, more recently, a review of innovative practice in housing and support. He is currently finishing research on the workings of social services complaints procedures. A key feature of all his work has been an attempt to include the views of people with learning difficulties themselves. Ken Simons has a long-standing interest in all forms of user participation. Until recently he acted as adviser to Avon People First, and he helped establish an experimental service brokerage project in Bristol.

Jeannie Sutcliffe

Jeannie Sutcliffe taught adults with learning difficulties for seven years, first at a large college in Essex, and then in the context of a small but flexible adult education scheme in Bedfordshire. She moved to her current post in 1988, becoming the development officer for adults with learning difficulties at the National Institute of Adult Continuing Education. She has written a number of books on education for adults with learning difficulties on topics which include self advocacy, integration and basic skills. She received the international J. Roby Kidd Award for innovations in adult education in 1990. Jeannie Sutcliffe is currently working on staff development packs funded by the Department of Health and the Baring Foundation and is hoping to develop a certificated course for tutors of adults with learning difficulties across agencies.

David Thompson

David Thompson is the team leader of the Sex Education Team, Horizon NHS Trust. There he has been developing sexuality work with people with learning difficulties since 1989. This work is described in two manuals for staff co-authored with Michelle McCarthy: *Sex and the Three R's* and *Sex and Staff Training* (Pavilion, 1993, 1994). One major aspect of his work has been the pioneering of safer sex interventions for men with learning difficulties who have sex with men. This is informed by his wider experience of gay men's health education as a volunteer at the Terrence Higgins Trust. Recently he was seconded to the Tizard Centre, University of Kent, to work with Hilary Brown on a research project funded by the Mental Health Foundation which is examining service responses to men with learning difficulties who have unacceptable or abusive sexual behaviour.

Alan Walker

Alan Walker is professor of social policy and chairperson of the Department of Sociological Studies, University of Sheffield. He has researched and written extensively in the fields of social policy and social gerontology including *Disability in Britain* (edited with Peter Townsend and Martin Robertson, 1981), *Community Care* (Blackwell, 1982), *Social Planning* (Blackwell, 1984) and *The Caring Relationship* (with Hazel Qureshi, Macmillan, 1989). He was co-director, with Carol Walker, of the research that monitored the community placements of ex-residents of long-stay hospitals in the North Western Health Region. He is chairperson of the European Union's Observatory on Ageing and Older People. He co-founded the Disability Alliance and, for 20 years, was its honorary secretary. He is patron of the National Pensioners Convention.

Carol Walker

Carol Walker is senior lecturer in social policy in the School of Health and Community Studies, Sheffield Hallam University. Her main research interests have focussed on the impact of policy on service users. She has researched and written in the area of social security including *Changing Social Policy: The Case of the Supplementary Benefit Review* (Bedford Square Press, 1983) and *Managing Poverty: The Limits of Social Assistance* (Routledge, 1993). She was co-director, with Alan Walker, of the research that monitored the community placements of ex-residents of long-stay hospitals in the North Western Health Region. She is currently conducting further research with Alan Walker and

Tony Ryan, funded by the Joseph Rowntree Foundation which examines the position of different groups of people with learning difficulties who are living in the community.

Jan Walmsley

Jan Walmsley is a lecturer in the School of Health and Social Welfare at the Open University. Her first degree was in history and she has brought this interest in the past to bear on her current work in learning disability. She recently completed her PhD thesis, *Gender, Caring and Learning Disability*, which looks specifically at the roles which women with learning difficulties have as carers. She is chair of the course team producing a unique new course, *Equal People*, addressed to parents, staff and people with learning difficulties on the subject of learning difficulties. She hopes through her research and writing to increase the visibility of women with learning difficulties, and encourage appreciation of the contribution they make to the welfare of others.

Linda Ward

Linda Ward is a writer, researcher and consultant. She is a senior research fellow at the Norah Fry Research Centre, University of Bristol and programme adviser (disability) to the Joseph Rowntree Foundation, which supports an extensive programme of applied research and innovative development projects in the UK. She has researched and written widely in the field of learning difficulties and has a particular interest in equal opportunities issues. Her publications include *People First: Developing Services for People with Mental Handicap* (1982) and (as co-author) *Double Discrimination: Issues and Services for People with Learning Difficulties from Black and Ethnic Minority Communities* (1990). She was a member of the course team which produced the original Open University/MENCAP course for parents and staff, *Mental Handicap: Patterns for Living*, and consultant to its successor course, *Equal People*, developed with the self-advocacy organisation, People First.

Andrea Whittaker

Andrea Whittaker is project manager, Building Inclusive Communities, which is part of the community care group at the King's Fund Centre. Her work covers user participation and self-advocacy, particularly with people with learning difficulties. She has had a major involvement in the King's Fund 'An Ordinary Life' initiative and is now developing work related to community participation. Andrea Whittaker has been closely associated with the self-advocacy organisation People First since it began in 1984 and was its adviser until October 1988, when People First moved out of the King's Fund Centre and set up its own office. She has been involved in a wide variety of user participation initiatives including joint user/staff training and user-led evaluation of services.

Christopher Williams

Christopher Williams is a research fellow at the Norah Fry Research Centre, University of Bristol. He is also a tutor for the Open University and serves as a magistrate. He is, at present, researching crime against people with learning difficulties and this two-year project is supported by the Joseph Rowntree Foundation. Other work has included employment of, and video use by people with learning difficulties, and human rights. He has recently been awarded a fellowship by the Economic and Social Research Council for a victim study relating to environmentally caused developmental disability. He worked in Egypt for two years, at Cairo University and also at a school for blind children. Whilst living in South Africa he co-founded Street-wise, an education project for street children. More recently he has made study visits to India, Turkey, Thailand, Hong Kong and China. Originally he was a professional trumpeter.

Jean Willson

Jean Willson's experience of profound and multiple disabilities comes from caring for her daughter Victoria, now aged 23. After qualifying as a social worker in 1983 she became the first director of Camden Society for People with Mental Handicaps, bringing people out of long-stay hospitals to live in the community, and opening a café run by people with learning difficulties. She was, for six years, director of One-to-One, a charity which provides friendship and advocacy schemes for people with learning difficulties who are living in hospitals and in the community. She has since continued to work in the voluntary sector and now manages a domiciliary respite service for carers who have children or adults with a physical or learning difficulty in Islington. She also does consultancy work on a whole range of issues connected with learning difficulties. Jean Willson works both locally and nationally to improve services for people with profound and multiple disabilities and their carers. With Pat Fitton and Carol O'Brien she has written *Home at Last* (1995), which gives a detailed account of the project set up for her daughter and that of Pat Fitton.

Liz Wright

Liz Wright is project co-ordinator at Skills for People, a post she has held for over two years. For over ten years she has worked in the field of advocacy with people who receive social welfare services. Her role has included acting as a formal advocate and campaigning for improved rights. An example of this was when she worked as legal advice officer for MIND. After a move to Newcastle in 1989 Liz Wright was involved in setting up a user-run drop-in and advice service for people with mental health problems. She acted as facilitator for the unique mental health consumer group which was funded to ensure the involvement of people with mental health problems in the planning and management of services. Skills for People is a registered charity which aims to promote self-advocacy among people with learning difficulties and physical disabilities. Most of the work of the project is carried out in the North East. Volunteers, most of whom have physical disabilities or learning difficulties plan and present training courses and conferences for people with disabilities.

The courses aim to encourage people to speak up for themselves, gain in independence and confidence, develop relationships and have more of a say in their lives. Volunteers also provide training for staff and other professionals in the field of disability. The project also gives support to some self-advocacy groups in the area and often provides training to new groups. Skills for People aims to make sure that users of services have a real say in what happens in their lives. People with learning difficulties and physical disabilities are responsible for the philosophy of the project and the direction of much of its work.

Preface

In 1993 Jackie Downer and Alice Etherington, two women with learning difficulties, were selected, in the face of stiff competition from a wide range of talented and committed professionals and carers, as the first winners of the Norah Fry/*Community Care* award. The award was established to recognise the achievement of an individual who, through their activities, had made the most significant contribution to developments in the field and helped to enhance the lives of people with learning difficulties. Jackie and Alice were chosen as joint winners for their work in self-advocacy and community care and particularly for their work on black and women's issues respectively. Their achievements epitomise the concerns of this book: the importance of celebrating positive achievements at a time of resource constraint, uncertainty and service change; the growing significance of users' voices (and of advocates for those who cannot speak up for themselves) and the increased recognition of the necessity and value of their contributions; the gradually increasing attention to equal opportunities issues in this field.

In putting together this volume we wanted to address some key questions. In the midst of the endless preoccupations with the administrative reforms brought by the NHS and Community Care Act, what are the important issues for service users, their families and the professionals with whom they are involved? What can research tell us about these topics? What are the experiences and views of service users themselves? What are the leading edge projects from which we can all learn? What, in short, are the practical possibilities for change?

In selecting the authors who have contributed to this book we have looked for people with a wide range of backgrounds and experience: people with learning difficulties, parents, a variety of professionals from the voluntary and statutory sectors, academics, researchers, consultants and trainers, from the UK and beyond. Their contributions are as varied as their subject matter but certain key themes embody, for us, the values and visions of our title which should inspire developments in the future. There is, for example, a significant shift away from thinking about the disabilities of the *individual* towards the changes that need to be made in the *society* in which they live, an issue taken up by Richler and Rioux in their account of the shift in focus of the activities of the Canadian Association of Community Living (see Chapter 26). There is a growing emphasis on making changes, not just in our services, but in the communities in which they are based (see Chapter 25), even for those people whose difficulties pose the greatest challenges (see Chapter 18). Increasingly, the shift is towards inclusion, more opportunities for people with learning difficulties (see Chapters 4 and 5) and better support for their families within the neighbourhoods where they live (see Chapter 2). Most significantly, perhaps, is the theme of rights not charity: a thread running through many of our chapters and including the rights of people with learning difficulties to their own sexuality and sexual relationships (see Chapter 19), to be parents (Chapter 20), to question the services they receive (see Chapter 13), to be accurately reflected in the media (see Chapter 24), and to push for legislation to outlaw discrimination against them and embody their equal citizenship within the law. There remains, of course, much that is distressing in the lives of people with learning difficulties in this country, not least the poverty in which most of them live (see Chapter 23) and their ready victimisation (see Chapter 22). But there is much to celebrate too, not least their increasing confidence. As Anya Souza of Young People First put it so eloquently 'my biggest problem is that people think I can't and I like to think I can' (Boston, 1994).

We hope that this book will help more people feel, like Anya, that they can bring about positive changes with and for people with learning difficulties in their communities.

Terry Philpot and Linda Ward

Reference

Boston, S. (1994). The upside of Down's. *The Guardian*, June 14.

Part One

Changing Lives

Chapter 1
Equal citizens: Current issues for people with learning difficulties and their allies

Linda Ward

> Our voice may be a new one to many of you, but you should better get used to hearing it.
> Many of us still have to learn how to speak up.
> Many of you still have to learn how to listen to us and how to understand us.
> (Barb Goode, 1992)

On 12 October 1992, Barb Goode, a Canadian woman, became the first person with a learning difficulty to address the General Assembly of the United Nations. The subject of her speech? The desire of people with learning difficulties to push forward their rights so that they could take their place as equal citizens, living and working in their own communities. In the 15 years since her chance introduction to self-advocacy (through a baseball game in her local park) Barb Goode has come a long way. Indeed, in the last few years she has spread the words of the self-advocacy movement in places as far flung as Amsterdam, Budapest, Bristol, Detroit, London, Germany, Italy, Jamaica, Kenya, Mexico and New Zealand. Though still diffident of her abilities, she is no longer the young woman whose parents were concerned at her restricted lifestyle; the woman who 'wasn't very vocal' (Ward, 1993). She now has her own apartment and a job; she has friends and interests and travels (more than most people!). There have been huge changes in her life – as there have been in the lives of many people with learning difficulties in her native Canada, in the UK and elsewhere. Yet obstacles to real equal citizenship remain. This chapter looks first at three major issues confronting people with learning difficulties and their allies in the UK today: institutional services; the NHS and Community Care Act reforms; abuse and discrimination; and then at areas of positive change along the road to empowerment and equality.

Institutional services

> There are more bad things than good things about living in the hospital. You have to be told what to do in hospital and you call people 'Nurse' or 'Sister'. You rely on the food being dished up to you and I don't like it. When I was young in hospital, we always had to go to bed early. I didn't agree with that. If I had still lived with my father I wouldn't have gone to bed that early. (Peter Stevens, 1990).

Government policy is to close long-stay institutions for people with learning difficulties and to ensure that people with learning difficulties have the same opportunities to live an ordinary life in the community as other people. The commitment stretches back to the 1971 White Paper, *Better Services for the Mentally Handicapped* (DHSS, 1971). It was confirmed by the community care White Paper, *Caring for People* (DoH, 1989) and, most recently, by two Department of Health circulars in October 1992 (DoH, 1992). Yet for more than 15 000 people in the UK alone, community living remains a dream (Collins, personal communication, 1995). Why?

Research by Jean Collins at Values Into Action sheds some light on this area (Collins, 1992; 1993; 1994 and Chapter 6). Her study of hospital closure found that the resettlement programme in England is haphazard and unco-ordinated, dependent on the personal commitment of individual officers and undermined by both lack of funding and the NHS reforms. She found that there were problems transferring money and staff from the NHS to social services departments, and that resources which should have been invested in community provision were being spent on maintaining institutions scheduled for closure. Moreover, the creation of NHS trusts was working against resettlement by encouraging the actual retention of some hospitals, since many trusts were committed to developing their on-site services to ensure business viability. As a result, the right of people with learning difficulties to enjoy life in the community, rather than in an institution, is proving slow to realise. And even where resettlement is going ahead, Collins' research shows that institutional values continue to dominate services, often at the expense of an ordinary life.

Ideally, community living means the opportunity to live in a small home, with a companion or companions of one's choice, in an acceptable neighbourhood, with the support that is needed to lead an ordinary domestic life and make use of the facilities available nearby. Those were the goals of the Ordinary Life movement of the 1980s (King's Fund Centre, 1980), pursued by many health and local authorities in the intervening decade. But recent research and experience suggest that financial and other pressures mean that 'small homes' are in fact getting larger (from 10 to 25 beds or even more) and that they are often becoming more institutional too, with centralised laundry and catering services, even in four-bed houses. In fact, 'the institution is dispersed, not disbanded' (Collins, 1992). In addition, institutional values may be transmitted directly from hospital to small home where there is extensive redeployment of existing staff. One manager in Collins' study acknowledged that 'It probably means transferring the institutional baggage of the hospital system into the community' but saw this as 'a price that has to be paid for the historical legacy' (Collins, 1993). Of course, deployment of staff need not necessarily lead to an institutional ethos in the community setting if intensive re-training opportunities are given before re-location and topped up by in-service training in the community and intensive management supervision. But current preoccupations with budgets make such expenditure of time and effort unlikely.

Janice Sinson's investigation of ten public sector group homes to see how far they promoted opportunities for learning and ordinary living for their residents paints a similarly depressing picture (Sinson, 1993). Indeed, her findings are summed up by the book's sub-title *Micro-institutionalisation?*. Here there is no shortage of evidence for those who have ever harboured doubts about how far group homes really are homes in the usual sense. Evidence, too, that even the term 'group home' can be infinitely elastic, stretching here to embrace units of more than 20 people and confirming that they may be as institutional in some ways as the hospitals they have sometimes replaced. In particular, Sinson draws attention to the huge impact of institutional management practices and the negative effects of contracting services – including catering, cleaning, laundry, gardening, hairdressing, chiropody, even clothing accounts at old-fashioned department stores – which effectively sabotage attempts at ordinary living. Sinson's work does include stories of two independent homes which did manage to deliver good-quality services to their residents, largely through the personal commitment and flair of their individual proprietors and their freedom to work within fewer constraints than their public sector counterparts. The work of at least one of those is now threatened by the new situation prevailing since the implementation of the NHS and Community Care Act, with purchasers being more concerned now about cheapness than value for money in relation to quality of life.

The NHS and Community Care Act reforms

> Our goal is to create a seamless service based entirely around the needs and wishes of users of care and their carers. Virginia Bottomley, Minister of Health. (DoH press release, 1991).

> Community care is finally here and the government paper says *users* (us) are to be asked about it.
> It will also have to be *user-led* (meaning *we* are in control).
> It has taken us many months to make some sense of community care and we are not very happy with what we found out (People First, 1993).

One of the biggest impediments to the achievement of better lives for people with learning difficulties is, ironically, the aftermath of the NHS and Community Care Act 1990. Ironically, because the Act laid emphasis on support in the community, rather than the former reliance on residential care; a wider variety of services from which consumers could choose; individual user-centred assessment and packages of care; the centrality of meeting user needs and encouraging user empowerment. But, the reforms were also driven by other agenda: the promotion of a market in health and social care and a commitment to curtail public expenditure by staunching the steeply rising social security bill which resulted from the previous automatic entitlement of people to move to residential accommodation with their fees paid by the state. Sadly, early research suggests that some of the key mechanisms introduced by the Act may not have the positive outcomes envisaged.

Contracting

In principle, a more mixed economy of care means more, different service providers. Local authorities withdraw from some direct service provision but have an increasing role purchasing services, monitoring and ensuring standards. This is achieved through contractual relationships. But Common and Flynn's study of some early contracts found no increase in choice for the users and no increase in innovative service provisions (Common and Flynn, 1992). Indeed, only one quarter of the contracts they looked at allow providers to develop innovative provision. In three quarters of the cases, innovation was explicitly not allowed. So it is possible that services, contrary to expectation, may become more rigid and less innovative and responsive to consumer views, unless attention is paid to bringing about positive change (see Chapter 10).

Assessment

Assessment is supposed to be the cornerstone of the new system, with users and carers being 'able to exercise the same power as consumers of other services', no longer subordinate to the wishes of service providers (SSI, 1991a). But Kathryn Ellis' research into assessment and disabled people, undertaken before the NHS and Community Care reforms were introduced, but in authorities specifically chosen as examples of good practice in the field, found that assessment was widely based on *professionals'* judgement of what individuals needed (regardless of what users themselves said) and according to services or supports the professionals knew were available (Ellis, 1993). This seems unlikely to change dramatically. How can even well-meaning practitioners accommodate people's individual needs within the constraints of local policy and resources? Can assessment really empower users and carers if there is not a menu of local services upon which they can draw? How meaningful can changes in the assessment process be in a situation of resource restraint, where local authorities are hesitant to record people's unmet needs for fear of legal challenges and ensuing obligations to provide services they cannot afford? The prospects do not look good (see Chapter 8).

Care management

Ann Richardson and Ray Higgins' early work on case management and people with learning difficulties sounds a similar warning (Richardson and Higgins, 1992). Care management may mean a better understanding of people's needs and wishes, with customised individual plans, and the promise of a better quality of life. But it cannot deliver what is outside its control and so can provide no solution to service shortages or budget constraints. In short, it is not a magic solution.

The purchaser/provider split

In theory, the separation of purchasing and providing functions in both health and social services provision should mean more competition between providers, a greater variety and better quality of services, better value for money and more choice for service users. Purchasers are supposed to buy services in the best interests of users, where users are unable to do this themselves. But the people now responsible for purchasing within both health and local authorities often have little knowledge of the kind of services which people with learning difficulties in particular may want. Services may be selected on the basis of costs alone, with no increase in quality, user choice or satisfaction at all. This is a particular problem within health authorities. Trusts have become both the assessor and the provider of their residents' requirements, with the result that some district health authorities are now in the position of having to pay for services with which they are dissatisfied, because they have no means of challenging the Trusts' views. Jean Collins' research shows that large and powerful trusts which monopolise resources in provision for people with learning difficulties in their local areas are particularly difficult for purchasers to influence to ensure more appropriate or individualised services for people with learning difficulties in their areas (Collins, 1993).

In practice, services for people with learning difficulties have been negatively affected by the implications of the NHS and Community Care Act in four key ways.

First, NHS trusts, through their monopoly of local resources, may discourage the development of alternative forms of provision. The tendency to develop on-site facilities to ensure their business viability works against hospital closure. Meanwhile, those which provide their own social care in the community are thwarting official community care policy, which designates social services departments as the lead agency. In both cases, people with learning difficulties are continuing to have their needs met in ways which the government has acknowledged is inappropriate.

Second, the effective collaboration between health and local authorities, which is essential to the delivery of good community care, remains elusive. The desired goal is a 'seamless service' resulting from joint planning. In practice, difficulties in collaboration, highlighted by the Audit Commission in 1989, continue (Audit Commission, 1989). Resettlement plans are frequently not made jointly. Parallel services,

NHS or social services led, continue to operate in some areas (Collins, 1992). There are squabbles over what constitutes health or social care and who should pay for what. The government's reliance on guidelines, which encourage the transfer of resources from health authorities rather than requiring them, means that health authorities can remain reluctant to hand over money to social services departments, the supposed lead agency in community care. The needs and wishes of the user scarcely figure in these debates.

Third, the implementation of the NHS and Community Care Act has been both prompted and accompanied by strict resource constraints. Whatever the rhetoric about user-centred and seamless services, the reality is that purchasers are watching their budgets and that services which are not viewed as essential or clients who are not deemed to be at risk of personal safety have low priority. For people with learning difficulties this is having manifold effects: a reduction in the availability of respite places for adults; an increase in the size of residential homes; targeting of services to those with severe needs at the expense of those with milder disabilities; the axing or vulnerability of innovative development projects or even routine community or family support.

Fourth, GP fundholders, who became eligible to purchase services for people with learning difficulties in April 1993, are a further wild card whose impact has yet to be determined. Research by Langan and colleagues (Langan *et al.*, 1993) shows GPs to be unusually ignorant about the service needs of people with learning difficulties and to be almost completely unaware of the contributions to be made by occupational therapists, physiotherapists and other members of community learning difficulty teams. They have little contact with professionals working in learning difficulty services. There is growing concern that GPs, unaware of the potential needs of individual patients with learning difficulties, and ways in which these can be most appropriately and effectively met, may be reluctant to commission the services of individual team members, unconvinced of the need of their services when it comes to balancing their books.

A particular casualty of the NHS and Community Care reforms may prove to be the community learning difficulty teams, which since the early 1980s have been the main means of support, and development of services, for people with learning difficulties in the community (see Chapter 7). Where they have functioned well, the teams, with their multi-disciplinary membership, have worked across agencies, involving different professionals, assessing individuals' needs and putting together appropriate packages of services across organisational and professional boundaries. Most significantly, they have been able to straddle the health/social care divide and ensure that previously fragmented services were brought together in one seamless whole. But research by the National Development Team and the Nuffield Institute (Brown *et al.*, 1992) suggests that the experience and expertise accumulated by these teams may now be at risk, their development work threatened by budget cuts, the emphasis on health versus social needs presenting a serious challenge to teams which have developed shared areas of responsibility. Community learning difficulty teams have been slow to develop systems of performance review by which their operations can be appraised and their value for money indicated. It is not at all clear how well they will survive in the brave new world nor what their demise would mean to the people with learning difficulties they once served.

Abuse and discrimination

> I think people with learning difficulties should have a campaign about being sexually abused. (Millard, 1994).

The 1990s will go down as the decade in which the abuse of people with learning difficulties was finally recognised as the widespread phenomenon that it is. Hilary Brown and colleagues' work at the University of Kent has provided us for the first time with some reasonably solid statistics on the reported incidence of abuse and much-needed guidelines on how individuals and agencies can work together to be alert to abuse, encourage its reporting, support effective prosecutions, protect whistle-blowers and develop adequate therapeutic services for those involved. Key findings from their study of reported cases of abuse in one regional health authority are as follows.

- Sexual abuse is a significant problem (perhaps 950 new *reported* cases alone in the United Kingdom as a whole per year).
- Both men and women are at risk (27 per cent of the victims in their first survey, and 43 per cent in their second, were men).
- People with communication problems are especially vulnerable.
- Abusers are most likely to be men and to be already known by the victims: this is no 'stranger danger'. (In over half the cases reported the perpetrators were other service users with learning difficulties; most of the remainder were family members, staff or other known and trusted adults.)
- Often more than one person is sexually abused by the same perpetrator

(which means that staff need to check for other potential victims, both men and women, if abuse is discovered).

- Distress, new sexual behaviour or language or other changes in behaviour or new fears of people or settings may indicate that abuse is occurring; staff need to be alert to these signals.
- Prosecutions are rare; intra-agency procedures are needed to investigate cases consistently and obtain reliable evidence. (Reorganisations resulting from the NHS and Community Care Act mean new guidelines need to be developed.)
- Therapeutic services are needed to help victims deal with their experiences and distress, regardless of whether criminal proceedings can be brought. (Turk and Brown, 1992; Brown et al., 1994).

It is clear from experiences and research on sexual abuse that the criminal justice system is generally failing to address the needs of people with learning difficulties and that police responses to incidents are inconsistent. The establishment of the pressure group VOICE by Julie Boniface in the wake of her own daughter's painful experience is one attempt to address these problems (Williams, 1993). Meanwhile, Chris Williams' research at the University of Bristol (see Chapter 22) has looked at the nature of victimisation of people with learning difficulties more broadly and explored what they, staff, carers and others involved with them can do both to reduce the incidence of victimisation and to achieve justice.

Abuse, victimisation and crime against people with learning difficulties have been a regular feature of life in institutions (see, for example, Ryan and Thomas, 1988). Sadly, life in group homes and day centres often host similar forms of victimisation. In addition, people may be at risk because they are expected to live in high crime areas (Flynn, 1989). There are some important lessons here for both purchasers and providers about where homes and services for people with learning difficulties should be located and about ensuring the services with which they are concerned pay due attention to appropriate strategies and guidelines for preventing and dealing with abuse and victimisation of any kind. On the positive side, there is now a wealth of strategies and ideas on how to prevent and combat abuse and victimisation by staff and people with learning difficulties themselves, including the proposed establishment of Powerhouse, a safe house by and for women with learning difficulties who have been attacked or abused (ARC/NAPSAC, 1993; Aspis, 1992; Brown and Craft, 1992).

Signs of change

Despite the obstacles created by institutional services, the NHS and Community Care Act reforms and the prevalence of abuse and discrimination, there are, nonetheless, signs of positive change and progress for people with learning difficulties and their allies, especially in the areas of supported employment (see Chapter 4), supported living and advocacy and empowerment.

Supported living

Few people with learning difficulties ever really choose where they live, with whom, their staff, their routines or how they spend their money (most of which is handed over to the agency running their home). People are fitted to programmes or particular houses that are available. If their need for support changes, they are too often transferred elsewhere, even back to an institution, in the absence of more flexible staffing arrangements which would allow them to stay put.

The flaws of this 'group home' model were recognised sooner in the USA than in the UK. Over the last few years there has been a strong movement away from group homes there, in recognition of the fact that no one model of service can work for everybody. In its place, there has been a growing movement towards supported living: individuals choose where and how they want to live and with whom, with a flexible range of supports built in. The movement has been supported by recent legislation and the award of pilot funding to nine states to develop community-supported living arrangements. These developments have been richly documented by Racino et al. (1993). The key characteristics of supported living (though how it is implemented varied enormously from one part of the States to the next) are as follows.

- The separation of housing from support. (The agency providing or co-ordinating support is not the landlord; this makes it easier for a person to move home or change support arrangements if they want to.)
- Focusing on one individual at a time. (Individual planning is used to find out what each person wants and to assist them to secure the accommodation and supports which are right for them.)
- Full user choice and control. (Individuals choose where they live, with whom (if anyone), who supports them and how. They hold their own tenancy or mortgage and are in control of their own money and household.)

- Rejecting no one. (Supported living assumes that everyone can live in the community. If someone has complex needs they should still have the chance to lead the lifestyle of their choice; attention is given to environmental adaptations and personally designed supports.)
- A focus on relationships, with maximum use of informal support and community resources. (The starting point is to build upon a person's existing relationships and connections. Paid help is used only when natural and informal supports are not available and paid supporters work to develop a person's social network alongside their other activities. Paid help may take the form of 'live-in' staff, 'come-in' or peripatetic staff. 'Paid neighbours' are also used as a source of flexible and informal support and links into the community (Kinsella and Ward, 1993).

There is now growing experience in the UK of supported living of this kind (see, for example, Chapter 3) with a new initiative spearheaded by the National Development Team to promote supported living across Britain in conjunction with purchasers and providers of services, those who use them and their carers (Kinsella, 1993). It has always been assumed that individually arranged services would cost more and that large organisations are cheaper because of economies of scale. But evidence from the USA points to the contrary. If purchasers here can be persuaded to take on an enabling and developing role, supporting small organisations to establish individualised supported living, then a real ordinary life, as opposed to an institutionalised one, could become a realistic option for people with learning difficulties in the future.

For people with moderate learning difficulties, there is already some experience of creating supported housing, through the innovative work of KeyRing in London. KeyRing creates neighbourhood and housing networks, occupying clusters of eight to ten flats, in partnership with housing authorities or housing associations in different neighbourhoods. The properties are taken from standard stock, the only special requirement being that each needs to be within easy walking distance of the others. Members of the network (people with moderate learning difficulties who can wash and dress themselves and have a basic grasp of money and cooking skills) pay their rent to the local council or housing association just like any other tenant, but, because they live so close to one another, they are able to make friends and offer neighbourly help when required. Equally important, they can call on the services of a part-time KeyRing worker who lives as part of their network in a self-contained flat, and is committed to offering a flexible ten hours of support a week to the KeyRing tenants. KeyRing had made it possible by the end of 1993 for nearly 45 people with moderate learning difficulties to enjoy independent housing with their support.

KeyRing has a number of positive features. It is innovative: its networks offer a much needed alternative to outreach social work, group homes and hostels. It is also successful: monitoring reveals a high rate of satisfaction among the tenants and a clear improvement in their quality of life. It is easy to set up: KeyRing networks make use of existing properties: And it is cost effective: an entire KeyRing network for ten people can be run for the same cost as a single place in a residential home. Moreover, it is good community care policy: Key-Ring gives people with learning difficulties a chance to lead independent lives in a home of their own, encouraging self-help and mutual support. Finally, it is adaptable: the housing networks have demonstrated a creative model of community care, which can be adapted to suit other client groups. KeyRing are currently developing a network which will cater for the needs of those who need more support (KeyRing, 1993; undated; Utting, 1993).

Advocacy and empowerment

> The rationale for this reorganisation is the empowerment of users and carers. (SSI, 1991a).

User empowerment is supposed to be one of the driving forces behind the reforms. The government, however, has shown some ambivalence on the issue, not least in its original exclusion of any users from the community care support force, set up to help local authorities in their preparation for the implementation of the Act and in the continuing quarrels which beset the National Users and Carers Committee established by the government on the support force's demise. Nonetheless, there is no doubt that local authorities are putting user involvement and empowerment higher on their agenda, and making efforts to change (Hoyes *et al.*, 1994) and there are increasing examples of innovative practice and even user-led services for all community care client groups (Beresford and Harding, 1994).

Self-advocacy has been the single most significant development for people with learning difficulties over the last decade or so. Throughout the country, there are now self-advocacy groups in adult training centres and other service settings as well as independent People First groups which cross agency boundaries. There is a full-time People First office in London (and a few similar offices elsewhere) responsible for a steady stream of work and training (see Chapter 12) and offering a timely user perspective on new initiatives and publications on assessment, sexuality and issues for people from black and ethnic minority groups. (People First, 1993; undated; Black People First, 1994). Elsewhere in the country, Advocacy In Action in Nottingham and Skills for People in Newcastle (see Chapter 9) are similarly energetic, productive and challenging to established views. Ken Simons' study (Simons, 1993) offers the most up-to-date review of current key issues in this area, based on the views of self-advocates themselves. He shows that people have clear ideas on the kinds of services they like and dislike and that the diversity of expectations of self-advocates means that it is difficult for any one kind of group to meet all their needs. Self-advocacy is clearly a vibrant movement with individual groups that are often fragile, being bombarded by demands from outside (for example, from the statutory authorities) to consult and give their views on everything. And there remains a continuing concern about representativeness. If self-advocates are articulate, they are dismissed as 'unrepresentative'. If they are not articulate, then it is difficult for them to put their case and bring about change. An impressive Catch 22 (Lindow, 1991).

For some people with learning difficulties, however, an independent representative or advocate is the best chance of ensuring that their views can be heard. The SSI guidance on care management and assessment (SSI, 1991b) makes many references to the potential scope for the involvement of independent representatives. However, the government has announced its intention not to implement Sections 1–3 of the Disabled Persons Act 1986 which would have enabled this to happen on a routine basis. Independent citizen advocacy organisations are, therefore, the main source of independent advocates for people with learning difficulties at the present time. Recent research shows that citizen advocacy is widely misunderstood by service providers (creating unrealistic expectations of what advocates will do) but continues to challenge services over a wide range of concerns including inappropriate forms of punishment, behaviour modification and medication (Simons, 1994).

Increasingly, people with learning difficulties are becoming involved in many other aspects of service planning, purchasing and provision which affect their lives in a variety of ways. There are positive examples and ideas for involvement in community care planning (Bewley and Glendinning, 1994); in evaluating services (Whittaker et al., 1991); in quality assurance initiatives like quality action groups (Milner et al.,

1991 and Chapter 11); as trainers and tutors on courses (see Chapters 9 and 12); on management and steering committees; in selection of staff (King's Fund Centre, 1991) and as conference or workshop planners, delegates and speakers. Belatedly, people with learning difficulties are now also becoming involved in planning and carrying out research on services and issues which affect their lives (Ward and Flynn, 1994). Most critical, perhaps, is the new emphasis on making information easy to understand. 'When we think of accessibility for people with disabilities, we think of ramps, lifts, etc. People with learning difficulties find their community inaccessible to them in many formats but none more powerful than inaccessible information' (People First, unpubl.). Hence People's First's initiative in this area.

Equal citizenship for all?

> It can be difficult for people with learning difficulties who are black. We are treated badly because of our learning difficulty and because of the colour of our skin. (Black People First, 1994).

So what are the prospects for people with learning difficulties and their allies? Despite the obstacles outlined and the continuing lack of resources, windows of opportunity for positive change do exist. There are chinks of possibility in the confusion of current circumstances which can be exploited for positive ends. The NHS and community care reforms may sometimes mean that local community-based opportunities will develop as, for example, training centres fill up. Supported employment opportunities look set to increase. The user voice is getting stronger and user involvement in every aspect of service planning, purchasing and provision will become more routine (Morris and Lindow, 1993). Information about services and benefits for people with learning difficulties will, gradually, become more accessible. Organisations of people with learning difficulties and their allies (including parent groups like MENCAP) will progressively, it is to be hoped, join forces to push for change as they have done so successfully in the Canadian Association for Community Living (see Chapter 26). As organisations of people with learning difficulties become stronger, alliances between them and organisations of other disabled people will continue to grow as they jointly campaign against the discrimination that all disabled people encounter in our society and push for the anti-discrimination legislation which is needed to ensure their rights. Increasingly attention will, hopefully, be given to equal opportunities for all people with learning difficulties. The dawning recognition that people with learning difficulties are as mixed and heterogeneous as the rest of us is spreading and, gradually, more attention will be given to the particular needs of older people, women, those from black and ethnic monority groups, those with profound and complex needs and those who are gay or lesbian (see, respectively Chapters 16, 15, 14, 17 and 19). Finally, there will assuredly be more and more emphasis on the *rights* of people with learning difficulties to equal citizenship with others underpinned by the comprehensive anti-discrimination legislation they have been seeking for so long.

'. . . we demand that you give us the right to make choices and decisions regarding our own lives.

We are tired of people telling us to do what they want. Instead, let us all work together as a team!' (Goode, 1992).

References

Aspis, S. (1992). 'Safe house for women'. *Disability Issues*, May/June.

Association for Residential Care/NAPSAC (1993). *It Could Never Happen Here! The Prevention and Treatment of Sexual Abuse of Adults with Learning Disabilities in Residential Settings*. Chesterfield & Nottingham, ARC and NAPSAC (National Association for the Protection from Sexual Abuse of Adults and Children with Learning Disabilities).

Audit Commission (1989). *Developing Community Care for Adults with a Mental Handicap*, HMSO, London.

Beresford, P. and Harding, T. (1993, eds). *Challenge to Change: Practical Experience of Building User-led Services*. National Institute for Social Work, London.

Bewley, C. and Glendinning, C. (1994). *Involving Disabled People in Community Care Planning*. Joseph Rowntree Foundation/*Community Care*, York.

Black People First (1994). *Conference report*. Black People First, London.

Brown, H. and Craft, A. (1992). *Working with the Unthinkable*. FPA, London.

Brown, H., Turk, V. and Stein, J. (1994). Sexual abuse of adults with learning difficulties. *Social Care Research Findings*, 46, Joseph Rowntree Foundation, York.

Brown, S., Flynn, M. and Wistow, G. (1992). *Back to the future. Joint Work for People with Learning Disabilities*. National Development Team and Nuffield Institute, Manchester and Leeds.

Collins, J. (1992). *When the Eagles Fly*. Values into Action, London.

Collins, J. (1993). *The Resettlement Game*. Values into Action, London.

Collins, J. (1994). *Still to be Settled*. Values into Action, London.

Common, R. and Flynn, N. (1992). *Contracting for Care*. Joseph Rowntree Foundation/*Community Care*, York.

Department of Health and Social Security (1971). *Better Services for the Mentally Handicapped*. HMSO, London.

Department of Health (1989). *Caring for People*. HMSO, London.

Department of Health (1991). 'Virginia Bottomley opens conference on community care training' press release. Department of Health, London.

Department of Health (1992). *Health Services for People with Learning Disabilities (Mental Handicap)*, HSG (92) 42. HMSO, London.

Department of Health (1992). *Social Care for Adults with Learning Disabilities (Mental Handicap)*. LAC (92) 15. HMSO, London.

Ellis, K. (1993). *Squaring the Circle. User and Carer Participation in Needs Assessment*. Joseph Rowntree Foundation/*Community Care*, York.

Flynn, M. (1989). *Independent Living for Adults with Mental Handicap*, Cassell, London.

Goode, B. (1992). Address to the U.N. general assembly. *ILSMH News*. **14**, 92. International League of Societies for Persons with Mental Handicap, Brussells.

Hoyes, L., Lart, R., Means, R., and Taylor, M. (1994). User empowerment and the reform of community care. *Social Care Research Findings*, 50. Joseph Rowntree Foundation, York.

KeyRing (1993). Community living for people with learning difficulties. *Social Care Research Findings*, 41, Joseph Rowntree Foundation, York.

KeyRing (undated). *Living Support Networks for People who have a Learning Difficulty*. KeyRing, London.

King's Fund Centre (1980). *An Ordinary Life*. King's Fund Centre, London.

King's Fund Centre, Community Living Development Team (1991). Involving service users in appointing staff. *Information Exchange on Self-advocacy and User Participation*, **1**, November.

Kinsella, P. (1993). *Supported Living – a New Paradigm*. National Development Team, Manchester.

Kinsella, P. and Ward, L. (1993). Supporting roles. *Community Care*, 22 July.

Langan, J., Russell, O. and Whitfield, M. (1993). *Community Care and the General Practitioner: Primary Health Care for People with Learning Disabilities*, University of Bristol, Norah Fry Research Centre (unpubl.).

Lindow, V. (1991). Experts, lies and stereotypes. *The Health Service Journal*, August 29.

Millard, L. (1994). Between ourselves: experience of a woman's group on sexuality and sexual abuse. In *Practice Issues in Sexuality and Learning Disabilities* (ed. A. Craft). Routledge, London.

Milner, L., Ash, A. and Richie, P. (1991). *Quality in Action. A Resource Pack for Improving Services for People with Learning Difficulties*. Pavilion Publishing, Brighton.

Morris, J. and Lindow, V. (1993). *User Participation in Community Care Services*. Department of Health, London.

People First (undated). *Everything You Ever Wanted to Know about Safer Sex*. People First, London.

People First (undated). *Making it Easy*. Project Proposal (unpublished).

People First (1993). *Oi! It's my Assessment*. People First, London.

Racino, J.A., Walker, P., O'Connor, S. and Taylor, S. (1993) (eds.) *Housing, Support and Community*. Paul H. Brookes, London.

Richardson, A. and Higgins, R. (1992). *The Limits of Case Management*. Nuffield Institute for Health Services Studies, Leeds.

Ryan, J. and Thomas F. (1988). *The Politics of Mental Handicap*, revised edn. Free Association Books, London.

Simons, K. (1993). *Sticking up for Yourself*. Joseph Rowntree Foundation/ *Community Care*, York.

Simons, K. (1994). *Citizen Advocacy: The Inside View*, Norah Fry Research Centre, University of Bristol.

Sinson, J. (1993). *Group Homes and Integration of Developmentally Disabled People*. Jessica Kingsley, London.

Social Services Inspectorate (1991a). *Care Management and Assessment: Managers' Guide*. HMSO, London.

Social Services Inspectorate (1991b). *Care Management and Assessment: Practitioners' Guide*. HMSO, London.

Stevens, P. (1990). About myself. In Atkinson, D. and Williams, F. (eds). *Know Me as I Am*. Hodder & Stoughton, London.

Turk, V. and Brown, H. (1992). Sexual abuse & adults with learning disabilities. *Mental Handicap*, **20**, June.

Utting, D. (1993). Ring of confidence. *Community Care*, Dec 30.

Ward, L. (1993). The Goode life is full of firsts. *Community Care*, Nov 25.

Ward, L. and Flynn, M. (1994). What matters most: disability, research and empowerment. In *Disability is not Measles: New Research Paradigms in Disability* (eds M. Rioux and M. Bach). Roeher Institute, Toronto.

Williams, C. (1993). Vulnerable victims? A current awareness of the victimisation of people with learning disabilities. *Disability, Handicap & Society*, **8**, 2.

Chapter 2
Supporting families

Philippa Russell

The past decade has seen major developments in terms of policy and practice for families with children who have disabilities and special needs. The principles of *family-based* services and *inclusion* are widely recognised but the rhetoric and the reality do not always match. Complex assessment systems and changes in the management of child health, education and social services have improved the actual commissioning of services but – in an increasingly contractual culture – have created major challenges to families in terms of understanding the system.

It is estimated that there are about 360 000 children with disabilities in the age range of 16 and under in the UK (around three per cent of the child population) (OPCS, 1989). Of these children, all but 5500 live at home. Of those living away from home, 33 per cent of the families felt the children's health or behaviour was too difficult to cope with. Fifteen per cent of children had been physically or sexually abused. The same study found, notwithstanding the increase in family support services, that 45 per cent of families felt that their own health had been adversely affected by caring. A similar number felt that the care of their *other* children had been adversely affected by the often competing demands; appointments and general levels of care needed by the disabled child. A contributory factor to parental stress was the financial impact of disability, with all families worse off than their counterparts and a large number of parents (particularly in single parent families) relying solely on benefits.

The Office of Population and Census Surveys (OPCS) study also noted that only around 38 per cent of parents belonged to or knew of a disability organisation which might help them. Respite care was available to around four per cent of families only, although there were strong messages about families' needs for additional practical support.

Subsequent to the OPCS study, it has become apparent that although the vast majority of children with disabilities will live in a family home, and the NHS no longer provides any long-stay residential services, there are nonetheless children with disabilities spending time away from home, particularly in residential education, where the reasons for their placement and the arrangements for the return home to local communities may be unclear. Some 16 550 children with special educational needs are currently attending residential schools, with the largest number – 8 000 children – in schools for children with emotional and behavioural difficulties. Many residential schools are under increasing pressure to provide 52 weeks a year residential care. This trend has to be offset against gradual but encouraging increases in mainstream school placements for all children with disabilities and a recognition that *parents* are expecting more community-based services which enable them and their children, in the words of the Children Act, to lead lives which are 'as ordinary as possible'.

Developing a policy of family support

Special child, special parents?

> Motherhood has a single long-term goal, which can be described as the mother's own eventual unemployment. A successful mother (and father) bring up their children to do without them. But if a child has a disability or special need, there may be no longer-term unemployment. In effect the life plan which all parents make for their children will be *different* for the child with special needs. Some parents, particularly if they have poor self esteem, low incomes, poor quality housing and little family support, may find the adjustment to disability too difficult to cope with. They are not bad parents. They do care. But somebody has to care for *them* as people before they can enter the wonderful new world of partnership between parents and professionals that we all hear so much about. Having a disabled child changes you for life! (Parent attending Parent Workshop, Russell and Flynn, National Development Team, 1991).

Successful parenting of a child with special needs will not only depend upon the quality of the early education or child health programmes which are available. A number of studies in the UK have shown the pressures placed upon young families by the *care* needs of their children. A study by Glendinning (1983) found that out of 361 young children with disabilities, 50.1 could not be left alone for even ten minutes in a day. A study by Wilkin (1979) on the lives of families with children with severe learning difficulties found that there was little significant help from relatives, friends or neighbours in terms of day-to-day caring. In the UK, the absence of support in local communities may, in part, be due to greater social mobility; few young families have grandparents in easy distance. There has also been a marked rise in the number of one-parent families and increased evidence of poor housing, low income and general problems relating to low income or unemployment. A number of studies of family life with a young child with learning difficulties describe the support networks of many as 'negligible in terms of the informal social network'. Recognition of dimensions of care is important, not only in seeking extended patterns of support (not least in involving fathers), but also in recognising that parental participation in any educational or child health programme must depend, not only on the parents' willingness to be involved in educational activities, but also upon other demands made upon the family's time and energy.

A study by Monique Robin and Denise Josse (1986) on parental reactions to the diagnosis of a learning difficulty hypothesised that all mothers develop a process of *anticipation* in interacting with their babies: 'Each mother has a plan for her child. It is a changeable plan, which is at the same time an interpretation of his behaviour and projection into the future.' Robin and Josse argued that children, as they develop new characteristics, may sometimes not fulfil the expectations of their parents. Illness, disability or changing family circumstances can interrupt the 'life plan', sometimes with disastrous results. Robin and Josse concluded however, that appropriate and non-judgemental information and support (with *positive* images of the child's future development) could have powerful impacts on family life and expectations and on the child's development. Cunningham and Davis (1985), in a study of children with Down's Syndrome in a Manchester health authority, similarly found that parents adapted to a diagnosis of learning difficulty at different stages. Traditional early intervention often focussed around the initial disagnoses reducing at around the child's first birthday – just when parents might become more aware of developmental delays and the importance of extra help. They concluded that structured early intervention and teaching programmes were both positive, but that many families also did very well with a regular and optimistic home visitor who would provide continuing support and encourage families to lead 'ordinary' lives and make connections with their local communities. Cunningham and Davis also believed that early intervention had positive effects on children and families and that children with these experiences were more likely to have better health and to go into integrated education than those without similar support. Both factors could be related to the parents feeling more confident and optimistic and having higher expectations for their children.

Interest in the problems of families with young children with learning difficulties and concern about the research findings have led to a number of initiatives to provide counselling, practical support and an educative role for parents. This concern with making parents effective, whilst being sensitive to the degree of partnership which they feel appropriate at a particular point in time, has important messages for other groups of vulnerable children and families in the community. There is growing interest in developing a care management approach for families to ensure consistent support and to encourage parents to sustain any education or other intervention programmes.

Cunningham and Davis (1985) at the London Hospital, found that trained home visitors, offering parents a menu of regular support, could make a major impact on parent involvement in education and in community activities. The menu of support may consist of highly structured home teaching programmes or of general friendship and counselling. Cunningham's evaluation of his service found that the *children* of *supported parents* were more likely to go into integrated education, to be healthier, and to have better social relationships in their local communities. Cunningham and Davis, working in a de-prived inner city area, found that many parents were quite incapable of using Portage or other services without sympathetic friendship and counselling. But with such support, parents went on to become confident and active in their child's care, education, and integration into the local community. Both Cunningham and Davis stressed the importance of informed, sympathetic and ongoing counselling and advice as parents come to terms with a disability and also for a comprehensive programme of support right from the start.

Right from the start: early identification and intervention

The idea of early intervention for very young children developed in the 1960s, with growing involvement of educational and clinical psychologists in behaviour modification and other training programmes using parents as co-workers and, most importantly, with the formal recognition that the family was the most effective and economical system for fostering and sustaining the development of a young child. The early home visiting programmes were initiated in the USA (and subsequently widely developed in the UK). Such schemes had certain common and important factors:

- They were non-selective, including all families who wished to participate.
- The partnership with the home visitor or teacher was seen as an integral part of the success of the programme – in terms of personal trust and relationships with other professionals.
- Most programmes started by working with the child and going on to involve the parent (usually the mother).
- Parental involvement was based on an initial agreement or contract, setting out what the programme could offer and ensuring that demands on the parents were commensurate with other family or personal commitments.
- Programmes taught success to parents who either felt inadequate or incompetent, or who were concerned that their child's special needs would inhibit progress. Demonstration, as well as written activities, was an integral part of such success.

Robert Cameron (1989), when evaluating a number of early intervention schemes and considering 'how to teach parents to teach children', noted the importance of acknowledging that parents have two primary educational roles when a child has a disability or special education need. First parents need to understand how to teach a child everyday life skills. Second, they need help in managing difficult or disruptive behaviour which the child may acquire. Since the mid 1970s, the Portage home teaching model has become increasingly popular and it has been estimated that there are now over 300 schemes in the UK. Portage is characterised by focussing upon helping parents to teach children with special needs within their own homes and, by involving families in selecting their own education goals. The strengths of Portage and other home-based learning programmes are shown below.

- Involve the strengths and knowledge which parents already hold.
- Involve a trained home visitor who is able to link back to a wider network of professionals.
- Provide an essentially private service, inasmuch as it can take place in a venue chosen by the parent.
- Enable parents to select their own priorities, not only in terms of cognitive development, but in seeking practical solutions for difficult behaviour.

- Match the actual level of parental involvement to individual family dynamics. Home-based learning programmes such as portage can be combined with other forms of provision, for example, nursery or school classes, day care arrangements, members of the extended family and so on.

Successful home teaching programmes, like Portage, offer flexible structures and approaches to meeting individual needs. They also acknowledge the interdependence of children's educational, social care and health needs and the importance of offering services which reflect children's and families' culture, lifestyle and other family commitments. In practice, portage is a process, not a single solution. As Cameron (1989) and others have emphasised, the central feature of portage is the home teaching process which has the three following features.

- Using direct contact people (especially parents) to teach the child.
- Using an individualised teaching programme which is based upon a realistic assessment of the child's existing skills.
- Providing positive monitoring and recording procedures.

One of the major benefits of a good Portage scheme is that it permits information to travel between parents and professionals, and, provides a detailed data base on a child which can be utilised by subsequent service providers. A major criticism of some early intervention programmes was that they frequently fail to manage the transfer of relevant information between families and different networks of professionals. Portage provides a key worker approach in offering support to parents through a familiar individual and in effectively co-ordinating often complex advice from multiple professionals and caregivers. One local authority has developed a Portage programme within a social services department to provide support and practical help to parents in caring for their children at home. In other authorities, the self-assessment skills of parents have been utilised in planning for children's wider needs and in ensuring that parents are aware of the full range of local services.

Part III of the 1993 Education Act replaced the 1981 Act in September 1994. The 1993 Act is accompanied by a Code of Practice, which gives clearer guidance on the identification, assessment and specification of provision for children with special educational needs (including the under fives). The Code of Practice offers important new opportunities to local authority social services departments and child health agencies allowing them to become more actively involved in a more proactive assessment process (which will also clearly involve pupils in the process of assessment and review of progress). The Children Act 1989 created new opportunities for joint assessment which have been little utilised – in part because of major structural changes within the education system. But for children with learning difficulties, the implementation of the 1993 Act and the procedures identified in the Code of Practice offer important new ways forward and, in particular, real possibilities for the development of assessment and care management systems which acknowledge the importance of holistic support for all children with special needs and, specifically, the need to develop integrated early intervention systems right from the start.

The Children Act 1989

The Children Act 1989 has been widely welcomed for bringing together most public and private law relating to children and for establishing a new and unified approach to local authority services for children and families in England and Wales. Many of the changes (and challenges) of the Act will be most apparent in services for children with disabilities and their parents. Historically, such services have been provided through health as well as local authorities, with confusing variations in local management and many conspicuous gaps in service. The Children Act restores the leadership to social services departments and importantly requires that every local authority has services designed to: minimise the effect on disabled children within their area of disability; and give such children the opportunity to lead lives which are as normal as possible (Schedule 2, para 6). Like the Education Act 1993 the Children Act has an integrationist principle underlying its provisions. But defining integration has always been a challenge in terms of identifying positive support for children with special needs and which provides appropriately for such needs.

Many children with learning difficulties will require health *and* social care, both at home and in educational contexts, if they are to achieve their full potential. However, a 'single door' approach to services can only happen if definitions of 'need' and assessment arrangements dovetail and inter-agency support systems for individuals are complementary, well organised, of good quality and convenient to user

The Children Act 1989

For the first time in UK legislation, the Children Act 1989 requires local authorities to provide services for children with disabilities which are designed to minimise the effects of the children's disabilities and to give them the opportunity to lead lives which are as normal as possible.

These requirements are based upon the 'five great principles' outlined below which must inform *all* local authorities working with children.

The welfare of the child
Local authorities have new duties to safeguard and promote the welfare of children in need, those they are looking after and those who are living away from home.
Partnership with parents
Local authorities should try and support parents without the use of compulsory powers.
The importance of families
Children should be brought up in their own families (immediate or extended) wherever possible.
The importance of the views of children and parents
Local authorities have duties to ascertain and take account of their wishes and feelings.
Corporate responsibility
The Children Act is addressed to the local authority *as a whole* and not just to social services departments.

Local authorities have new duties to provide a range of services for children 'in need' (see page 29) and their families. These include the following.

- Advice, guidance and counselling.
- Practical and financial assistance by grant or loan.
- Occupational, recreational or social activities.
- Home help (including laundry services).
- Help with travel in order to use a service.
- Day care and supervised activities (including after-school and holiday programmes).
- Accommodation (which includes respite care).

The local authority has a duty to prevent neglect and abuse and to avoid court proceedings if possible. The authority has new powers to provide for young people who are over 18 but under 21 if they have continuing needs.

families with no waste of resources. (The general duties of local authorities to identify and assess children in need are set out below.) But they will only be effective for children with a range of disabilities if there is genuine collaboration and co-ordination of working practices across agencies. There is growing interest in joint purchasing strategies with shared operational and strategic guidelines across the three main statutory agencies. But such an approach requires careful negotiations at local level, to reconcile different priorities and cultural differences between agencies, and to create incentives to work together in the future.

Four years of implementation of the Children Act has made it clear that the majority of local authorities are seriously addressing new models of services for children and young people with learning difficulties. In many instances this means adult service providers (for example, some community learning difficulties teams) having to rethink their 'all-age' approach to learning difficulty and work with children's services on new approaches which reflect child care practice. But the majority of children's services lack awareness of disability and may underestimate the very complex needs of some children with profound or multiple disabilities or challenging behaviour who need expert, regular and local support in order to remain in their local communities.

For the first time in the history of child care in the UK, the Children Act 1989 integrates provision for children with disabilities within mainstream children's legislation. The Act introduces a new concept of 'children in need'. A child will be regarded as being 'in need' if:

- 'He is unlikely to achieve or maintain, or to have the opportunity of achieving or maintaining, a reasonable standard of health or development without the provision for him of services by a local authority under this Part (of the Act).
- His health or development is likely to be significantly impaired, or further impaired, without the provision for his services.
- He is disabled.'

A key theme in the Children Act is that of partnership with parents. The principles of welfare and of parental responsibility require new partnership arrangements between the local authority and parents of children in need (which will include children with disabilities). The concept of partnership is not new, but is based on the following well-established beliefs.

- The family is the natural and most appropriate home for the majority of children.
- Families are already caring for children and supporting them to do so is in the best interests of the child and the allocation of resources in the local authority.
- The family has a unique and special knowledge of a child and can therefore contribute significantly to that child's health and development – albeit often in partnership with a range of service providers.
- Families provide continuity for children throughout the life cycle, and, in the context of the Children Act, 'families' are recognised as being more widely defined than 'parents', (that is, including grandparents and other relatives).

The Children Act has been widely welcomed in providing a new legal framework for the provision of services for children with a range of disabilities, and, in particular, for including children with disabilities within a wider framework of legal powers, duties and protections which relate to the welfare of *all* children and in that context see all children are literally children first. Section 17(1) of the Children Act sets out the general duty of every local authority to safeguard and promote the welfare of the children within their area who are in need, and, so far as it is consistent with that duty, to promote the upbringing of such children by their families, through providing a range and level of services appropriate to their individual needs.

The Children Act makes a number of specific requirements with reference to children with disabilities which are as follows.

- Schedule 2, paragraph 6, requires local authorities to provide services for children with disabilities which are designed to minimise the effect of their children's disabilities and to give them the opportunity to lead lives which are as 0 normal as possible.
- Schedule 2, paragraph 3 provides that a local authority may assess a child's needs for the purpose of the Children Act at the same time as any assessment under certain other Acts (for example the 1993 Education Act, the Disabled Persons Act 1986, the NHS and Community Care Act 1990).
- Schedule 2, paragraph 2, sets out the requirements on local authorities to open and maintain a register of children with disabilities in their area.
- Section 23(8) requires that where a local authority provides accommodation (that is residential, respite or foster care) for a child whom they are looking after, they shall, so far as is reasonably practicable, secure that the accommodation is not unsuitable to his particular needs.

For the first time in UK child care legislation, local authorities must take account of the religious persuasion, racial origin, culture and linguistic backgrounds of children and must ensure that these issues are taken into account when assessing children's needs. The Children Act gives local authority social services departments a lead role in planning for children but it expects them to work collaboratively. Local authorities are encouraged to 'facilitate the provision by others', in particular the voluntary sector, and are expected to publicise and disseminate information about the full range of services in their areas.

The Children Act has a strong integrationist principle. Schedule 2, paragraph 6, does not explain to local authorities *how* they may provide services for children with disabilities which will minimise the effect of their disabilities upon them, nor does it attempt to describe an *ordinary life*. But the ordinary life principle runs through all the Act's procedures, including those relating to the courts, where children have new rights to emphasise their own preferences about where they wish to live; whom they wish to live with and how their lives should be organised. The Act assumes that local authorities will 'promote access for all children to the same range of services' but volume 6 of the guidance on *Children with Disabilities* (DoH, 1991) notes the importance of avoiding simplistic notions of integration and acknowledging that some children can use ordinary services, but may need support to do so.

In the majority of local authorities the notion of including children with learning and other disabilities within a common child care framework has created major challenges. Initially many authorities proposed to totally integrate services for children with disabilities within generic child care provision. But practice sometimes challenged policy and there is currently an increased awareness that effective integration or inclusion nonetheless requires appropriate specialist advice and input in order to ensure that children are included and not merely 'placed' within a generic child care environment. Historically the majority of services for children with learning difficulties were located within all-age disability-specific specialist services. Such services had expertise and usually ring-fenced budgets but they were not well equipped to encourage the use of ordinary services and, working in general with adults, were not necessarily familiar with the very rapid changes and developments in services for *children* in the 1980s. In the 1990s the emerging management structures seem more likely to favour provision and management within children's services – but with the appointment of senior managers with specific responsibility for children with disabilities and with inter-agency responsibilities to ensure that assessment and care management reflect both individual needs for specialist services and access to good quality provision that as far as possible is within mainstream children's services. There is also a marked trend to integrate disabilities under one senior manager rather than fragment services under categories of sensory, physical or learning disabilities.

John O'Brien (1987) has defined the key components of a community service as *five service accomplishments*, that is, services should try to achieve community presence, choice, competence, respect and community participation.

All these goals are implicit in the Children Act. But there are issues about how best to address the needs of children with a wide range of special needs whose effective inclusion will be heavily dependent upon the availability of a range of appropriate, local and well resourced services. The Mansell Committee (1992), in considering a range of issues relating to challenging behaviour and adults, identified three different approaches to working with people with disabilities in local authorities. These are 'removers' (a heavy reliance on specialist and out-of-area services); 'containers' (seek to provide local services, but often with inadequate resources and little creativity in increasing the capacity of existing provision or attempting new models of care or support); and 'developers' (try to provide a good range of individual local services by prioritising training and staff development; consulting with consumers and ensuring that management structures encourage change and innovation whilst sustaining existing good practice).

Many local authorities (and parents) will recognise these approaches; indeed many local services combine the three, with children with challenging behaviour most likely to rely on out-of-authority provision and least likely to have access to a range of *local* support services.

Access to good quality local services for families with children with learning difficulties has always been problematic, not least because children with learning difficulties will inevitably constitute a minority within any local authority planning system and because their needs will equally inevitably be met through a multiplicity of different agencies. The Children Act lays down a crucial *new* duty on social services departments to publish information about services provided by themselves and others (Schedule 2, para 1) and to ensure that information reaches those who might benefit from such services. Many parents who agreed to their children being included within the new registers of children with disabilities (Schedule 2) consider that registration is worthwhile if it only achieves access to good, regularly updated and relevant information on all services available through social services, child health and education, the voluntary sector and the social security system. In one local authority such information made available to parents listed all sources (voluntary and statutory) of advice on welfare benefits and resulted in a 15 per cent increase in take-up of disability benefits, with a 30 per cent increase in parents winning at appeal. Although the Children Act places no conditions upon access to information, which should be freely available and actively promoted for all who might need it, the existence of an accurate, regularly updated and generally accepted register clearly facilitates information exchange and sensible planning decisions. But, as the Social Services Inspectorate (1994) noted in the first report of a national inspection of services for children with disabilities:

> The lack of effective registers in many of the Authorities up to the time of the Inspection has resulted in no reliable information on the numbers of disabled children in those communities. . . . Services were being provided, therefore, on an historical basis rather than using current information to help with the planning and monitoring of services. . . . The DoH commissioned national monitoring survey revealed that by June 1992 one third of Local Authorities had yet to complete their arrangements for maintaining a register of children with disabilities . . . most of the parents and carers consulted by SSI as part of this inspection held no objections to the establishment of a register . . . these parents suggested that the register could be used as a planning tool for services and also as a mailing list for the circulation of information.

As Baldwin and Carlisle (1994) in a review of the research literature on services for disabled children and their families noted, any support system for families with children with disabilities must be based on the following five key criteria.

- The availability of accurate information for families, practitioners, planners and for the purchasers and commissioners of services.
- A recognition of the emotional and social context of assessment and use of services and any special provision.
- An acknowledgement of the stress under which some parents live on a day-to-day basis.
- The active involvement of those parents whose personal circumstances make it difficult for them to use parent networks and other community support systems for information, advice and practical help without additional support.

- A commitment to the principle of maximum integration in good quality children's services, but with specialist support available when required.

Family support

Respite and short-term care

Access to regular and emergency short-term or respite care is considered an essential service by almost all parents with a child with a disability or special needs. Historically, respite care developed as an emergency service, frequently providing care within a hospital or institutional setting and usually seen as crisis intervention. But in the past decade respite care has been seen increasingly as one aspect of an integrated support service for families with children with special needs. The most commonly available and acceptable form of respite care in the UK is now provided through family-based schemes. Robinson *et al.* (1991) estimated there were currently 265 family-based respite care schemes in the UK, of which 53 were for adults. The OPCS surveys (1989) estimate that there are around 360 000 children with disabilities of whom 165 000 have disabilities in the higher severity levels. Of these children only 3.7 per cent currently have access to family-based respite care, although an average of 50 per cent of parents of children in all the disability categories felt that their quality of life was adversely affected by restrictions on going out or giving time to other family members.

Family-based respite care is generally much reduced in terms of availability for older children and young adults. It has been estimated that only 1 500 adults with disabilities receive family-based respite care, out of a potential user group of 6 000 000 (OPCS 1989).

At present virtually all schemes have some kind of waiting list. The average length is 14 people. Adult services tend to have higher percentages of people on a waiting list than do children's services (38 per cent and 27 per cent, respectively). In addition to the general shortage of respite carers, several studies have suggested that there may be particular problems in recruiting families for children with very challenging behaviour. However, Robinson *et al.* (1991) found that 42 children's and seven adult schemes said they did cater for service users with very difficult behaviour. Stalker (1990) found that high degrees of physical dependency in older children could also cause difficulties but that some carers specifically wished to care for children with high dependency needs.

Respite carers are recruited, trained and paid in very different ways according to the local authority concerned. Some carers have a semi-professional status. Others provide a service as volunteers with expenses only being paid. There are wide variations in local authority policies for charging parents using respite care, with many choosing not to do so because of the likelihood of respite care helping to prevent family breakdown.

The Children Act and respite care: the legal framework

The Children Act 1989 makes new and special provision for short-term placements of children with special needs within schemes which are variously known as respite care, short-term care, phased care, or family link schemes. Under these schemes, the SSD or voluntary agency makes arrangements for a child who normally lives with his or her family – and whose family continues to exercise full parental responsibility – to spend short or sometimes longer periods of time with either an approved family or in a residential home.

An important principle of the Children Act is that parents and children should be actively involved in any decisions to be made about a child's care. Regulation 3 of the Arrangements for Placement of Children gives a new statutory duty to local authorities or voluntary organisations to prepare a written plan for any child whom they propose to accommodate; parents and children and any relevant individuals or agencies must also be consulted. The plan will be expected to give details of the accommodation to be offered and the purpose and timescale of the arrangements. Respite carers must now be approved under the same regulations as foster parents and children will be expected to have a medical examination and a written health assessment prior to placement.

The Children Act and the regulations on foster placements and residential care all emphasise the importance of planning and review in safeguarding and promoting children's welfare. Developing an effective planning and review process which is economical in terms of resources but effective in terms of supporting children and families will be a challenge to many authorities. The Children Act requires workers to develop a new approach to working with parents which acknowledges parents as key partners, but which places the welfare of the *child* at the heart of any decision-making. Respite care schemes will need to become more child-centred and less orientated to giving respite to parents. This is likely to mean changing attitudes and practice and may create considerable pressure on services in terms of more creative consultation with consumers, as well as with additional planning and record-keeping for all children using respite care.

The rationale for more specific planning for respite or short-term care lies in growing concern about children with disabilities using multiple sources of respite care and sometimes spending considerable periods of unplanned time away from home without any overall assessment of their needs. Initially a number of individuals and organisations expressed concern about the administrative complexity of the new arrangements and the strain which they will place upon scarce resources. For example, if a family uses two respite carers (perhaps making a differentiation between term-time and holiday care), the procedures had to be carried out twice. Social Service departments also found the arrangements for occasional use of respite care (e.g. a weekend) unnecessarily bureaucratic. After wide consultation the Department of Health is issuing more flexible guidance for short-term breaks.

Most importantly, family-based respite care's great strength has been its inherent flexibility coupled with its ability to engage a very diverse range of carers from local communities (including minority ethnic groups). There has been considerable concern that the new and more formalised arrangements under the Children Act may deter some potential carers from coming forward and, indeed, that arrangements designed primarily for children living away from home may be too regulatory for children who are merely staying for a short period of time. But these concerns have to be put in the broader context of growing awareness of the risks to children with a disability in terms of sexual, emotional and physical abuse. For all short-term care schemes, the challenge of balancing safeguards for children will need to be balanced against avoidance of unnecessary bureaucracy and a reduction in the numbers of families offered a service.

Other forms of respite care

Figures are difficult to obtain for the use of non-family-based respite care, although residential homes and schools, holiday schemes and NHS provision, and children's hospices may all provide support. Although children are no longer admitted to hospitals for residential care, some long-stay 'mental handicap' hospitals continue to provide short-term placements. It is declared DoH policy that such hospitals are inappropriate placements for children. New guidance on the welfare of children in hospital (DoH, 1991(6)) states that the use of any form of NHS provision for respite care should be justified on specific medical or other special needs and be part of a coherent process of assessment and planning for the children concerned. Department of Health guidance notes that if respite care is provided by the NHS, it should generally be in 'small homely units' which take account of the child's overall needs. The best known example of such a unit is Honeylands attached to the Royal Devon and Exeter Hospital. An evaluation of Honeylands (Brimblecombe and Russell, 1987) showed a high degree of user satisfaction with a service which placed great emphasis on high standards of child care, flexibility and a strong emphasis on parent participation. Parents of sick or vulnerable children appreciated the availability of specialist help. Similar views have been expressed about the growing use of children's hospices for respite care, such usage usually also reflecting complex or multiple disability or terminal illness.

The amount of residential respite care provided by local authorities appears to be declining as policies turn to family-based provision. There are no figures for the numbers of residential homes providing respite care and indeed many local authorities use provision in the voluntary or private sectors. Oswin's study (1984) of a number of residential respite care provisions gave rise to considerable concerns about the training, support and monitoring of such provision. An evaluative study of residential respite care in selected settings currently being undertaken by staff at the Norah Fry Research Centre provides helpful data on the implementation of the Children Act within the residential respite sector (Robinson *et al.*, 1994).

Hubert (1991), looking at the needs of teenagers and young adults with severe and profound learning difficulties and behavioural problems, found that young people who were incontinent, physically disabled, had little speech and could be aggressive or destructive were the most likely to have no respite care or care which was considered inappropriate and inadequate because of their difficulties. She found major stresses in parents who felt that the switch from children's to adult units at 16 was much too early and that the poor care offered made some parents so guilty that the use of respite care was associated with little relief. The absence of family-based care for these young people may have reflected problems in recruiting carers. Stalker (1990) found that older children with physical disabilities or difficult behaviour were the most likely to remain on waiting lists. Robinson *et al.* (1991) found similar evidence of problems in placing older 'difficult' children but noted that some schemes did successfully recruit families for these groups and that some carers were interested in looking after children or young people with high dependency needs.

Respite care on its own is not a universal panacea. Stalker and Robinson (1991) found that 55 per cent of parents interviewed in Croydon and 65 per cent of parents interviewed in Sheffield wanted other kinds of help apart from respite care. These included day-care for young adults; holidays and holiday play schemes and sitting services. Robinson (1987) evaluating the Avon Family Based Respite Care scheme similarly noted the importance of assessing families' total needs and avoiding any assumption that respite care on its own would change parents' lives.

In recent years there has been growing concern to provide flexible short-term care which offers the services listed here.

- A local service, where the child can continue to attend school as if he or she were living at home.
- Good quality child care which ensures that the child is not treated as a sick patient, but as any child who happens to have a disability.
- Availability on demand. Research into different models of respite care has clearly indicated the importance of parents choosing patterns of use and being able to use a service flexibly. There is good evidence that many families prefer to use respite care services for short periods of time (sometimes during the day only) rather than in longer term block bookings.
- A service which meets the needs of all children. Concern has been expressed about the lack of respite care for children with the greatest need, for example, emotional and behaviour difficulties or complex medical problems and multiple disabilities.
- Age-appropriate care – so that young children and adolescents are given relevant care and occupation.
- An integrated programme of family support which sees respite care as part of a wider range of professional support services to meet family needs. Escalating use of respite care may indicate a need for preventive services to avoid some children slipping into long-term care.

Some issues for the future of respite care

All studies of respite care (whether in substitute families, residential or health provision) confirm the importance of the careful planning of placements and of the first introduction to the service. Stalker (1990) found that the majority of families wished for a number of visits prior to any actual overnight stay. These visits created mutual confidence and trust. Evaluations of the health service respite care facilities of Honeylands and Preston Skreens (Brimblecombe and Russell, 1987) similarly found that parents who were particularly stressed might need the greatest help in actually agreeing to use a service. The same studies also found that parents had very varying patterns of use, some parents making heavy demands when family circumstances required, others using respite care on an occasional basis.

Despite waiting lists and heavy demand, some respite care services have noted occasional under-use by referred families. The Honeylands evaluation (Brimblecombe and Russell, 1987) and an SSI study (1984) of respite care in Oxfordshire and Norfolk found that parents needed to go through different stages in using respite care. The latter identified three hurdles, namely using a service for the first time, leaving the child overnight and placing a child for a longer period while the parents went away on their own. Oswin (1985) and Hubert (1991) have also described the ambivalence of parents who were desperate for relief but felt that the provision was inadequate or who worried about how their child would be cared for when they were not there.

Family-based respite care has been, and will continue to be, a key service for families with disabled children. It provides important opportunities to support and integrate children within their local communities and all studies show high levels of parental appreciation. However, respite care cannot exist in isolation and should be seen as one of a range of options for children and families. Evidence about the ability of respite care to alleviate family stress is inevitably subjective. However the Honeylands and Preston Skreens evaluations and Robinson et al. (1991), in their final report on a study of family-based respite care schemes in the UK, all found a high degree of satisfaction with a good quality service. However, all the above evaluations noted that parents were concerned by waiting lists; and that families would have welcomed a broader range and availability of support services for families with a disabled child. There is continuing concern about the development of acceptable respite care for children from minority ethnic communities and for older children and young adults from all backgrounds. As the DoH guidance on children with disabilities notes (1991) 'respite care should be provided in the context of a package of care for families', an integrated programme of family support which sees planned respite care as part of a wider range of professional support services to meet family needs.

The role of child health services

Although the lead role for the care of children with learning difficulties now rests firmly with social services departments, child health services will continue to play a key role in determining how these children achieve maximum progress, and to ensure that their learning difficulties are not compounded by additional health care needs or secondary disabilities. Key issues for future debate and development in the context of major NHS reforms are as follows.

- The development of effective surveillance and early identification programmes whose outcomes are shared with parents and education and social services in an intelligible and helpful way.
- Clarification of the specific contribution of child health services to the wider packages of care which will be important components in any 'care in the community' policies. Such clarification will include clear policies for district handicap, child development or community learning difficulty teams and their contribution to children's services.
- Agreed procedures for sharing information about special health care needs with other agencies, whilst protecting confidentiality where necessary.
- Promotion of parent involvement in assessment and care (with the use of parent held child health records and partnership arrangements) with education and health services.
- The provision of medical advice and support to community services (including schools) on the special health care needs of children with complex needs.
- Clarification of the continuing role of the NHS with regard to respite and longer term health care.
- Wider discussion about the contribution of child and adolescent mental health services to the care and development of children with learning disabilities.

As noted earlier, effective implementation of the changes to both social and health care as a consequence of the recent legislation will necessitate integration of services, as well as the individual children who use them. Community care for children is not a new concept, but its effective interpretation means considerable changes in terms of financial, organisational and cultural approaches to needs-led assessment; service provision through care-management and review and clarity about the respective contributions of health, education and social services. Although social services will be the lead agency in terms of children's services, district health authorities and family health services authorities will increasingly be required to work together to provide a 'seamless service' which transcends traditional agency divides. As a response to the need to integrate medical and social models of care, some local and health authorities are producing joint purchasing strategies for children's services.

The Children Act requires local authorities to consider children's general health and welfare as part of any planning and care management. There has been growing awareness that many services for children with learning difficulties have focussed upon the child's difficulties and have not necessarily looked at wider issues of health and development. The Welsh Office (Welsh Health Planning Forum, 1992) has published a *Protocol for Investment in Health Gain for People with a Learning Disability*. Although prepared for a wider audience than special educational needs, the protocol has nonetheless been very helpful in assessment in an education setting. The initiative was triggered through the All Wales Mental Handicap Strategy and sets goals to be achieved by 1993. These goals are also shared with the education service, which has a major responsibility for identifying any potential problems such as secondary disabilities in the school years.

The role of child health and nursing services will be crucial to those parents who are caring for a child with multiple disabilities at home. More children are surviving neonatal difficulties; trauma and serious infectious illnesses, and living longer with some of the rarer metabolic and genetically determined diseases – but with very significant medical and nursing needs. A number of health authorities are beginning to provide community outreach schemes but there has been no direct replication of some of the support programmes for 'medically fragile' children which are developing in the USA. The Jackson, Florida, medical care programme provides an individualised nursing care plan as well as a child care plan (Hochstadt and Yost, 1991). There is an energetic programme of involving the natural parents in as much of the child's care as possible, with respite carers recruited who have the necessary skills to carry out any special procedures. The programme provides the loan of any specialist equipment and has guaranteed access to advice when required. In the UK some similar initiatives are developing, with parents in some health authorities being trained to administer rectal valium, manage tracheostomies and perform other nursing procedures. However, some families are finding themselves confused by the new purchaser/provider arrangements in some health authorities. Divisions of opinion about who pays for nursing care (such as injections or tube feeding) have meant some children being refused respite care in a local authority or voluntary care setting. Ultimately the otherwise welcome shift from a 'medical' to a 'social' model of care poses the important question as to how children with very complex health care needs can best be supported and the extent to which joint commissioning arrangements between local and health authorities can be achieved.

The last ten years have seen major developments in creating more family-based services for children with disabilities and special needs. Integration – or inclusion – has become a primary objective, but the ultimate challenge remains the balance between meeting special needs in the most natural environment for child and family. As one parent commented at a National Development Team workshop:

> The most important thing to any family is the birth of a child, *their* child. Disability can spoil the celebration and set parents and child apart. But all families need their own support. Let's stop talking about *special* families and just ask what *all* families want for themselves and their children. (Russell and Flynn, 1991).

References

Baldwin, S. and Carlisle, J. (1994). *Social Support for Disabled Children and their Families: A Review of the Literature*. Social Work Services Inspectorate (Scotland), HMSO, Edinburgh.

Brimblecombe, F. and Russell, P. (1987). *Honeylands: Developing a Service for Families with Handicapped Children*. National Children's Bureau, London.

Cameron, R. (1989). *Portage: Ten Years of Achievement*. NFER, Slough.

Cunningham, C. and Davis, H. (1985). *Working with Parents: Frameworks for Collaboration*. Open University Press, Milton Keynes.

Department for Education (1994). *Code of Practice on the Identification and Assessment of Special Educational Needs*. Department of Education, London.

Department of Health (1991). The Children Act 1989: guidance and regulations, Volume 6, *Children with Disabilities*. HMSO, London.

Department of Health (1991). *Welfare of Children and Young People in Hospital*. HMSO, London.

Fish, J. (Chair) (1985). *Report of Committee of Enquiry into Special Educational Needs in the ILEA; Equal Opportunities for All?* Inner London Education Authority, London.

Glendinning, C. (1983). *Unshared Care: Parents and their Disabled Childen*. Routledge and Kegan Paul, London.

Hochstadt, N. and Yost, D. (1991). *The Medically Complex Child: The Transition to Home Care*. Harwood Academic Publishers, New York.

Hubert, J. (1991). *Home-bound-Crisis in the Care of Young People with Learning Disabilities*. King's Fund, London.

Mansell, J. (Chair) (1992). Services for people with learning disabilities and challenging behaviour or mental health needs. *Report of Committee of Enquiry*, HMSO, London.

O'Brien, J. (1987). A guide to personal futures planning. In *A Comprehensive Guide to the Activities Catalogue: An Alternative Curriculum for Youth with Severe Disabilities* (eds E.T. Bellamy and B. Wilcox). Paul H. Brookes, Baltimore.

Office of Population and Census Surveys (1989). OPCS surveys of disability in the UK: Report 3 *Prevalence of Disability among Children*, Report 5 *Financial Circumstances of Families*; Report 6 *Disabled Children: Services, Transport and Education*. HMSO, London.

Oswin, M. (1984). *They Keep Going Away*. King Edwards Hospital Fund/ Blackwells, Oxford.

Robin, M. and Josse, D. (1986). *Working with Parents*. Unpubl.

Robinson, C. (1987). *Avon Short Term Respite Care Scheme: Evaluation Study*. Department of Mental Health, University of Bristol.

Robinson, C., Orlich, C. and Russell, O. (1991). *A Survey of Family based Respite Care Schemes in the United Kingdom*. Norah Fry Research Centre, University of Bristol.

Robinson, C., Weston, D. and Minkes, J. (1994). *Quality in Services to Disabled Children under the Children Act 1989*. Norah Fry Research Centre, University of Bristol.

Russell, P. and Flynn, M. (1991). *Future Services for Families with Children with Learning Disabilities*. Report of Parent Workshop, National Development Team, London.

Social Services Inspectorate (1994). *Services to Disabled Children and their Families: Reports of the National Inspection to Disabled Children and their Families*. HMSO, London.

Stalker, K. (1990). *Share the Care: An Evaluation of a Family-based Respite Care Service*. Jessica Kingsley, London.

Stalker, K. and Robinson, C. (1991). *The Non-users of Respite Care Services*. Third Interim Report, Norah Fry Research Centre, University of Bristol.

Welsh Health Planning Forum (1992). *Protocol for Investment in Health Gain. Mental Handicap (Learning Disabilities)*. Welsh Office, Cardiff.

Wilkin, D. (1979). *Caring for the Mentally Handicapped Child*. Croom Helm, London.

Chapter 3

A home of their own: Achieving supported housing

Pat Fitton and Jean Willson

It is natural and normal for young people to leave their parents and set up home independently. If people with profound intellectual and multiple disabilities are to do this successfully, clear aims and meticulous attention to detail will be required. No one should underestimate the amount of work involved in conception and planning. If the project is to run successfully, clear structures of management and accountability must underpin the philosophical commitment to the venture. The project described below has been running since April 1991 and provides a home of their own for two young women with profound intellectual and multiple disabilities. Its successes and problems are outlined to help those planning similar ventures.

If such a project were to be initiated now, the process would need to start with an assessment of care needs under the NHS and Community Care Act 1990. This project began before this Act came into force, and those involved in the planning process had to evolve their own rules and methods. It was essentially a collaborative experience between the parents as representatives of the two women and the professionals. There were some very positive aspects with this way of working and it remains to be seen whether the new Act throws up methods of planning that allow such a degree of participation by service users and their representatives.

When planning started, Kathy was aged 26 and Victoria 20. They had much in common. Both had profound intellectual and multiple disabilities; Victoria's condition was caused by a rare condition, tuberous sclerosis; the reason for Kathy's original disabilities was not known. Both suffered severe and complex epileptic attacks. Victoria walked a little with assistance, Kathy could only shuffle on her side along the floor. Neither communicated verbally. Both needed regular medication. Both were doubly incontinent although Victoria was learning to use the toilet. Each was closely involved with a loving family. The two had known each other for many years, and both sets of parents were closely bonded through years of campaigning to improve services and sharing one another's problems. Both women loved music – opera, classical, jazz, folk – food and outings. Both could feed themselves with supervision. Both had strong personalities, a sense of humour, no need for assertiveness training and a determination to communicate with eyes, arms and sounds. Kathy had become more frail in recent years and suffered from a group of auto-immune conditions which exacerbated her existing disabilities and gave her much pain and discomfort. Since 1984 she had been using a naso-gastric tube for taking medication and fluids.

Both women had previously lived in settings that were not suitable. They had to fit into an institutional framework with meals, bedtimes and so on determined by staff. Often the women's emotional and social needs were neglected. Certainly their relationships with family and friends became fragmented. By early 1989, the care situations in each of the residential units where Kathy and Victoria were living were totally unacceptable due to staff shortages, unsympathetic attitudes, poor management and accountability and incompatibility with other residents. The families discussed informally the idea of the women sharing a home, which would be staffed for 24-hour care. Their social workers were excited by the idea. Parents and social workers met Simon Palmour, principal officer for learning difficulties in Islington Council, and put the idea to him. He responded enthusiastically, seeing it as a trail-blazing project. He asked the parents to write to him formally requesting independent living schemes for Kathy and Victoria. The assistant director gave his agreement to continue meeting to see if the project was feasible.

The philosophy underpinning the project for their own home was based on the belief that these two women had fundamental rights as people with learning difficulties, however severe those difficulties, to have a decent life and to be treated with respect. This meant it should be their home, shared by compatible people, living in an ordinary house with arrangements made to suit them.

The planning process

The parents had worked together previously in joint planning groups. We expected to be fully involved in the planning of this new venture. The project team consisted of the parents as representatives of the two women, their social workers, the agency already providing care for one of the women, the lettings officer from the council's neighbourhood office and Simon Palmour. Simon Palmour convened the meetings which took place from late 1989. We met at least monthly, and during busy periods, more frequently. In addition, individuals and sub-groups took items of business away to work on and reported back to the main group. Everyone had to fit in the meetings and consequent work on top of their normal workload; the parents worked full-time in demanding jobs, and had to get time off to attend meetings, then do any consequent work in the evenings or at weekends.

Discussions were open and frank; the working relationships were direct and informal, but Simon Palmour ensured that meetings were businesslike and kept to agendas. We shared minute taking and always specified who was going to take action on which issues. Individuals such as the welfare rights officer or the occupational therapist were invited to meetings for specific topics.

It was not possible to deal with issues one at a time and then move on to the next. Issues constantly overlapped. An obstacle or crisis would need to be resolved such as when the Independent Living Fund initially turned down Kathy's application. When we thought we had the housing sorted out, there were further problems about the care costs. When the care costs were settled, there were problems with the benefits. When all that was on course, there were further problems with the adaptations to the house.

Financing the project

The big financial issue was the care costs. Both women would need 24-hour care and could not be left alone in the house for even a few minutes. The care agency costed up the optimum package (details are given later). Tough discussions then followed with the assistant director of social services. The borough insisted that it would contribute no more than was already being paid out for the two women's current residential placements. Because of the way these payments were calculated, a large shortfall was left. We had already approached the

Independent Living Fund (ILF) to assess Kathy and Victoria. It now became clear that they would need the maximum contribution from the ILF if the project was to work. Even then, we had to agree to cut the original care package to the bone. We agreed to a sleep-in worker rather than one on waking night duty. We also had to accept that each woman would have only the one worker, even at crunch times such as bathing. This may sound generous until you look at the pattern of daily life, for example with one worker going out with Kathy and the other having to cope with Victoria's severe fitting with no one else around. Workers were also doing all shopping, cooking and cleaning.

The total cost of the package for each woman was roughly £50 000 per annum. Recent enquiries show that this figure is less than the cost for places in two local authority units, a home run by a charitable foundation and a long-stay hospital.

The Independent Living Fund

Each family applied on behalf of its daughter and by the autumn of 1990 the ILF agreed to give each woman her maximum grant of £400 per week. It was agreed at the project meeting that the parents should write accepting this offer on behalf of the women, giving a provisional start date of 25 February 1991. Our relief at clearing this hurdle changed to shock on learning that the ILF would reduce their contribution to the total care costs by the amount of the Severe Disability Premium and half the amount of the Attendance Allowance (now the Disabled Living Allowance, care component) for each of the women. The meeting re-calculated the personal budget and decided that with these deductions the women could manage – just. We felt at this stage that we were taking a great risk on their behalf, and Simon Palmour asked the meeting if we still felt able to go ahead with the project. After further discussion we agreed unanimously to go ahead. The parents were still anxious, but we could see no better solution.

Acquiring the house

At the same time as we were exploring council and ILF finance, both sets of parents wrote formally to the housing department asking for a joint tenancy for their daughters. Kathy and Victoria were also nominated to a housing association.

We soon received an offer from the housing association but it was not suitable. We were very despondent, but soon after we received an offer to view a council property. This was a new purpose-built bungalow on a large, older housing estate near King's Cross. The surroundings were not as congenial as the previous offer, and shops, markets and transport were not quite as convenient. However, when we got inside we immediately felt this was it. The design was spacious, with wide corridors and large rooms making wheelchair access easy. There were two large bedrooms, one with *en suite* facilities. A smaller room would accommodate the sleep-in worker. There were large wardrobes and storage cupboards. Some details had been left to be finalised according to the particular needs of the tenants. There was a small garden at the front. The offer was accepted.

We then had to meet the architect and the occupational therapist and specify particular requirements. The bath had to be raised; we wanted a sluice installed in the utility room to deal with soiled clothing and bedding; the *en suite* toilet and shower had to be adapted; a hoist was needed in the bathroom and an intercom system had to be installed. There were some hold-ups; Simon Palmour had to go back to committee to get extra finance agreed. The delays meant the start date had to be moved to 1 April. We hoped it was not a bad omen! The chairperson of the housing committee had been notified about the project and had asked for more information. The lettings officer was now able to arrange for tenancy agreements to be drawn up and signed by the parents on behalf of the two women.

The care package

The ideal arrangements for the care package had to be pared down considerably during discussions in 1990 and the following points and questions considered.

- Sleeping-in or waking night duty.
- What role day care would play in reducing the need for care workers at that time.
- Should periods at home with parents be built into the calculations?
- Should there always be two support workers, one for each of the two women, during waking hours, or was it possible for one to manage at times?
- What would happen if day care arrangements failed or either woman became unwell and needed to stay at home?
- What would the back-up be if staff were sick or became ill on duty?
- It had to be established that neither woman could be left alone in their

home for even a few minutes, (for example, if a support worker failed to turn up to take over a shift).

The final agreed package was three workers for Victoria's team (including the sleep-in worker), and two for Kathy's team. That way there would be one worker on duty with each woman during waking hours, and one sleeping in at night. It was agreed that the care package had to sustain arrangements independently of the parents.

Workers would be on 13 weeks probation and note would be taken of the reactions of each of the women to individual carers. Some of the workers had worked with Kathy before. All were very enthusiastic and the care agency set up induction arrangements. Parents took part in this initial training.

When it came to personal finance the benefit income would be: Severe Disablement Allowance; Income Support top-up; Severe Disability Premium; Attendance Allowance (now DLA care component); Mobility Allowance (now DLA mobility component); Housing Benefit; and community charge (now council tax) benefit. Out of this, Severe Disability Premium and half of Attendance Allowance would be counted as a contribution to care costs.

Once the project started the two women would be responsible for paying for food and drink; cleaning materials; toiletries; clothing; household bills (gas, electricity, water, telephone); furniture, furnishings, appliances (and their repair); redecoration; garden maintenance and equipment; outings and holidays; personal expenses like greetings cards, presents; and household insurance. There were many problems with actually obtaining the benefits, and Victoria's were not sorted out until a year after she moved in.

We set up two new accounts for each woman: a building society account to receive the ILF money, with a facility for cheque payments to be paid to the care agency; and a bank or separate building society account to receive benefits and to be used to make withdrawals for personal expenses. Setting up these two accounts was hard work. After a few visits the building society staff grasped the issues and set up accounts 'in re. of . .XYZ'; the parents signed as appointees.

The house had a kitty for food and household expenses (an agreed amount would be paid in for each woman on Sunday night. Simple accounts were to be kept by staff), and a personal kitty for each to cover toiletries, personal items, outings, and so on with a simple account book.

There were the usual problems with explaining to the gas, electricity and water companies what the set-up was. Parents had to provide evidence of their own good payment record and underwrite the accounts. A joint account was set up for payment of bills and Kathy and Victoria made regular payments into this to cover this expense. The building society had got the message by now and sorted this out very quickly.

Because the two women could not be left alone in the house they were entitled to free installation and rental of a telephone. This was arranged by one of the social workers and soon installed. However, communication problems in the local authority neighbourhood office meant they did not arrange their payments, and threats of disconnection followed swiftly. We were very worried about this as the telephone was essential to guarantee the safety of the two women. It was sorted out eventually after much effort by the parents.

We were less worried when there were muddles and misunderstandings over housing benefit and community charge (now council tax) exemption. Both women were entitled to full housing benefit and exemption from the community charge. Rent arrears notices nevertheless arrived from the very office which was dealing with the housing benefit application. We decided to let them get on with it. Similarly, it took ages before the community charge exemption was sorted out. We said, half-jokingly, that if Kathy and Victoria were summoned to court we would take them there, and let the magistrate and the council discuss it directly with them. We also had to arrange household contents insurance, which could have been sticky, but the path was smoothed by a friend taking this on for us.

Getting the house ready

Even when all the alterations had finally been completed and new equipment installed, there was much still to be done before moving in day. The entire bungalow had to be cleaned and polished, and a new washing machine, tumble drier and fridge freezer purchased, though we were given a second-hand cooker. (Social Fund grants for furniture and equipment of £330 for Kathy and £700 for Victoria just about paid for the washing machine and tumble drier.)

Family and friends rallied round with second-hand furniture, lamps, rugs, curtains and a music system. MENCAP City Foundation and the North London Spastics Society made generous donations. We produced a booklet describing the project and circulated it to local businesses and organisations, asking them for donations or to sponsor a specific item. We had a memorable visit to Ikea with both women to buy kitchen equipment and basic furniture and we also had to equip the sleeping-in room.

When the great day came the bungalow was basic but could be lived in. Gradually gifts have made the interior more comfortable and attractive. Setting up their home cost about £8000 eventually.

One continuing problem was the slow response by the council to basic repairs needed. We had to take the iron security grilles off the windows and doors ourselves, as no one came as promised. The heating was essential yet it sometimes took days for someone to come when it broke down. Some of the sliding cupboard doors came out of their fixings, and the response of the neighbourhood office was 'we don't fix cupboards'. There were some difficulties over rubbish collection. Disabled parking markings have still not been done and parents had to install a chain barrier themselves. These problems raised questions of whose responsibility it was to chase these things. As the two women could not do it, the support workers would make the initial calls but did not have time to keep chasing. It had to be the parents.

Information, documentation, communication

Once Kathy and Victoria moved in the house

- Diaries were set up to record the women's activities, well-being, any problems, medication, food and drink intake, output, and so on.
- Care books were prepared by parents for each woman. These gave a brief history of their condition, described their personalities, likes and dislikes, methods of communication, and covered all their basic care needs, including emergencies such as severe fitting. They included photographs which showed Kathy and Victoria in a variety of moods and situations.
- More detailed information sheets on dealing with fits, Kathy's special diet, and the like were also supplied. When support workers started they would often be working by themselves with one of the women, and would not have the back-up of a larger institution. So we drew up basic care and activities guidelines covering 24-hours to be used initially until all workers knew the women really well.
- Information sheets and booklets were prepared for all household appliances, including the intercom, and on the security of the house as it was situated in a high-crime area.
- A house book contained copies of all the information sheets on household appliances and equipment, and guidance on all aspects of running the

household, from ordering incontinence supplies, to fire safety procedures, to giving medication.

Simon Palmour drew up a service agreement on behalf of the council which outlined the agreed care package, specified the arrangements for the tenancy and specified action in eventualities such as one tenant moving out. This was to be signed by the council, the care agency and the parents on behalf of the two women.

An operational policy was largely drawn up by parents, but in consultation with the social workers and the care agency. It was intended to give policy guidance on care and daily routines, drawing attention to the practical implications to be found in the house book. It stated the underlying philosophy of equal rights to a meaningful life, and gave guidance on issues such as risk-taking, sexuality and family relationships.

Issues raised by this project

Management

Because neither woman can direct her own care, her representatives do so on her behalf. The framework for this is the operational policy which underpins the whole care package, providing directions and ground rules, and outlining the agreement on what the purchasers require.

It is now agreed by all parties that the care agency's management model may need to be modified in a project serving people with profound learning difficulties. There is some confusion about the varying roles of parents, social workers, advocates and care managers. As eventually parents wish the project to be capable of surviving in the event of their incapacity or death, these various roles need to be sorted out. The parameters of the social worker's role need to be clarified and the local authority needs to decide whether it is going to appoint care managers to oversee day-to-day management of such projects. The care agency now recognises that there needs to be a senior support worker for each team, to be responsible for communication between all concerned, and to have overall responsibility for matters concerning each woman.

Parents accept that in the long-run their daughters should have citizen advocates. At present, they feel their knowledge and experience of many years is essential in enabling the project to work. It is not easy to get advocates, and they do not always stay for long periods. An advocate would not carry out hour by hour, day by day detailed management of the care of his or her partner.

So advocates are needed who would be willing to give a reasonable time commitment. Their role would need to be carefully defined in relation to those managing day-to-day details. To do this job effectively they will need the back up of a support and supervision system independent of the care agency.

Accountability

The women purchase their individual care packages (using local authority and ILF money) from a voluntary organisation which is a limited company with charitable status. At present their parents act as their representatives in directing their care. They, with the local authority, act as purchasers on behalf of the two women.

The operational policy was intended to set the ground rules for how the home would be run. The document still remains unsigned because of unresolved discussions about advocates' roles. There have been no reviews of how the project has worked. Meetings between the purchasers and the organisation to try and resolve any difficulties were agreed initially as necessary but do not always take place when needed. There is no one representing the needs of people with learning difficulties or their representatives on the agency's committees. When a decision or action of major importance is required, such as a decision about the health of one of the users, putting the wheel back on a wheelchair or a breakdown in machinery in the house, everyone always turns to the parents. The local authority still needs to sort out a mechanism to ensure accountability in its role as purchaser.

Staff team and on-going training

The staff team was stable for the first 18 months. Regular supervision sessions, fortnightly team meetings concerning the individual women, and monthly team staff meetings are organised by the care agency. What is lacking in these arrangements is a formal or informal way of the women's representatives' views or wishes to be heard or addressed.

Inevitably there have now been staff changes. Current practice is for induction to be done by the manager, and training is by shadowing present workers on shift. Due to financial constraints, there are few opportunities for workers to attend outside training. Some internal training is offered by the organisation, but this is not always on topics seen as most important by the women's representatives. Continuing training is essential to maintain staff morale and expertise.

Financial security for the future

There will be regular expenses in redecorating and replacing furniture and equipment. The women's income does not allow much margin for saving for these items and parents are already considering fundraising for this purpose.

The other worry is over the long-term financial security of the project itself. Will the criteria change? Will the local authority and ILF funding keep pace with increases in staff costs? This could have an effect on the quality of staff recruited. This year has seen a wage freeze for staff on this scheme.

Conclusion

Kathy died in August 1991, four months after the project opened. Her parents were devastated, but her death also had a profound effect upon Victoria and her family. There was a difficult period when Victoria was on her own, and both she and the reduced staff experienced some isolation. Eventually Kathy's place was taken by Lisa, another young woman with profound intellectual and multiple disabilities, who had known both Kathy and Victoria for many years.

This project involved much hard work, but also great stress not only for the parents, but also for the two young women. This was a huge upheaval in their lives with changes in their home, carers, GP and daily routines. It undoubtedly had effects on their behaviour and put great demands on their ability to cope with change.

Could this project happen now? There is now a new Independent Living Fund (1993), and the rules are different. The funding allocated to Victoria and Lisa is secure under the old rules, but the contribution available from the new ILF for anyone applying now would not make up the shortfall between actual care costs and the amount the local authority is prepared to pay. If this type of project can no longer be repeated because of funding problems, where will people like Kathy, Victoria and Lisa go when their parents become incapable or die?

With all the difficulties and anxieties, there is still no doubt that this project provided for the first time in their lives, a life style geared to the needs and wishes of the two women, instead of them having to fit into the framework of an institution. Leisure opportunities were opened up and they began to make more use of London's museums, art galleries, concert halls, theatres and cinemas. They and their carers became regular visitors to local pubs and restaurants and gradually became part of the local community.

For an expanded account of this project with supporting documentation see: Fitton, P., O'Brien, C. and Willson, J. (1995). *Home at Last: How two young women with profound intellectual and multiple disabilities achieved their own home.* Jessica Kingsley, London.

Chapter 4
Real jobs and supported employment

Stephen Beyer

One of the central themes in the development of services for people with learning difficulties in recent years is that help should be provided to people in environments, and in ways, which are culturally valued by other citizens (Wolfensberger, 1972). This perspective has led to a continuing critique of service designs which have segregated people with disabilities from the rest of society. Employment is one of the most significant areas of normal life that has been largely denied people with learning difficulties, and in recent years commentators have argued that services should refocus their efforts towards the inclusion of people with disabilities in ordinary work settings.

Helping people to gain and keep employment in ordinary settings has been a major feature of service development in the USA and much of the recent growth has been achieved through the funding and development of supported employment schemes. In the British context, this model is emerging as an alternative to provision through day centres and associated leisure and recreation schemes, and it is timely to review the role supported employment can play in fulfilling the expectation of a wide range of people for a real job.

The growth of supported employment in the USA

By the late 1970s the USA had created a national system of vocational rehabilitation which had people with learning difficulties as its main recipients (Buckley and Bellamy, 1985). The network of mainly private and voluntary sector rehabilitation facilities provided a continuum of vocational services consisting of adult day care programmes, work activity programmes, sheltered workshops, and placements in employment enclaves and transitional employment schemes. The system assumed that people would move along the continuum, receiving progressively less support as they become 'ready' for each stage, hopefully ending in open competitive employment (Bellamy *et al.*, 1986). Pay and the level of work-related activity varied as a person passed along the continuum. Adult day programmes generally provided pre-vocational, recreational and basic skill training for those labelled as having severe or profound learning difficulties. Work activity programmes tended to serve those viewed as unable to perform at the rates of production required in sheltered workshops. Sheltered workshops offered time limited vocational training and evaluation, along with extended employment in activities such as industrial subcontracting, renovation of used materials, and manufacture of new goods.

The continuum or 'readiness' model of vocational services came under severe criticism in the USA, the most fundamental charge being that these vocational services failed to move people along the various stages of the continuum to full competitive employment (Gardner, 1981). Bellamy *et al.* (1986) found:

> . . . if each consumer had an equal probability of movement along this continuum and was placed in a day activity programme, he or she would require an average of between 47 and 58 years to move through programme levels before realising community employment; for clients in work activity centres it would take, on average, 10–19 years to obtain a job.

It became clear that people entering sheltered workshops and work activity centres were not being moved on, throughput being only in the order of 12 per cent of those attending each year (USA Dept. of Labor, 1977; 1979). On the one hand these facilities operated as businesses providing products through sheltered workshops, while on the other they provided time limited transitional employment services. This led to conflicts between ensuring the facility's income, and moving people through into competitive employment. Rehabilitation facilities have also been criticised for the poor outcomes they achieved for those who continue to work in them, particularly the low level of wages they generated (Conley, 1985), and their lack of integration (Mcloughlin *et al.*, 1987; Nisbet and Callahan, 1987).

As dissatisfaction with traditional vocational rehabilitation models grew, research was confirming that gainful employment was a realistic aim for a wide range of people with a learning difficulty. Primary influences were the use of applied behaviour analysis in training practical work skills (that is, breaking jobs down into a series of small tasks, each to be learned in turn) (Gold, 1981) and the realisation that being in a job was not an aim, but an essential component of effective training (Kiernan and Stark, 1986; Rusch, 1986). The technology for teaching people the tasks required in real jobs had been developed initially in sheltered settings and was championed and made widely available through the work of Gold (1981) and the organisation he founded. This accessible application of applied behaviour analysis served to demonstrate the ability of people with moderate and severe learning difficulties to undertake complex work tasks (Bellamy *et al.*, 1979). The extension of this teaching technology into integrated employment settings came through a number of demonstration projects set up by researchers where people with varying degrees of learning difficulty were taught a variety of ordinary jobs (Rusch and Mithaug, 1980; Wehman, 1981). Direct placement into real work-places and training on the job have been defining features of the supported employment alternative, a number of authors arguing for the desirability of this 'place and train' approach over the traditional 'train and place' model (Pomerantz and Marholin, 1977; Rudrud *et al.*, 1984).

The significant progress made by early pilot programmes maintaining people in ordinary jobs was reflected in legislation (The Developmental Disabilities Act, 1984 and The Vocational Rehabilitation Act, 1986). Supported employment was defined as competitive work in integrated work settings, in work groups of no more than eight individuals with disabilities, having regular contact with non-disabled colleagues and receiving continuing training and support at the job site. Four models of supported employment have been funded in the USA: individual jobs, work crews, enclaves and structured small businesses (Mank *et al.*, 1986). The individual jobs model provides for on the job training and continuing support from a job trainer for an individual placed in an ordinary company. The work crew model is usually based on a business activity, typically gardening or cleaning work, and involves a small group of people with learning difficulties working as a team with a shared job trainer. The enclave model places a small group of people together into a company with a shared job trainer to carry out industrial or commercial work. Finally, the small business (or work-bench model) provides systematic training to a small group of people with more severe learning difficulties to carry out work in a single purpose business, an example being electronic assembly. This model differs from the enclave model by virtue of the fact that groups are often segregated from ordinary work settings and support needs are often high (Mank *et al.*, 1986).

Opinions differ over the relative merits of the various forms of supported employment that have emerged. It has been argued that the four models of supported employment represent a reformulation of the continuum approach operated by traditional rehabilitation facilities and that work crew, enclave and small business options discriminate against those with more severe disabilities who continue to find themselves separated from non-disabled people. The individual jobs model, it is argued, offers better integration potential, access to higher incomes, and better associated company benefits, such as company pension schemes and health insurance.

The growth of supported employment in Britain

Supported employment has largely developed since the late 1980s in the UK, with the individual jobs model being the dominant form developed here. Those employment initiatives, which concentrated on people with learning difficulties, operating in the UK prior to 1987 generally did so without the benefit of extended support on the job. In 1987 a small group of British professionals were funded by the Joseph Rowntree Foundation to learn from the American Marc Gold and Associates the task training methods that were the driving force behind supported employment in the USA. From this initiative Training in Systematic Instruction Ltd was formed to deliver the training technology within the UK, and this training has played a significant part in fuelling the development of supported employment since that time. According to the survey by Lister *et al.* (1992), the number of services offering some form of supported employment grew steadily from 24 in 1988 to 79 in 1991, 31 of these being independent agencies, 48 part of larger organisations such as a social services day centre. One thousand six hundred and nineteen people with learning difficulties were employed in total, the survey showing that a significant number were employed on a full-time basis (29 per cent working 35 hours a week or more), but many were working on a part-time basis (45 per cent less than 16 hours a week).

By 1991 the number of services providing supported employment had reached a size sufficient to make the formation of a national organisation to represent the interests of supported employment services and the people they served a realistic possibility. The Association of Supported Employment Agencies (ASEA) was formed in 1991 under the auspices of the National Development Team's 'Real Jobs Initiative' (Wertheimer, 1992) and was formally constituted in October 1992. By 1994 ASEA had 120 member organisations. The Association of Supported Employment Agencies aims to act as a focus for continuing improvement of supported employment practice and for the development of national policies by government and other organisations that promote the paid employment of people with learning difficulties and the provision of the support they need to succeed.

What makes for effective supported employment?

As the number employed through supported employment schemes has risen considerably, attention has been given to the identification of key elements that are required for supported employment to be effective (Lagomarcino, 1986; Vogelsberg, 1986; Wehman, 1986; Trach and Rusch, 1989). Wehman and Kregel (1985) identified the following stages applying equally to the various models mentioned above: job placement; job site training and advocacy; continuing monitoring; follow-up and retention. Considerable attention has been given to detailing the elements within each of these vital areas required to achieve the best outcomes for those supported in work.

Job placement

This involves finding the right job for the person, ensuring practical details such as transport are arranged, the impact of the job on welfare benefits are understood and agreements reached with the Benefit Agency, and that any worksite adaptations needed are tackled. Comprehensive information about the person seeking employment is needed, including the person's work or work related interests and connections with work, as well as their basic abilities and needs. Much thought has also gone into describing the techniques for marketing supported employment to employers and obtaining jobs. This has increasingly included creating jobs through bringing together entry level aspects of existing jobs to create one job for a person with a learning difficulty. Collecting detailed information about the social and physical environment of potential job sites in addition to job descriptions has also been viewed as crucial for an effective match between the prospective worker and a job (Mcloughlin *et al.*, 1987). The emphasis placed on job match reflects research which identifies worker motivation and interest in the job as key determinants of successful placement (Annable, 1989; Lister *et al.*, 1992). The need for good inter-agency planning to ensure that practical arrangements outside of work are in place to support people in work has also been highlighted. It is particularly important that expectations at home support the view that successful work is possible and desirable so that the worker's motivation is not undermined, that transport to work is consistently available or the person is trained to get to work themselves, and that appropriate dress codes, personal hygiene and social behaviour are reinforced. The characteristics of workplaces have become a more important consideration. While the preferences of the workers must remain paramount, a stable workforce with potential for the development of lasting relationships, the availability of supportive co-workers and jobs which promote valued images of people with disabilities have become important stepping stones to achieving good outcomes for workers (O'Bryan, 1992).

Job site training and advocacy

This involves analysing the tasks of the job, the design and implementation of training for that job, and effective communication with supervisory and other co-workers in the workplace. While much attention has been paid to task training, a number of studies have pointed to failure on the part of people with learning difficulties in adapting socially as a factor in the breakdown of work placements (Foss and Peterson, 1981; Greenspan and Shoultz, 1981; Hanley-Maxwell *et al.*, 1986). Helping people fit in socially has in the past been seen as a key role for the job coach. However, the involvement of the job coach, and any specialist training techniques they adopt, can disrupt natural processes of interaction and the natural support of other workers that can flow from it (Hagner, 1989). It has become increasingly clear that successful job placement comes through achieving a balance between competent learning of the tasks involved in the job, and minimising the social distance between the new worker and his or her colleagues. In the area of task training this balance has been pursued through the use of decision making protocols such as The Seven Phase Sequence to ensure training only moves away from what is natural for the workplace if the worker needs more powerful forms of instruction (Callahan, 1992).

Continuing monitoring

This involves monitoring of the worksite, the review of worker performance, retraining if needed, and communication with company personnel. One of the principle concerns is to identify problems stemming from the performance of the worker or challenges coming from the workplace before they threaten the worker's continued employment. A swift response by supported employment service personnel to any requests for assistance has been found to be crucial in maintaining the job. Regular reviews covering issues such as job performance, attendance and appearance, with views taken from the worker and workplace supervisors, can play a useful part in heading off potential problems.

Follow-up and retention

This includes a range of services to ensure the continued employment of the worker. Whether the source of support is a job coach or co-workers, improving the person's competence in the whole range of job and job related activities, thereby reducing the worker's dependence on others, is an important long-term goal in the follow-up phase. As with any worker, it must not be assumed a job is for life and career counselling and development is an additional long-term consideration. As many placements fail through the collapse of external support systems, the co-ordination of planned support systems such as transport, and working with families and professional carers are important continuing tasks.

Research on outcomes from supported employment

Researchers have looked at what supported employment produces for its clients, sometimes in comparison to traditional vocational services, at other times drawing comparison between the individual job, work crew, enclave and structured small business models of supported employment. In the main, the outcomes of supported employment have been measured in terms of wages earned, length of time the job was retained for, financial benefits in relation to costs and quality of life.

Vogelsberg (1986) reported that all salaries paid to workers in three supported employment programmes were at or above the national minimum wage and far exceeded payments to those in sheltered workshops. Average hourly wage rates in supported employment have been found to be approximately double those in sheltered workshops in two national USA surveys (Schalock *et al.*, 1989), reflecting a general finding that wages are higher in these schemes (Hill *et al.*, 1987a). Average hourly wage rates also vary between the four different models of supported employment, in one study wages in individual placement models being approximately 40 per cent higher than enclave or work crew models (Ellis *et al.*, 1990; Kregel *et al.*, 1990).

A six year study found that the length of time over which jobs were retained compared favourably with turnover rates for non-disabled people in similar industries in the first year (Wehman *et al.*, 1985). However, larger data sets reveal that after two years 48 per cent of people placed were no longer working (Kregel *et al.*, 1990). In the face of this problem there have been calls for job placement by agencies to be accelerated to ensure that people do not have prolonged waits for re-employment, or the creation of alternative schemes for those whom supported employment is currently unable to support (Kregel *et al.*, 1990). Others argue for more attention to be focussed on the instructional strategies being used (Ellis *et al.*, 1990), failure in work performance and ability to meet social expectations in the workplace being significant causes of people losing their jobs (Martin *et al.*, 1986).

Cost studies of supported employment schemes have looked at the financial benefit–cost equation at three levels: the individual worker, the taxpayer and society as a whole. The general conclusion from these studies has been that the benefits of supported employment schemes outweighed their costs, primarily due to the increased wages generated in supported employment programmes (Hill *et al.*, 1987a,b; Moss *et al.*, 1986; Rusch and Mithaug, 1980; Wehman, 1981). In many cases, the cost of support for specific individuals reduced over time as their need for on-the-job support decreased, the result being that supported employment programmes soon become cheaper than the long-term fixed costs expended in sheltered workshops. Moreover, the reduction in welfare benefit rates and tax income largely offset government spending on supported employment programmes after a critical number of workers had been placed. More recent studies suggest that increases in the income of workers placed through supported employment may be lower than previously found, and that programme costs may be higher, particularly in programmes that have emerged later in the movement's history (Conley and Noble, 1990; Tines *et al.*, 1990; McCaughrin *et al.*, 1991; Thornton, 1992). Some of the early schemes were designed 'model programmes' and, as such, tended to attract highly motivated and innovative staff whose performances were closely scrutinised. These schemes were also provided with intensive training and technical support from university departments, and were able to demonstrate significant reductions in the cost of support over time as they moved from a training to a maintenance phase. While the majority of second generation schemes still perform better than traditional day services, the implication is that when model schemes are widely replicated, more effort will be required to maintain the intensity of performance achieved in the earlier schemes. Any reduction in financial benefit for workers, or any increase in time and resources needed to reach the point where the worker is independent on the job, is reflected in less dramatic cost–benefit results.

Integration with non-disabled co-workers is one of the primary aims of supported employment (Mcloughlin *et al.*, 1987). Integration has been defined as comprising work settings which are not specifically designed for people with disabilities where people with disabilities are represented at proportions roughly comparable to the proportion of disabled people in the general population (Brown *et al.*, 1983). Others relate integration more specifically to the level and quality of social interaction with co-workers. Nisbet and Hagner (1988) noted that significant levels of social interaction and support took place between co-workers in workplaces, and cited these as potential sources of long-term on-the-job support.

Research across individual job, enclave and work crew models revealed more interaction between disabled and non-disabled workers for individual job and enclave programmes than for work crew programmes (Storey and Horner, 1990). Comparison of the interaction patterns for disabled and non-disabled workers have revealed few differences in interaction between supervisors and disabled workers, but co-workers do seem to interact more frequently with non-disabled colleagues than with disabled colleagues, the difference occurring mainly during breaks (Chadsey-Rusch and Gonzalez, 1988; Chadsey-Rusch *et al.*, 1989).

Feedback from supervisors has been used to determine the success of placement. Hill *et al.* (1980) looked at supervisors' opinions of the way workers worked and the way they fitted in socially and found generally high levels of satisfaction. Shafer *et al.* (1988), in a longitudinal study of written employer evaluations, concluded that these were valid predictors of whether people would stay in employment with attendance, punctuality and consistency of task performance having the strongest influence.

In the British context there have been few studies that have looked at outcomes, particularly at outcomes compared with other forms of day activity. Published case study material has emphasised the positive impact supported employment has had on people's lives (Wertheimer, 1993). A descriptive study of ten agencies in the UK identified 20 operational features which seem to facilitate successful and enduring placement (Pozner and Hammond, 1994). The report concluded: 'Supported employment agencies are effective in achieving their aims and objectives, and are supporting large numbers of people with disabilities into ordinary paid employment'. The outcomes that have been described in the USA have been achieved in a particular context and, while the potential for a broad range of positive outcomes is clearly shown, research is still needed to demonstrate the extent to which these are achievable in the British social care, welfare benefit and employment policy contexts.

Policy issues for supported employment

Although the growth of supported employment in the UK has been impressive, it has taken place in a harsher environment than that which supported its growth in the USA. Until recently, there had been no consistent approach to funding supported employment from mainstream employment sources. Its growth has been funded largely by social service departments (Lister *et al.*, 1992) and in the current climate of tight financial control on local government expenditure, activities not perceived as key responsibilities remain susceptible to cut backs. The announcement that one-to-one support on the job can be funded as part of the employment department's 'Access to Work' scheme to aid people with disabilities into work gave supported employment a place in mainstream government funding for the first time (DoE, 1994). This is, however, unlikely to provide core funding to enable agencies to provide the continuing support that is central to the supported employment model, and finding a source for such funding remains a challenge for policy makers.

The current welfare benefits system is a major restraint on potential outcomes from supported employment agencies (Pozner and Hammond, 1994). The fear of losing one's entitlement to welfare benefits should one become unemployed appears to have acted as a major barrier to people taking up jobs, or led many to take on only part-time work up to a limit allowed under 'therapeutic earnings' rules. This fear reduces the number of people who may be able to move away from state benefits entirely and achieve the increased financial independence that may result. The potential outcomes for people over and above any financial benefits appear to be substantial and constitute a strong argument in favour of supported employment being made more widely available. Many of the successful cost–benefit outcomes of supported employment reported in the US have, however, been achieved with 20 hours per week as a minimum working week being a requirement of funding. The emphasis has, therefore, been on finding full-time work and those working for 20 hours or more tend to earn enough to pay income tax and often generate a significant cost saving because of reductions in use of other day services. The extent to which the same degree of cost–benefits at the taxpayer level are achievable in the UK will be limited, not by what the model can deliver, but by the current welfare benefit regulations which tend to restrict many to part-time work where little or no tax is reclaimed and costs are still incurred in other forms of day service.

Practice issues for supported employment

Natural supports

There are a number of areas of practice where experience in the USA is already pointing to ways of improving outcomes which remain relatively untried in the British context. One of the most important changes to accepted practice is the move to promote co-workers as natural supports for disabled workers to enhance integration outcomes. A number of studies have demonstrated that non-disabled co-workers readily involve themselves with their disabled colleagues, but differences in interaction patterns have been found from those common between non-disabled workers. For example, workers with disabilities are greeted more frequently but are less likely to be asked for information or to be included in workplace banter. (Lignugaris/Kraft et al., 1988). They are also less likely to be included in any interaction away from work, during lunch or coffee breaks (Chadsey-Rusch et al., 1989; Parent et al., 1990). These studies and others emphasise the fact that there are strong workplace cultures with their own rules for behaviour that need to be addressed by new comers if they are to integrate successfully with their colleagues.

The importance of insiders in helping new recruits to negotiate their way into the workplace culture has been emphasised and the fact that job coaches are often outsiders without this essential and subtle knowledge has been used to criticise the traditional supported employment approach (Hagner, 1992). The job coach is an obstacle to the development of naturally occurring 'mentors' in the workplace and contributes to the development of a mystique around the expertise needed to teach a person with learning difficulties a job. They may reinforce the social distance between the person and the workforce. Hagner (1992) identifies five strategies to ameliorate this.

- Allowing flexibility in the training of job tasks to create a need for other workers to get involved and help out.
- Choosing jobs which require the collaborative effort of a small team.
- Identifying workplace customs and helping people perfect these.
- Looking from the beginning to involve co-workers in direct training with only indirect support from job coaches in order to reduce social distance.
- Involving the prospective worker's own or family networks in finding jobs to help promote the likelihood that the person is located in a situation where there is an internal sponsor who will aid with the introduction to the informal culture.

Callahan (1992) highlights the tension between encouraging and supporting 'natural' co-worker training and the need to ensure people with significant learning difficulties learn the job effectively. He notes that reliance on co-workers can itself leave the worker in a permanently dependent situation that can be damaging to the person's dignity and self-esteem and argues for a carefully considered continuum of responses. Training may range from that which is natural to the workplace, through 'naturally referenced' enhancement of interventions following advice from job coaches and, where these are ineffective, to intensive instructional procedures if success remains elusive. The challenge for those involved in supported employment will be to find practical ways to maximise integration outcomes without sacrificing job performance.

Transition from school or college to adult working life

Helping young people with disabilities to make successful transitions from school or college to an independent life has been a major focus in the USA spanning three administrations from the early 1980s. The implications for the whole range of agencies involved in the development and support of people with learning difficulties have been profound. Transition from school or college to adult life has been defined as 'the life changes, adjustments, and cumulative experiences that occur in the lives of young adults as they move from school environments to more independent living and work environments.' (Wehman, 1992). It involves adjustment to the whole gamut of adult experience and is not just focussed on employment. There are implications here for school or college curricula and their relationship to future workplace skills and knowledge (Edgar, 1987). There is a need for much improved co-ordination between school or college and post-school or college agencies and community leaders and institutions, a concept described as the principle of shared responsibility (Steere *et al.*, 1990). There is also a need for greater involvement of families and crucially, of young people themselves. Promoting choice and self-determination of young people through their involvement in personal planning, in deciding what type of job skills are to be developed and what career paths are to be taken through structured work experience need to be high on the future agenda (Turnbull *et al.*, 1989). Once again the whole area of transition from school to college remains largely undeveloped in Britain. It is likely that transition will be the next significant stepping stone towards real jobs and employment for people with learning difficulties.

Ensuring the inclusion of people with multiple disabilities in supported employment

While supported employment has proved successful in placing people with learning difficulties in real jobs, programmes have less frequently placed people who have additional physical and multiple disabilities (Wehman *et al.*, 1988). The definition of supported employment put forward by ASEA in the UK suggests a concept of 'full participation' namely that all people, no matter what their level of disability, should have the same opportunities to participate in real work as anyone else. If people are to be helped to experience work, there appears to be a need for greater effort to be made to increase the scope of supported employment. While many aspects of the general supported employment model are relevant, there is a need for processes to be modified and adapted (Wood, 1988).

Critical adaptations needed in nine key areas have been identified (Everson *et al.*, 1990; Callahan, 1990; Sowers and Powers, 1991). 'Job carving' has been used to create a job by combining managable tasks taken from the jobs of other non-disabled workers, who can then concentrate on more complex duties. Government financial incentives have been used in the USA to compensate employers for the reduced productivity of some severely physically disabled workers. Using work experience placements to train real job skills has proved to be a favoured strategy with systematic instruction being the favoured training method; its use being extended to teach the motor skills required in a job. For people with high support needs the natural method of doing a job, more often than not, has to be adapted through the use of assistive devices, and agencies have had to develop skills in this area. Effective co-ordination between schools, adult support services and families is even more important where people have multiple disabilities to ensure a consistent approach to support and training and a smooth transition from school to adult working life.

Supported employment has its roots in the belief that employment plays a crucial role in our society and that people with learning difficulties have a right to participate in it. It is clear that supported employment can make a major contribution to fulfilling this aim for many people with learning difficulties. There remains much that can be done within supported employment to refine and adapt procedures to improve outcomes and to move closer to the ideal of 'full participation' irrespective of the level of disability. Without significant change in the areas of welfare benefits and employment policy, however, it will prove more difficult to achieve the full potential of support employment.

References

Annable, G. (1989). *Supported Employment in Canada: final report.* Canadian Council on Rehabilitation and Work, Winnipeg, Manitoba.

Bellamy, G.T., Horner, R.H. and Inman, D.P. (1979). *Vocational Rehabilitation of Severely Retarded Adults: A Direct Service Technology.* University Park Press, Baltimore.

Bellamy, G.T., Rhodes, L.E., Bourbeau, P.E. and Mank, D.M. (1986). Mental retardation services in sheltered workshops and day activity programs: Consumer benefits and policy alternatives. In *Competitive Employment: Issues and Strategies* (ed. F.R. Rusch). Paul H. Brookes, Baltimore.

Brown, L., Ford, A., Tisbet, J., Sweet, M., Donnelan, L. and Grunewald, L. (1983). Opportunities available when severely handicapped students attend chronological age appropriate regular schools. *Journal of the Association for the Severely Handicapped*, **8**, 16–24.

Brown, L., Shirago, B., York, J. *et al.* (1984). *The Direct Pay Waiver for Severely Intellectually Handicapped Workers.* Unpubl. University of Winsconsin, Iadison.

Buckley, J. and Bellamy, G.T. (1985). Day and vocational programs for adults with severe disabilities: A national survey. In *Issues in Transition: Economic and Social Outcomes: Report from the Consortium for Youth with Disability* (ed. F. Ferguson). Eugene, University of Oregon, Specialized Training Program.

Callahan, M. (1990). *National Demonstration Project on Supported Employment.* United Cerebral Palsy Association, Inc., Washington DC.

Callahan, M. (1992) Job site training and natural supports. In *Natural Supports in Schools, at work, and in the Community for People with Severe Disabilities* (ed. J. Nisbet). Paul H. Brookes, Baltimore.

Chadsey-Rusch, J. and Gonzalez, P. (1988). Social ecology of the workplace: Employers' perceptions versus direct observation. *Research in Developmental Disabilities*, **9**, 229–245.

Chadsey-Rusch, J., Gonzalez, P., Tines, J. and Johnson, J.R. (1989). Social ecology of the workplace: Contextual variables affecting social interaction of employees with and without mental retardation. *American Journal of Mental Retardation*, **94**, 141–151.

Conley, R.W. (1985). Impact of Federal programs on employment of mentally retarded persons. In *Strategies for Achieving Community Intention for Developmentally Disabled Citizens* (eds K.C. Lakin and R.H. Bruininks). Paul H. Brookes, Baltimore.

Conley, R. and Noble, R. (1990). Benefit–cost analysis of supported employment. In *Supported Employment: Models, Methods and Issues* (ed. F.R. Rusch). Sycamore Publishing Company. Sycamore, Illinois.

Department of Employment (1994). Press release 33/94, 28 February.

Edgar, E. (1987) Secondary programs in special education: are many of them justifiable? *Exceptional Children*, **53**(6), 555–561.

Ellis, W.K., Rusch, F.R., Tu, J. and McCaughrin, W. (1990). Supported employment in Illinois. In *Supported Employment: Models, Methods and Issues*, (ed. F.R. Rusch). Sycamore Publishing Company, Sycamore.

Everson, J., Callahan, M., Hollohan, J. *et al.* (1990). *Getting the Job Done: Supported Employment for Persons with Severe Physical Disabilities.* United Cerebral Palsy Association, Washington DC.

Foss, G. and Peterson, S. (1981). Social interpersonal skills relevant to job tenure of mentally retarded adults. *Mental Retardation*, **19**, 103–106.

Gardner, K.A. (1981). The nonprofit work-orientated rehabilitation facility. In *Annual Review of Rehabiliation, Volume 2.* (eds E.L. Pan, T.E. Backer and C.L. Vash). Springer Publishing Company, New York.

Gold, M. (1981). *Try Another Way.* Research Press, Champaign, Illinois.

Greenspan, S. and Shoultz, B. (1981). Why mentally retarded adults lose their jobs: social competence as a factor in work adjustment. *Applied Research in Mental Retardation*, **2**, 23–38.

Hagner, D. (1989). *The Social Integration of Supported Employees: A*

Qualitative Study. Center on Human Policy, Syracuse University, New York.

Hagner, D.C. (1992). The social interactions and job supports of supported employees. In *Natural Supports at School, at Work, and in the Community for People with Severe Disabilities* (ed. J. Nisbet). Paul H. Brookes, Baltimore.

Hanley-Maxwell, D., Rusch F.R., Chadsey-Rusch J. and Renzaglia A. (1986). Reported factors contributing to job termination of individuals with severe disabilities. *Journal of the Association for Persons with Severe Handicaps,* 11, 45–52.

Hill, M., Hill, J.W. and Wehman, P. (1980). An analysis of supervisor evaluations of moderately and severely retarded workers. In *Vocational Training and Placement of Severely Disabled Persons* (eds P. Wehman and M. Hill). Commonwealth University, Richmond, Virginia.

Hill, M., Banks, P., Handrich, R., Wehman, P., Hill, J. and Shafer M. (1987a). Benefit–cost analysis of supported competitive employment. *Research in Developmental Disabilities,* 8, 182–189.

Hill, M., Wehman, P., Kregel J., Banks, P.D. and Metzler, H.M.D. (1987b). Employment outcomes for people with moderate and severe disabilities: an eight year longitudinal analysis of supported competitive employment. *Journal of the Association for Persons with Severe Handicaps,* 21, 128–189.

Kiernan, W. E. and Stark, J. A. (eds.) (1986). *Pathways to Employment for Adults with Developmental Disabilities.* Paul H. Brooks, Baltimore.

Kregel, J., Wehman, P., Revell, W.G. and Hill, R. (1990). Supported employment in Virginia. In *Supported Employment: Models, Methods and Issues* (ed. F.R. Rusch). Sycamore Publishing, Sycamore, Illinois.

Lignugaris/Kraft, B., Salzberg, C., Rule, S. and Stowitschek, J. (1988). Social-vocational skills of workers with and without mental retardation in two community employment sites, *Mental Retardation,* 26, 297–305.

Lister, T., Ellis, L., Phillips, T., O'Bryan, A., Beyer, S. and Kilsby, M. (1992). *Survey of Supported Employment Services in England, Scotland and Wales.* National Development Team, Manchester.

Lagomarcino, T.R. (1986). Community services: using the supported work model within an adult service agency. In *Competitive Employment: Issues and Strategies* (ed. F.R. Rusch). Paul H. Brookes, Baltimore.

Mank, D., Rhodes, C.F. and Bellamy, G.T. (1986). Four supported employment alternatives. In *Pathways to Employment for Adults with Developmental Disabilities,* (eds W. Kiernan and J. Stark). Paul H. Brookes, Baltimore.

Martin, J.E., Rusch, F.R., Lagomarcino, T. and Chadsey-Rusch J. (1986). Comparison between nonhandicapped and mentally retarded workers: Why they lose their jobs, *Applied Research in Mental Retardation,* 7, 467–474.

McCaughrin, W.B., Rusch, F.R. and Conley, R.W. (1991). *A Three Year Benefit–Cost Analysis of Supported Employment in Illinois.* The Secondary Transition Intervention Effectiveness Institute, University of Illinois at Urbana–Champaign.

Mcloughlin, C.S., Garner, J.B. and Callahan, M.J., (eds.) (1987). *Getting Employed, Staying Employed.* Paul H. Brookes, Baltimore.

Moss, J. Dineen, J. and Ford, L. (1986). University of Washington Employment

Training Program. In *Competitive Employment: Issues and Strategies* (ed. F.R. Rusch). Paul H. Brookes, Baltimore.

Nisbet, J. (ed.) (1992). *Natural Supports in School, at Work, and in the Community for People with Severe Disabilities*. Paul H. Brookes, Baltimore.

Nisbet, J. and Callahan, M.J. (1987). Achieving success in integrated workplaces: critical elements in assisting persons with severe disabilities. In *Community Integration for People with Severe Disabilities* (eds S.T. Taylor, D. Biklen and J. Knoll) Teachers College Press, New York.

Nisbet, J. and Hagner, D. (1988). Natural supports in the workplace: Reexamination of supported employment. *Journal of the Association for Persons with Severe Handicaps*, **13**, 260–267.

O'Bryan, A. (1992). *Evaluating Elements of Quality in Supported Employment Services*. National Development Team, Manchester.

Parent, W., Kregel, J., Twardzik, G. and Metzler, H. (1990). Social integration in the workplace: an analysis of the interaction activities of workers with mental retardation and their co-workers. In *Supported Employment for Persons with Severe Disabilities: From Research to Practice, Volume III* (eds. J. Kregel, P. Wehman and M. Shafer). Virginia Commonwealth University Rehabilitation Research and Training Center, Richmond.

Pomerantz, D. and Marholin, D. (1977). Rehabilitation: a time for change. In *Educational Programming the Severely and Profoundly Handicapped* (ed. E. Sontag). Council for Exceptional Children, Division on Mental Retardation, Reston, Virginia.

Pozner, A. and Hammond, J. (1994). *An Evaluation of Supported Employment Initiatives for Disabled People*. Employment Department Research Series No. 17, Sheffield.

Rudrud, E.H., Zarnik, J.P., Bernstein, G.S. and Ferrara, J.M. (1984) *Proactive Vocational Habilitation*, Paul H. Brookes, Baltimore.

Rusch, F.R. (ed.) (1986). *Competitive Employment: Issues and Strategies*. Paul H. Brookes, Baltimore.

Rusch, F.R. (ed.) (1990). *Supported Employment: Models, Methods and Issues*. Sycamore Publishing, Sycamore, Illinois.

Rusch, F.R. and Mithaug, D.E. (1980). *Vocational Training for Mentally Retarded Adults: A Behavioural Analytic Approach*. University Press, Champaign, Illinois.

Schalock, R.L., McGaughey, M.J. and Kiernan, W.E. (1989). Placement into nonsheltered employment: Findings from national employment surveys, *American Journal of Mental Retardation*, **94**, 80–87.

Shafer, M.S., Kregel, J., Banks, P.D. and Hill, M. (1988). An analysis of employer evaluations of workers with mental retardation. *Research in Developmental Disabilities*, **9**, 377–391.

Sowers, J. and Powers, L. (1991). *Vocational Preparation and Employment of Students with Physical and Multiple Disabilities*. Paul H. Brookes, Baltimore.

Steere, D., Pancsofar, E., Wood, R. and Hecimovic, A. (1990). *The Principle of Shared Responsibility*. Institute of Human Resources, Hartford, Connecticut.

Storey, K. and Horner, R. (1990). Social interactions in three supported *employment options: a comparative analysis. Journal of Applied Behaviour Analysis*, **24**, 349–360.

Thornton, C. (1992). *Uncertainty in Benefit–Cost Analyses of Supported Employment*. Mathematica Policy Research Inc., Princeton, New Jersey.

Tines, J., Rusch, F.R., McCaughrin, W. and Conley, R.W. (1990). *Benefit–Cost Analysis of Supported Employment in Illinois: A Statewide Evaluation*. University of Illinois, Urbana-Champaign.

Trach. J.R. and Rusch, F.R. (1989). Supported employment program evaluation: evaluating degree of implementation and selected outcomes. *American Journal on Mental Retardation*, **94**, 134–140.

Turnbull, H.R., Turnbull, A.P., Bronicki, G.J., Summers, J.A. and Roeder-Gordon, C. (1989). *Disability and the Family: A Guide to Decisions for Adulthood*. Paul H. Brookes, Baltimore.

USA Department of Labor (1977). *Sheltered Workshop Study: A Nationwide Report on Sheltered Workshops and their Employment of Handicapped Individuals: Volume I*. Department of Labor, Washington DC.

USA Department of Labor (1979). *Sheltered Workshop Study: Volume II*. Department of Labor, Washington DC.

Vogelsberg, R.T. (1986). Competitive employment in Vermont. In *Competitive Employment: Issues and Strategies* (ed. F.R. Rusch). Paul H. Brookes, Baltimore.

Wehman, P. (1981). *Competitive Employment: New Horizons for Severely Disabled Individuals*. Paul H. Brookes, Baltimore.

Wehman, P. (1986). Competitive employment in Virginia. In *Competitive Employment: Issues and Strategies* (ed. F.R. Rusch). Paul H. Brookes, Baltimore.

Wehman, P. (1992). *Life Beyond the Classroom: Transition Strategies for Young People with Learning Disabilities*, Paul H. Brookes, Baltimore.

Wehman, P. and Kregel, J. (1985). A supported work approach to competitive employment for individuals with moderate and severe handicaps, *The Journal of The Association for Persons with Severe Handicaps*, **10**, 3–11.

Wehman, P., Hill, M., Hill, J.W., Brooke, V., Pendleton, P. and Britt, C. (1985). Competitive employment for persons with mental retardation: a follow-up six years later. *Mental Retardation*, **3**, 74–81.

Wehman, P., Wood, W., Everson, J.M., Goodwyn, R. and Conley, S. (1988). *Vocational Education for Multihandicapped Youth with Cerebral Palsy*. Paul H. Brookes, Baltimore.

Wertheimer, A. (ed.) (1992). *Real Jobs.* National Development Team, Manchester.

Wertheimer, A. (1993). *Changing Lives: Supported Employment and People with Learning Disabilities*. National Development Team, Manchester.

Wolfensberger, W. (1972). *Principle of Normalization in Human Services*. National Institute on Mental Retardation, Toronto.

Wood, W. (1988). Supported employment for persons with physical disabilities. In *Vocational Rehabilitation and Supported Employment* (eds P. Wehman and M.S. Moon). Paul H. Brookes, Baltimore.

Chapter 5

Choice and change: Opportunities and issues in continuing education for adults with learning difficulties

Rob Hancock and Jeannie Sutcliffe

The development of education for adults with learning difficulties has progressed rather like a game of snakes and ladders. Opportunities to learn within continuing education have been patchy in terms of both the quality and quantity of provision available. The most recent national survey by Sutcliffe (1990) found 'significant inequalities' in provision to which there are no 'ready made solutions' or 'universal answers'. Yet Sutcliffe also identified a range of leading edge projects, which were each addressing the fundamental challenge of providing people with learning difficulties with the opportunities they wanted. As one adult learner commented 'I used to be made to learn, but now I choose which course I want to go to and when I want to go. It's great' (Quoted in Hancock, 1990, unpubl.)

Opportunities for adults with learning difficulties to determine and structure their own learning are still far too rare. It is common for learners to find not ladders but snakes, leading to segregated learning opportunities where the choices are few, and where people have their needs assessed and learning prescribed without regard to their views, rights or needs. Inequalities are often amplified and multiplied because of the age, gender, race or class of the person with learning difficulties:

> It is not the same thing to be a white disabled person and to be a black disabled person. Disability settles upon anyone, but the effect on any individual is very largely modified, minimised or exacerbated by who that person is in terms of their age, race and class. (Mason and Rieser, 1992).

The last two decades have witnessed changes in the range and purpose of learning opportunities for adults with learning difficulties. More choices are now available in terms of what to learn, where to learn and how to learn. The network of providers includes further education colleges, adult education centres and distance learning providers, such as the Open University. There is a wider curriculum choice for those who are learning for work, for leisure or for personal development.

Changes in attitude, legislation and society have influenced and shaped the learning opportunities available. The issues of equality of opportunity, inclusion versus segregation, empowerment, normalisation, entitlement and advocacy provide a framework for discussing current opportunities and are central to the shaping of future provision. Amongst the elements outlined are some of the factors which determine the snakes and ladders which are daily facts of life for people with learning difficulties. This chapter will explore the issues under the following headings.

- Change – looking at the concepts and context of continuing education.
- Opportunities – an outline of what is available, with examples of learning opportunities.
- Issues – identification and discussion of some key issues within continuing education.
- Choice – consideration of the choices available for future planning.

Change

> For those who wish to know where they are going, it may not come amiss to know something about the map on which they rely. (Pollard, 1968).

The concept of continuing education is a recent addition to the map of the educational world in the UK. What is continuing education? It has been described as a conjunction of policies, funding, provision and attitudes which affect changes in all the present educational sectors to the advantage of a rapidly growing number of adult learners (Jarvis, 1983). It is the door through which adults with learning difficulties have gained increasing access to education.

Further education colleges and adult education centres run by local education authorities have been the main providers of learning opportunities to adults with learning difficulties. However, as a recent survey has shown, there is a broader network providing continuing education for adults with learning difficulties (Sutcliffe, 1990). This extended network includes social services day centres, community living schemes, long-stay hospital provision, voluntary organisations, therapy professionals, parents, carers and the local community.

The map of continuing education is not, then, a well ordered landscape such as the schools system or higher education but a diverse network of providers. For some adults with learning difficulties, these providers have met their needs and offered progression routes to further skills and knowledge. For others, they have not met or even attempted to meet complex needs, or addressed the challenges of ethnic background, gender or different communication needs. For these learners, continuing education has led to cul-de-sacs, segregation in discrete classes, the attachment of negative labels and the only chance (if any) to move on, is to further inappropriate provision (Whittaker, 1994).

In recent years, there has been a commitment from central government, local education authorities and further/higher education to encourage the development and range of opportunities to learn for all adults. Opportunities have included access courses for so called 'second chance learners', accreditation of prior learning, educational advice and guidance, and other initiatives. However, in this drive to increase access and entitlement to learning for adults, the needs of those with learning difficulties have been a low priority. Despite this, pockets of good practice have flourished and hence the map is not devoid of high spots. First rate learning opportunities have been developed by providers in further education colleges, adult education and other agencies. Such developments have been possible mainly through the growing number of highly skilled and committed individuals working within the diverse networks providing continuing education (Sutcliffe, 1990; NATFHE, 1993b). Practitioners have been supported in their work by organisations such as the National Institute of Adult Continuing Education, the Further Education Unit and SKILL (the working name of the National Bureau of Students with Disabilities). Learners have been supported by these organisations and others to become partners in the process of continuing education (Sutcliffe and Simons, 1993).

It will be of great interest to both learners and educators to see whether the recent positive steps can be strengthened and developed within the context of the 'silent revolution' (Griffiths, 1993) which has recently taken place in all sectors of education in England and Wales. In both schools and continuing education (which includes colleges of further education, adult education centres and the university sector), the map of the world has changed more rapidly and more fundamentally than at any time in the last hundred years. Change has been driven and directed by central government during the 1980s and early 1990s through a series of Education Acts: those of 1981, 1986, 1988 and 1993 and the Further and Higher Education Act 1992. The reorganisation of education has resulted in three major changes. The curriculum is now controlled centrally, as in the example of the National Curriculum. Financial management is devolved from local education authorities to individual schools and colleges, which are now free to act and spend independently. Market forces are now the driving force in shaping and reshaping the map of education in all areas.

For adults with learning difficulties, it is not only educational legislation that is influencing and altering the structure and delivery of continuing education. The NHS and Community Care Act 1990 has set out a new pattern of resourcing the services delivered to adults with learning difficulties by social services departments, health authorities and voluntary agencies (Lavender, 1993). However, it is the Further and Higher Education Act which has brought major changes to the delivery of education. The changes as they affect adults with learning difficulties are many and complex.

Further education colleges are now independent, which means that they are no longer funded or controlled by local education authorities. They are now funded by the Further Education Funding Council (FEFC) in England. There is a separate FEFC for Wales. The FEFC will only fund certain types of designated courses. Particular reference is made to the education of adults with learning difficulties in the Further and Higher Education Act 1992. The courses listed under Schedule 2 include 'independent living and communication skills for students with learning difficulties'. This provision must demonstrate progression to other courses listed under Schedule 2, which include basic skills, vocational and academic courses. Other provision for adults with learning difficulties is now known as 'non-Schedule 2' and includes the sort of general adult education classes often provided by local education authorities, who have 'a duty to secure further education for adults with learning difficulties where the Council has no such duty' (SKILL, 1992). Within the new framework set by the NHS and Community Care Act, continuing education will be purchased for individuals if their assessed needs so dictate. Alternatively, it can be purchased by individuals from their personal budgets if they so wish. The network of providers of continuing education already outlined and the range of learning opportunities on offer may fluctuate, depending on the market.

What then of the future? An optimistic view of the possible outcomes from the new legislation has been expressed by Lavender (1993).

- 'New structures can be developed in collaboration.
- New and existing course development.
- Development of community support for adults and young people with disabilities or learning difficulties.
- Establishment and development of inter-agency collaboration.
- Contributing to an existing entitlement philosophy'.

The FEFC has expressed its commitment to future developments. Indeed, to drive and support developments, the FEFC has set up a review committee to respond to a number of issues (Maddison, 1993). The committee is chaired by Professor John Tomlinson of Warwick University and will meet for three years. The committee will be establishing assessment procedures and reviewing provision, as well as considering inter-agency collaboration. It will also advise on developing a funding structure which enables progress and integration and will explore opportunities for growth.

The reaction to recent legislation has not been well received by all educators (Whittaker, 1994). In the initial stages of implementation, practitioners quoted by Sutcliffe (1993) were in a state of some chaos. One said 'It's a time of confusion and uncertainty – it's a muddle.' Others stressed the positive: 'More than ever collaboration is essential. To support collaboration effectively, we need planners and managers to work together, as well as staff at grass roots level.'

For many adults with learning difficulties, past legislation has led only to 'rhetoric land' rather than to practical action to improve services, largely due to a lack of resources, collaboration and strategic planning. The new continuing education framework is structured by market forces, and key themes include producing an efficient work force, meeting attainment targets and being commercially oriented. It is hard to see how these values sit with the needs of the widely varied group of individuals who are labelled as people with learning difficulties. Is the current ethos compatible with entitlement, empowerment or equality of opportunity for them particularly when we know that those from ethnic minorities, or with complex needs have not been able to access many learning opportunities which match their needs?

Opportunities to learn

> I want to learn about Jesus and history and thunder and lightning. (Sutcliffe, 1990).

Within the network of continuing education providers, there is a wide range of excellent opportunities: examples of innovative practice are described in publications by NIACE, FEU and SKILL. Table 5.1 provides a guide to some of the opportunities available, including who offers them and who can provide personal and financial support. Details are also given of the access requirements, the duration of courses and the qualifications on offer. It will also draw on examples that offer a range of opportunities, delivered in a variety of settings by different providers, which enable access to all learners. These include learning for leisure, for personal development, for independence and for work. The following access grid is adapted from the Wales Council for the Disabled qualifications matrix (Burns *et al.*, 1993). It outlines access to continuing education opportunities available through colleges of further education, adult education, social service departments and voluntary organisations.

Learning for independence

An empowering approach to learning is offered by the pack *A New Life* (Cowan and Rolph, 1992). The pack offers a good model for others to replicate. The values are based on the principles of self-advocacy and self-assessment is used to determine the learning programme for each person. The primary purpose of the pack is to offer a framework for transition programmes for people moving from long-stay hospitals into the community. Its approach, however, serves as a framework for good practice in most areas of continuing education. It was designed and developed through a multidisciplinary approach, demonstrating the value of learning together. The learner is at the centre of a working partnership with the three following key elements (taken from Cowan and Rolph, 1992).

- A learner-centred approach, by means of self-assessment. Self-advocacy is at the centre of the process.

Table 5.1 Access to continuing education opportunities

Type of course	Providers	Financial support	Personal support	Duration of course	Possible qualifications	Entry requirements
Independent living	Local education authority. Adult education. Adult training centre. Social education centre. Further education college. Voluntary organisation.	Social services dept. Community care. Benefits. Personal finance.	Further education Funding council. Funded support. Social services dept. Support worker. Volunteer. Friend. Family.	Short course. Weekly class.	Course certificate. Personal portfolio. Open College Network Certificate.	None.
Adult basic skills. Numeracy. Literacy. Communication skills.	Local education authority. Basic skills service. Further education college.	Local education authority. Social services dept. Community care. Benefits. Further Education Funding Council.	Further Education Funding Council. Funded support. Social services dept. Support worker. Volunteer. Friend. Family.	Short course. Weekly class.	Course certificate. Wordpower. Numberpower.	None.
Vocational skills	Further education college. Adult Education. Specialised employment. Service run by voluntary organisations. Social Services.	Training & Enterprise Councils. Local education authority. Benefits. Further Education Funding Council.	Further Education Funding Council. Funded support. Social services dept. Support worker. Volunteer. Friend. Family.	1 year FT. 1 year PT. 2 years PT. Short courses.	GNVQ. National vocational qualification. Open College Network Certificate. Specific vocational qualifications.	None. Access course.

Table 5.1 Access to continuing education opportunities (*continued*)

Type of course	Providers	Financial support	Personal support	Duration of course	Possible qualifications	Entry requirements
Personal relationships	Location education authority. Adult education. Adult training centre. Social education centre. Family Planning Association. Further education college.	Social services dept. Community care. Benefits.	Further Education Funding Council. Funded support. Social services dept. Support worker. Volunteer. Friend. Family.	Short course. Weekly class.	Course certificate. Personal portfolio.	None.
Access course to prepare for entry to other course	Local education authority. Adult education. Further education college. Adult education centre.	Social services dept. Community care. Further Education Funding Council.	Further Education Funding Council. Funded support. Social services dept. Support worker. Volunteer. Friend. Family.	Short course. Weekly class.	Course certificate. Personal portfolio. Open College Network Certificate.	None.
General education	Local education authority. Adult education. Further education college.	Local education authority. Grant. Social services dept. Community care. Benefits. Further Education Funding Council.	Further Education Funding Council. Funded support. Social services dept. Support worker. Volunteer. Friend. Family.	1 year FT. 2 year PT.	GCSE certificate. Course certificate.	Pre-GCSE course or none.

Leisure courses. Arts and crafts.	Local education authority. Adult education. Arts centres. Adult training centres. Social education centre.	Social services dept. Community care. Benefits. Personal finance.	Social services dept. Support worker. Volunteer. Friend. Family.	Short course. Weekly class.	Course certificate. Personal portfolio. Open College Network Certificate.	None.
Leisure courses. Fitness.	Local education authority. Adult education. Leisure centres. Sports clubs. Voluntary organisations.	Social services dept. Community care. Benefits. Personal finance.	Social services dept. Support worker. Volunteer. Friend. Family.	Short course. Weekly class.	Course certificate. Personal portfolio. Open College Network Certificate.	None.
Leisure courses. Language. Communication.	Local education authority. Adult education. Distance learning. Further education college.	Social services dept. Community care. Benefits. Personal finance.	Social services dept. Support worker. Volunteer. Friend. Family.	Short course. Weekly class.	Course certificate. Personal portfolio. Open College Network Certificate.	None.
Self-advocacy group	Local education authority. Adult education. People First or other voluntary organisations. Adult education centre. Social education centre.	Social services dept. Community care. Benefits. Personal finance. Further Education Funding Council.	Social Services dept. Support worker. Volunteer. Friend. Family	Short course. Weekly class.	Attendance record. Course certificate. Personal portfolio.	None.

Adapted from Burns *et al.*, 1993.

- Negotiation – the individual learning programme is negotiated between learner and professional.
- Advocates are used for those learners unable to communicate easily.

The programme comprises self-assessment by the learner, and a joint assessment by the professional and learner, which leads to an individual learning plan and contract. Learning activities and outcomes are summarised in a menu, and the process is completed by evaluation and review.

Learning for leisure

Although most areas offer a wide variety of leisure activities through adult education, they often exclude adults with learning difficulties. Segregated classes are often all that is available. In contrast, Llanover Hall in Cardiff is a major arts centre with a policy of arts for all. Access initiatives for adults with learning difficulties have been jointly developed with community education. At the centre, the regular day and evening programme features over 50 different arts sessions and activities including ceramics, dance, theatre projects, music workshops, video, weekend workshops and regular exhibitions. Learning at the centre often leads to other community-based activities within the arts world of Cardiff.

Learning for personal development

Opportunities for self-advocacy have mushroomed in recent years (see, for example, Sutcliffe and Simons, 1993) but self-advocacy has not always been accessible to people with profound and multiple learning difficulties. The Information Exchange on Self-Advocacy and User Participation (King's Fund 1993) gives both an example of a leading project in Mid Glamorgan and evidence that, so far, we have not always made the right assumptions about the ability or suitability of individuals to learn.

Mid Glamorgan People First was asked to explore working with people in a special needs unit, in order to enable the people there to develop skills in expressing themselves. The King's Fund (1993) outlined the outcomes from the experience:

> Mid Glamorgan People First have learnt a lot from the people in the Special Needs Unit; most importantly that the people there want the

same as other people: nice houses, friends and relationships, an active social life etc. Also they have the same problems with their parents that most people have – never allowed to grow up, used as a scapegoat for serious problems in other members of the family, unable to confront parents on an equal basis.

People showed clearly how they communicated and what they wanted, once the learning opportunity had been made accessible to them.

Learning for work

Education for work is one of the choices students with learning difficulties can make at Coleg Glan Hafren in South Glamorgan within the computer workshop. The aim is to improve the employment opportunities for people with learning difficulties by a combination of college-based vocational training and working links with local employers. The workshop has developed a continuum of work opportunities that includes college-based training work visits, work placements, longer term work experience and part or full-time employment. This has proved very successful in allowing a step-by-step progression into mainstream college vocational courses and open employment which caters for individual students' abilities and support needs.

Issues

> It is of great importance that people with learning difficulties should be helped both practically and imaginatively to take their place in the community. Education provides the opportunities for integration, development of self-advocacy skills and attainment of independence. (Sutcliffe, 1990)

Current issues in continuing education may be similar to those confronting other services but they are set within a particular context or culture. As with most cultures or subcultures, education has its own language. Table 5.2 compares and contrasts how issues in continuing education are described and defined using O'Brien's (1987) five accomplishments which are often used as bench marks in community services and service plans.

Issues of partnership

It is clear from the comparison of perspectives that there is much common ground between agencies and a shared vision which should support and enable people with learning difficulties in the community.

Table 5.2 How issues in continuing education are defined*

The five accomplishments (O'Brien)	*A continuing education perspective*
Participating in the community	Integration/inclusion in all learning opportunities.
Increasing competence	Learning for work, leisure, independence or personal development.
Exercising individual choice	Being able to select from a wide range of learning opportunities within full-time and part-time continuing education which match individual needs.
Gaining self-esteem	Personal growth through progression and achieving accreditation through chosen learning opportunities.
Sustaining and widening friendships	The opportunity to learn and make relationships with other adult learners.

*Using O'Brien's (1987) five accomplishments.

Yet in some areas, there is a complete absence of an agenda for discussing and developing joint strategies and a lack of networking and information dissemination between services. Other common gaps include a lack of relationships on which to build joint planning, with no regular contact between senior managers. Often there is not an identified contact point between services. Joint consultation with consumers and joint training of staff is still rare.

There are documented examples of productive partnerships (Sutcliffe, 1990; 1992; Bradley and Maychell, 1991). However, constructive partnerships are still the exception rather than the rule. Until strategic partnerships are developed, continuing education can offer only limited opportunities. Partnership strategies must be forged, put into operation, evaluated and then improved. Only full partnerships between agencies, with education as an equal partner, can enable people with learning difficulties to participate to the maximum in the community.

Assessment: an issue in partnership

From April 1993, when the Further and Higher Education Act 1992 and the National Health Service and Community Care Act 1990 came into force, agencies had a duty to ensure the shared assessment of individual need and the identification of appropriate learning provision. It is hoped that all agencies involved will consider it a duty to include the person with learning difficulties as an equal partner within the assessment process (Cowan and Rolph, 1992). Whenever possible, the person with learning difficulties should be involved in determining both the process and the outcomes of the assessment.

Under the new legislation, assessment will not only be the basis for individual planning, but will also be the trigger for funding. The Further and Higher Education Act 1992 has caused a split of responsibility in funding and planning between adult education, which is the responsibility of the local education authorities, and the elements of continuing education which are the responsibility of the FEFC. The additional support each person requires will now be financed from three possible sources. The FEFC will fund learners in colleges and adult education if the course comes under Schedule 2 of the Further and Higher Education Act (1992). The local education authorities will fund courses described as 'leisure' adult education classes. Lastly, funding can be allocated through the community care budget.

The right assessment process is vital for the dignity of the person with learning difficulties. It is still too often a process leading to discrimination and segregation within education (Whittaker, 1993a). If the assessment process cannot fulfil its purpose, it can lead to the 'disabling of learning' (Vaughan Huxley, 1993), instead of the enabling of learning. Given the new complexities in the funding and organisation of continuing education, it is vital that comprehensive assessments should be carried out in full partnership. Shared assessment must become the cornerstone of individual planning, and not the optional extra it has often been in the past.

Integration: an issue or a right?

Integration sets up a 'virtuous circle' leading both to the acquisition of new skills and acceptance and respect from members of the public (Brown, 1993).

Is continuing education offering integrated learning opportunities? A survey of further education revealed that 88 per cent of colleges run discrete (segregated) courses for young people with learning difficulties (NATFHE, 1993b). In answer to the question 'Has adequate staff time been allocated to co-ordinate and support integrated learning?', 61 per cent of respondents answered no. There is no equivalent survey of adult education, day services and other providers, but it is reasonable to assume from what we know that the pattern within further education colleges is replicated by other providers.

The debate regarding the rights of people with learning difficulties to access mainstream learning opportunities is well rehearsed and recorded (Hegarty, 1982; Booth, 1988; Sutcliffe, 1992). Only a minority would nowadays offer any justification for segregated learning on educational or moral grounds. There remains, however, a complex debate which centres around choice for adults with learning difficulties. Sutcliffe (1992) and Brown (1993) have justified the need for both integrated classes (where adults with and without learning difficulties learn alongside each other) and for peer group learning opportunities (where adults with learning difficulties learn in a separate group) to be offered. The rationale is that there is a need for people with learning difficulties to have the opportunity to share common experiences through self-advocacy groups, women's groups, black groups or other groups if they so choose, in the same way that other oppressed groups have met for support. Peer groups offer a secure spring board, from which people who have been stripped of self-respect and esteem can build confidence, skills and knowledge to use to enter the wider community. While there is a need for people with learning difficulties to have the right to integrated learning opportunities, enshrined in policy charters and legislation, their right to choose the learning environments which match their personal needs is also important.

In the debate on integration, as in other debates regarding important issues in their lives, adults with learning difficulties are either not consulted or else their views are accorded less weight than professional judgements. Continuing education, with its networks and contacts with self-advocacy groups, is in a position to consult with users and to adapt provision accordingly. In a situation where there is little to argue with in the rhetoric of integration, but where the contrast with practice is stark, there is room for another view from those who have been, at best, a small voice in the discussion so far. There is little doubt that integration sets up a 'virtuous circle', but it is, as yet, far from complete.

Issues of progression – finding a starting point

Under the Further and Higher Education Act 1992, there is a duty of providers to 'secure provision of adequate facilities' for students aged

16 and over part-time and for full-time students with learning difficulties aged 19 and above. However, under Schedule 2 of the Act, the
ability of providers to secure funding is dependent on being able to
demonstrate that a learning programme will provide progression to
another course within Schedule 2. A link between funding, curriculum,
progression and perhaps integration is, in theory, established. However, as many young people and adults with complex needs, language
disorders or challenging behaviour have not yet been able to access
discrete courses, it is difficult to conceive how they will fit into the new
system. In addition to such possible exclusions, there is the mismatch
between the achievement level of many students with learning difficulties and the entry requirements of many courses, including those leading
to work related qualifications such as National Vocational Qualifications, known as NVQs (NATFHE, 1993b).

Many students with learning difficulties will enter pre-NVQ or other
courses only to find that progression to the 'real' courses is not possible.
Some colleges have overcome such a lack of progression to courses
offering nationally recognised qualifications by having their own
courses validated by the Open College Network. Open College
Network courses are locally designed and delivered, and are available
in many parts of the country. However, Open College accreditation
does not automatically ensure access to mainstream progression
routes.

Such dilemmas and dual standards could be a threat to provision if,
in the future, courses do not fit into funding patterns set by the FEFC.
More importantly, there is a threat to integration into mainstream
courses.

Real integration through progression can lead to self-esteem which
has been generated by personal achievement. Genuine empowerment
of this kind has rarely been attainable within an education system
where low expectations and segregation have prevented opportunities
for progression for most students with learning difficulties. Let us hope
that the FEFC educational managers and validating bodies can use
vision and creativity to unblock the log-jam, thus preserving provision
as well as enabling the growth of integration and personal progression.

Issues in managing learning support

Are tutors within continuing education able to design curricula, with
complementary teaching strategies, to effectively meet the learning

strategies of individuals? The answer is that they do it every day. However, Whittaker (1993b) concluded from a number of detailed evaluations within colleges that they were failing to meet the needs of students with learning difficulties because they lacked adequate learning support structures and strategies. Indeed, it was Whittaker's view that the 'colleges had learning difficulties'. Vaughan Huxley, senior inspector with the FEFC, has said:

> The transformation in quality and style of provision in further education colleges has been frustratingly slow since the changes to be made beyond the confines of your own (the special needs co-ordinator) responsibility necessarily required the approval and commitment of staff across the college. (Vaughan Huxley, 1993).

Yet a variety of 'non-traditional' learners have been absorbed into the mainstream further education system. Examples of institutions with models which promote effective support for learners in integrated settings are well recorded (Sutcliffe, 1990; 1992) and rich in the variety of successful strategies adopted. Within the further education system there is adequate knowledge of curriculum, teaching strategies and systems of learning support. Why then, are there so many institutions with 'learning difficulties'?

A research project into support for learning in an integrated setting (Corbett and Myers, 1993) has identified a possible cause of such widespread institutional learning difficulties. The authors suggest that 'despite the impact of external forces, it is the inevitable messiness of institutional polices which tend to determine how individuals think and behave'. Unless management constructs a working system, co-ordinated across all college provision, students with learning difficulties will remain outside of the mainstream. Whittaker (1994) outlines a number of measures. He suggests that there should be a centralised admissions system with careful personal course guidance for prospective students. A full range of learner support should be complemented by different modes of attendance to accommodate individual circumstances. A wide variety of teaching methodologies should be used to gain the maximum benefits from the diversity of student abilities. Courses should be modularised, with a system for credit accumulation and transfer. Lastly, the whole system should be underpinned by a clear statement on equality of opportunity.

One of the tasks of the FEFC specialist committee on provision for students with learning difficulties might be to explore how colleges and adult education can be encouraged or assisted with their learning difficulties. A lead through funding mechanisms could give incentives so that all adults with learning difficulties have an equal opportunity to learn in the most appropriate setting.

Choices for the future

Delegates repeatedly asserted their right to experience life, for them this meant having the power to make choices. (*Community Living*, 1993).

Self-advocacy has acted as a catalyst in spotlighting curriculum issues which are of concern to people with learning difficulties. It challenges the deficit model of learning (which focusses on what people cannot do) by demonstrating how people's strengths can be developed. It demands that individual learning styles and preferences are taken into account within all learning opportunities. The practice of not providing equal opportunities to those people who are black or from other ethnic minorities, those with little or no speech or those with complex needs has been highlighted within continuing education by self-advocacy. Self-advocacy has also solved the complex and much debated question on language and terminology by simply stating that most labels are offensive to those who are labelled, yet there is little evidence that the viewpoint is being listened to.

Since the Education Act 1971 first entitled school-aged people with learning difficulties to a right to education, we have learnt very slowly how people thus labelled, learn. Self-advocacy has helped us to see that all people have their own learning styles, but there are both learning and teaching strategies which work, and which are transferable to a range of other learning situations. Self-advocacy provides a process for developing continuing education which is based on realism and is responsive to needs.

Choices are most powerful when those selecting their preference and those offering the selection are in harmony. It is then that realistic and appropriate choices are more likely to be made. The likelihood that Hobson's choice is all that is on offer is also diminished. There is a need to strive for at least a balance of power between the providers and the consumers of continuing education. A quest to optimise the learning process through a more equitable relationship between learners, planners and providers is vital. Self-appraisal and self-determination are far too rarely part of the process through which adults with learning difficulties determine their needs.

We know that much has been done by a range of providers.

However, there are still many people with learning difficulties whose needs are not even addressed, let alone met. Many do not even know where to seek advice and guidance. People with learning difficulties are still a small voice when it comes to planning future provision or determining needs.

Continuing education is one of the keys to participation in the full life of the community. The key to enabling education to be visible and available to all is

> to ensure that opportunities are not lost and co-operation between providers and colleges, local education authorities, social services departments etc is established to make sure that provision is continued and provides a seamless garment. After all, a chain is only as good as its links. (NATFHE, 1993b)

Returning to the snakes and ladders analogy used at the start of this chapter, we must ensure that continuing education will provide a ladder leading towards a fuller life in the community.

References

Baxter, C., Poonia, K., Ward, L. and Nadirshaw, Z. (1990). *Double Discrimination: Issues and Services for People with Learning Difficulties from Black and Ethnic Minority Communities*. King's Fund Centre/Community Relations Commission, London.

Booth, T. (1988). Challenging conceptions of integration. In *The Politics of Special Educational Needs* (ed. L. Barton). Falmer Press, Lewes.

Bradley, J. and Maychell, K. (1991). *Preparing for Partnership. Multi-agency Support for Special Needs*. National Foundation for Educational Research, Slough.

Brown, H. (1993). Issues in normalisation and empowerment. In *Leisure: A Serious Business*. Standing Conference of Voluntary Organisations for People with a Mental Handicap in Wales, Cardiff.

Burns, E., John, H. and Low, M. (eds) (1993). *Aiming for a College Education, A guide for disabled people*. Wales Council for the Disabled.

Community Living, October, 1993.

Corbett, J. and Myers, L. (1993). Support for learning in integrated settings. *Educare*, SKILL, No. 46, June 1993.

Cowan, S. and Rolph, S. (1992). *A New Life*. Further Education Unit, London.

Griffiths, M. (1993). The silent revolution. *Mencap News*, September.

Hancock, R. (1990). *Access to Adult Education for Students with Learning Disabilities*. Committee Report to South Glamorgan local education authority.

Hegarty, S. (1982). *Integration in Action*. NFER-NELSON, Slough.

Jarvis, 1983. *Adult and Continuing Education*.

King's Fund (1993). *Information Exchange on Self Advocacy and User Participation: No. 6.* King's Fund, London.

Lavender, P. (1993). *Incorporation and Community Care.* Further Education Unit, London.

Maddison, L. (1993). The Further Education Funding Council. In *Learning Difficulties and Disabilities.* National Association of Teachers in Further and Higher Education, London.

Mason, M. and Rieser, R. (1993). *Disability Equality in the Classroom. A Human Rights Issue.* Disability Equality in Education, London.

National Association of Teachers in Further and Higher Education (1993a). *Adult Education: A Survey Report.* NATFHE, London.

National Association of Teachers in Further and Higher Education (1993b). *Learning Difficulties and Disabilities,* NATFHE, London.

O'Brien, J. (1987). A guide to future planning. In *A Comprehensive Guide to the Activity Catalogue: an Alternative Curriculum for Youth and Adults with Severe Disabilities.* (eds B. Wilcox and G. Bellamy). Paul H. Brookes, Baltimore.

Pollard, S. (1968). *The Idea of Progress.* C.A. Watts Co., London.

SKILL (1992). *Further and Higher Education Act 1992: Students with Disabilities and Learning Difficulties,* SKILL.

Sutcliffe, J. (1990). *Adults with Learning Difficulties: Education for Choice and Empowerment.* National Organisation for Adult Learning. Open University Press, Milton Keynes.

Sutcliffe, J. (1992). *Integration for Adults with Learning Difficulties.* National Organisation for Adult Learning, Leicester.

Sutcliffe, J. and Simons, K. (1993). *Self Advocacy and Adults with Learning Difficulties.* National Organisation for Adult Learning, Leicester.

Sutcliffe, J. (1993). The Further and Higher Education Act and Adults with learning difficulties and disabilities: workshop reflections from the 'Strategies for Collaboration Conferences' *Adult Learning,* April 1993.

Vaughan Huxley, M. (1993). Part II of the Walter Lessing Memorial Lecture. *Educare,* No. 46, June.

Whittaker, J. (1993a). I just want to be a real student. Segregation in colleges of further education. *Community Living,* Vol 7 No. 2, October.

Whittaker, J. (1993b). Colleges have the disabilities. *Times Educational Supplement,* 8 October.

Whittaker, J. (1994). Rhetoric removed from reality. *Times Educational Supplement.* 14 January.

Part Two

Changing Practice

Chapter 6

Moving forward or moving back? Institutional trends in services for people with learning difficulties

Jean Collins

Public and professional concern about the inadequacies and inappropriateness of long-stay hospitals has become a tangible force in the UK over the last three decades. Fanned by a series of scandals and public inquiries in the 1960s and 1970s, and given a voice by the founding, in 1971, of the Campaign for People with Mental Handicaps (now Values Into Action), the movement to close the hospitals grew steadily stronger and more influential. The recognition that hospitalisation represents a degrading and inhumane treatment of vulnerable people was given additional weight by the increasing evidence of successful community support schemes.

By the end of the 1980s the path of hospital dissolution was beginning to be well trodden. Most hospitals were undergoing a process of retraction and were working towards closure dates; some had already closed. Despite this progress there were nearly 19 000 people still living in such hospitals in England alone in 1993. Moreover, there remains a lingering belief that people with profound or multiple disabilities, who have complex needs or who present severe challenging behaviours continue to need a lifestyle separate from the rest of society.

Nevertheless the resettlement programme received crucial governmental support and reinforcement from the NHS and Community Care Act 1990. This set in motion for other groups of people the move away from institutionalisation that had already benefited many people with learning difficulties. The route to deinstitutionalisation almost seemed assured. The most recent official guidelines for the social and health care of people with learning difficulties have gone further than any previous government pronouncement towards securing for them ordinary life opportunities. One government circular, for example, (DoH 1992a) states that 'few, if any, need to live in hospitals' (para 1), and that 'living arrangements need to be outward looking, closely associated with the general community, and limited in size . . .' (para 27). The emphasis throughout the circular is on arranging services 'on an increasingly *individual* basis . . .' (para 9, emphasis in the original). Another circular (DoH, 1992b) reiterates the fact that 'the large majority of people with learning disabilities not living with their families can be cared for in residential accommodation arranged through the relevant social services authority,' (Annex A); and furthermore that 'purchasers should . . . ensure that wherever possible people with learning disabilities are enabled to use ordinary health services.' To facilitate the implementation of these two circulars the government reissued, with substantial clarification, the regulations for the transfer of resources from health authorities to local authorities (DoH, 1992c). This is to enable the latter to fulfil their duties in respect of people who would once have been the responsibility of health authorities.

The publication of these three circulars followed the publication of the first report (Collins, 1992) from the research on which this chapter is based, and preceded the second report (Collins, 1993). Undertaken by Values Into Action, and supported by the Joseph Rowntree Foundation, the research studied the progress of resettlement and the development of replacement provision in nine areas of England. Carried out between 1991 and 1993, the research was a response to the growing suspicion that hospital closure and resettlement programmes had run out of steam, and that institutional structures and values were re-emerging both in the new community schemes and on the old hospital sites. The research has confirmed the presence of these tendencies.

Residual hospitals and centres of expertise

The NHS and Community Care Act 1990 placed a resounding emphasis on supporting people in the community rather than in institutions. It appeared to place community care for everyone firmly in the main frame of national policy. At the same time, however, it created the new status of NHS trust, for hospitals and other health service bodies which wished to become self-governing and semi-autonomous entities.

The division of the NHS into 'purchasers' (usually the district health authorities) and 'providers' (the hospitals and other units providing health-related services), together with the scope for self-determination provided by NHS trust status, has encouraged almost all remaining long-stay hospitals to apply to become trusts. The business plans of most NHS learning difficulties trusts either envisage the continuation and development of services on the old hospital site or foresee the trust closing down its old site as it transfers its operations into the community. Learning difficulties trusts which become wholly community-based often specialise in both residential support and behavioural support services.

While some trusts have seized the change to control their own finances and operating strategies with a view to expediting the transfer of people and resources back into the community, others have grasped the opportunity to re-establish the long-stay hospital as an essential facility, albeit under a different name. These trusts generally identify three categories of people with learning difficulties for whom segregated residential facilities are considered to be necessary: those people who also have mental health problems; those who display challenging behaviour; and those who have a further differentiating characteristic such as a physical disability, a sensory deficiency or who are elderly.

The latter category often includes people who, after a life-time of deprivation, sometimes express uncertainty at the prospect of returning to a world of ordinary social experiences, choice and freedom. The first two categories may also include people identified by the courts as requiring secure accommodation, and indeed a number of NHS trusts are developing their provision specifically to meet that perceived need. The Mansell report (1993), however, recommends that people with learning difficulties who also have challenging behaviour or mental health needs, including offenders, should have their needs met by local services using multidisciplinary services.

One NHS trust anticipates that about one-quarter of its resident population will remain on-site. Some of these are older people who have stated a preference to remain. When a villa had to be closed in 1990 it was replaced with four bungalows in the hospital grounds to house 19 of these older people. The trust is also building a medium secure unit in the grounds for 26 people. This investment is considered to be worthwhile because, as the trust readily admits, the treatment service makes money. The profit is then ploughed back into the facilities on-site to improve, upgrade and extend, and thus enable the trust to sell its services to more purchasers.

The other people remaining on-site will be diagnosed as having challenging behaviour or mental health problems. They will be the recipients of the treatment and assessment service bought by purchasing authorities which have ignored calls to develop or utilise local facilities. The trust is open in its intention to sell its services as far afield as possible, publicising itself as a 'centre of expertise'. This is despite the fact that manifestations of disruptive or challenging behaviour are now widely recognised as often being the result of environmental factors, rather than the consequence of either learning difficulties or mental ill-health.

By contrast the managers of an NHS trust elsewhere, which is totally committed to community-based services, argue that the essence of a treatment service lies not in a hospital setting but in equipping staff with specialist skills. Specialist staff need to work with people in their own homes if long-lasting improvement is to be achieved: 'It's lack of skills that produces the need for the security of a building'. Where staff maintain control through the paraphernalia of institutional trappings their clients' problems are exacerbated by loss of power, loss of choice and loss of self-respect.

Another NHS trust has constructed a business plan around a range of services which, as a hospital, it has traditionally provided and in which it sees potential for expansion. The services include community support, child development, language, assessment and treatment. The trust admitted that the particular assortment of services included in the plan was due to its current operations rather than to an objective assessment of what may sensibly be structured together. The residential assessment and treatment service is supposedly short-term only, but the question of what constitutes short-term is an open one. Weeks can turn into months and months into years: as one manager said 'All it takes is the consultant's signature.' The same reservations apply here as previously: assessment and treatment services need to be locally based and person not building-centred. The high fees charged by these small, residual hospitals will not always deter purchasers who lack the commitment to encourage local and appropriate provision.

This NHS trust also intends its residual hospital to house existing long-stay residents who are deemed either too old or in too poor health to cope with resettlement, plus those people who do not want to leave. In other areas, of course, people in their 70s, 80s and 90s have moved into ordinary community houses after a life-time in hospital; people suffering ill-health have moved into ordinary nursing homes; and worried people have received extra support before, during and after the move; all with considerable personal achievement and satisfaction. This trust is now exploring the possibility of expansion into on-site residential provision for people who carry a second label besides learning difficulties, such as visual or hearing impairments, impaired mobility, epilepsy and so on.

An NHS trust in another part of the UK has already developed two units on existing hospital sites for people with learning difficulties who also have either a mental health problem or challenging behaviour. People are increasingly being separated into their respective categories as defined by hospital culture, and depending on their physical and mental characteristics. It seems that once a residual hospital becomes an established fact its potential for gradual expansion becomes almost limitless as it constantly redefines its own need.

The nature of the continuum between people who have most needs and those who have least makes it inevitable that any division between those considered suitable for community care and those considered unsuitable will be entirely arbitrary. Different people will draw the line in different places according to their perception of humanity and their notion of human rights. Belief in the universality of human rights means that there can be no distinction between people who should be included in the community and those who, because of the severity of plurality of their disabilities, might not. One NHS trust, however, is prepared to consider permanent exclusion of some people:

> Bearing in mind that most of the people with fewer needs have already been resettled, and that the people still in hospital have very high, often nursing, needs, there is one argument that they are as well-off being moved into high-quality hospital accommodation as into the community. (Collins, 1993)

The continued closure of hospitals is not, therefore, by any means assured while NHS trusts continue to wield considerable power and autonomy.

NHS trusts may argue that it is the purchaser, and not the provider of the service, which dictates the course of future provision. It is, of course, within the remit of a purchaser to take their business elsewhere if the service being provided is not to their liking. Many purchasers, however, are too dependent on a single provider to make adequate use of such potential power. Where purchasers still depend on block contracts with one provider for several hundred people they are in no position either to take their business elsewhere or to stipulate conditions. This is particularly so where the purchaser lacks expertise in the learning difficulties field, which is often the case now that health authorities' learning difficulties units have become trusts. With little contribution to hospital assessments from social services departments, despite the NHS and Community Care Act 1990, the NHS trust, in many cases, is both assessor of need and provider of service.

Institutional services in community settings

The research has shown that people returning from long-stay hospitals to live in the community do not always leave the institution behind. Sometimes this is because the NHS trust which now manages their hospital also manages and staffs their new community support service. Although some trusts intend that their community services should *not* be institution-oriented, others do not acknowledge their institutional focus or do not accept that users benefit from a non-institutional value system. Other community support services may also exploit institutional models and structures despite not having a health service origin or perspective. Private companies, voluntary organisations and social services departments may all construct services on an institutional model.

There appear to be two forms of community-based institution with which people who have learning difficulties are now commonly being faced. The most obvious form, perhaps, is the large residential home. It has long been recognised that when a large number of people live together there must be structures and rules if there is not to be chaos. The imposition of regulations and routines helps to ensure that everyone living in the home has equal access to facilities and opportunities, and that people are not sidelined because they may find it difficult to compete with others. Yet the degree of control which is necessary takes its own toll of people's freedoms and individuality. The need for routines and recognised decision-makers limits the extent to which individual residents can exercise and express their own preferences and idiosyncracies. Since there has to be a structure, and the structure has to be approved by those in authority, the degree to which personal spontaneity can be countenanced is restricted.

Life in a small, shared house must also be subject to a certain amount of routine and control, but in small groups such arrangements become negotiable. Every family home, or house shared by friends, has an established, basic standard or outline of behaviour and activities which is commonly recognised and accepted. The regime within the home adapts to make allowances as new opportunities occur, as people develop, change their minds, take up new interests or make new friends. Where power resides within the group, even where the group has an acknowledged leader, there is more give-and-take, more spontaneity and more recognition of individual taste and need than is possible where power resides in a hierarchy which extends beyond the group.

Although structures inherent to the large residential home, whether called hostel, group home or care home, are inevitably institutional in nature it cannot be assumed that the small group home will automatically be free from institutional pressures. Small-scale living arrangements have the *potential* to escape the institutional frame, but if the support agency carries out its task in an institutional manner the home will still suffer institutional blight. It is the nature of the support provided in the home, and the relationship between the three parties of service user, support worker and managing agency that determines whether the home will actually run on institutional or ordinary lines.

At the present time provision of residential support services in the community appears to be increasingly dominated by these two institutional forms: the large-scale residential home and the small-scale shared or group home managed by a bureaucratic hierarchy. The larger scale home is rightly avoided by many purchasers and commissioners of services although others perceive in it, often quite erroneously, the potential for cheaper provision. Some providers regard it as potentially more profitable, and many as more manageable and controllable.

The research has shown, however, that an increasing number of purchasers and providers are investing in new provision which follows a now well-established pattern. Typically, a three or four bedroom house or bungalow is owned by a housing association and let to a group of tenants, who are supported in their daily living by a care agency. This agency may be the social services department, a for-profit or not-for-profit private company, a voluntary organisation or an NHS trust.

Many care agencies are expanding their operations by replicating the same model of provision many times over, establishing in each house the same user–staff and staff–manager relationships. As the agency grows so its hierarchy grows correspondingly, and its management becomes further removed from the users of its services. Many of the problems of inherent institutional structures, values and expectations reappear. Vertical structures inevitably breed inequalities in the vertical line but expect homogeneity at each of the rankings. So users once again tend to be denied their own individuality; support workers are limited in the extent to which they can be flexible and innovative in their work; and each small home becomes merely one cog in a larger whole instead of the centre of its own universe.

The first casualty in such a system is the notion of a service being individually designed and constructed to meet the wishes and the needs of the user. The emphasis of the system is not on serving individuals but on providing a series of vacancies which can then be filled. Within those parameters efforts may well be made to satisfy residents' requirements, but not to an extent which would disrupt or disturb the equilibrium of the system. People who may fit the service tolerably well at first may find themselves being ousted when their circumstances change. Whether their level of need increases or decreases there is seldom scope within the system to respond appropriately.

A health authority in one part of the UK recently contracted with a private company to provide supported accommodation for 50 people leaving a long-stay hospital. The company was provided with a list of hospital residents from whom to make its selection. It could find only 40 people who would suit its service, however, and was therefore permitted to trawl through a second hospital to find another ten. Although the people concerned are probably much better off than in hospital, and although attempts were doubtless made to create compatible groupings within the houses, and to meet people's preferences where that was possible within the terms and structure of the scheme, it cannot be claimed that this is a service designed to meet individual needs and wishes. Small, dispersed housing may be as limited in its response and scope and as restrictive in its authority structures as any campus-based institution.

Some NHS trusts appear content to transfer in this way their whole institutional baggage along with their residents from the old hospital site into the community. In one case, for example, a trust has already moved the majority of its residents into its own houses. Most of the houses accommodate about ten people although a few are larger: one, for example, is used as an old people's home for over 50 residents. On several of the sites there are self-contained units for two, three or four people.

Although the residents' quality of life has undoubtedly improved since leaving the old hospital building they cannot be said to have left hospital. They live with large numbers of other trust residents, are supported by trust staff and attend day facilities provided and staffed by the trust. Although they are better placed to use shops and other community facilities, for most of the time they interact only with NHS trust personnel on trust property. However skilled and experienced staff may be they, too, remain embedded within the trust's institutional frame. Residents of this trust are not even discharged: they are being kept as NHS patients.

Some NHS trusts are developing extensive community support services while simultaneously planning the retention of a residual hospital, as previously described. This gives them a foot in both institutional camps: the traditional and newly emerging. Some of these trusts are developing their community support services along the lines described above; lip-service is being paid to ordinary life principles by the use of houses which are then tied into a bureaucratic hierarchy. Usually people are discharged from hospital and have tenant status in their new homes. Some trusts own community houses where they place people with a history of challenging behaviour, or who have profound or multiple disabilities, without discharging them. These people may then be returned to the on-site 'centre of expertise' at the trust's discretion.

One NHS trust has a range of hospital and community provision. Most of its community housing is managed by housing associations but it provides the support. Current provision ranged from three and four-person houses to large units of over 20. It expects to continue to resettle a large number of its hospital population but it accepts the arguments, set out in the previous section, that where people with learning difficulties also carry a second label, such as mental illness or challenging behaviour, they may require specialist, segregated provision. The trust is also sympathetic to the view that a range of people with very profound or multiple disabilities may be as well catered for in hospital as in the community.

The purchasing authority of many of this trust's residents has not been able to influence the trust's views on provision. The local social services department has little or no input into assessments of the trust's residents. As a consequence the trust is able to move people virtually as it sees fit: no one else has the necessary knowledge or power to make positive interventions. Within its range of provision, therefore, the trust seeks to find the placement best suited to each resident. Again, it is not a question of designing a service to meet individual wish or need. It is a question of fitting people into vacancies. In this case, however, unlike the example cited earlier where the private company accepts only those people suited to its very limited range of provision, this NHS trust will not exclude people. It simply places them in the most appropriate, or least disruptive, placement it can find within its own provision.

Options for purchasers

The research has shown that institutional trends in provision for people with learning difficulties have by no means been eliminated. Ways are being found to perpetuate specialist residential accommodation on segregated sites, and many community services are being constructed within an institutional value system.

Two arguments are commonly put forward in defence of an institutional framework: feasibility and finance. Some professionals continue to argue that certain degrees or combinations of disabilities can only be dealt with in segregated settings; or that a paternalistic approach is an inevitable requirement in services for people with learning difficulties. Such perspectives disregard not just our responsibility for ensuring the best possible outcomes for people, but also the fact that professionals elsewhere are achieving precisely what is claimed to be impossible. In respect of the argument on finance, various community schemes around the country are demonstrating that much can be achieved within current funding levels. Individualised services in the community need not be more expensive than well-staffed institutional ones. Indeed, small, specialist, residual hospitals are often the more expensive option.

Within the current health and social services arrangements responsibility for procuring the best value service rests with the purchaser. It is the purchaser, therefore, who holds the key to the provision of services which actually meet the needs and wishes of people with learning difficulties. As far as people leaving long-stay hospitals are concerned, their purchaser often continues to be their district health authority instead of their local authority, despite the provision of the NHS and Community Care Act 1990 and the three Department of Health circulars referred to earlier. The research suggests that many health authority purchasers are continuing to buy directly from NHS trusts, and that in most cases it is the trust itself which determines the kind of provision it will make for each resident. There is often little or no social services department involvement.

If the interests of residents are to be put first then they cannot be left to the discretion of an existing or potential provider, or to a purchasing authority which may lack the necessary knowledge, skills and expertise in the field of learning difficulties. The deliberate arrangement or creation of services to meet the needs and wishes of individuals almost always requires the involvement of an active, independent third party. The research indicates that resettlement teams which are at arms length from both providers and purchasers, and which consist of personnel who jointly possess considerable experience in both the health and social services sectors are most likely to achieve outcomes which avoid the perpetuation of paternalistic and institutional structures.

This means that health and local authorities must be prepared to co-operate in the setting up of such teams, and to develop a positive approach to the joint commissioning of services in the interests of people waiting to leave, or who have recently left, hospitals. This sharing of responsibilities will ease the transition of the social care of people with learning difficulties from health authorities to local authorities, where it belongs. And by emphasising not just the desirability but the essential nature of planning for individuals, and not for groups, then it will be possible to leave institutional services where they should stay: in the past.

References

Collins, J.A. (1992). *When the Eagles Fly – A Report on Resettlement of People with Learning Difficulties from Long-Stay Institutions*. Values Into Action, London.

Collins, J.A. (1993). *The Resettlement Game – Policy and Procrastination in the Closure of Mental Handicap Hospitals*. Values Into Action, London.

Department of Health (1992a). *Social Care for Adults with Learning Disabilities (Mental Handicap)*, LAC(92)15. HMSO, London.

Department of Health (1992b). *Health Services for People with Learning Disabilities (Mental Handicap)*, HSG(92)42. HMSO, London.

Department of Health (1992c). *Health Authority Payments in Respect of Social Services Functions*, LAC(92)17. HMSO, London.

Mansell, J.L. (1993). *Services for People with Learning Disabilities and Challenging Behaviour or Mental Health Needs: Report of a Project Group*. HMSO, London.

Chapter 7

A seamless service? Developing better relationships between the National Health Service and Social Services Departments

Bob Hudson

In the community care White Paper (DoH, 1989), one of the main aims was said to be the delivery of a service in which 'the boundaries between primary health care, secondary health care and social care do not form barriers as seen from the perspective of the user'. It is a message which ministers have repeatedly emphasised. In a keynote address to the Association of Directors of Social Services in June 1992, for example, Health Minister, Dr Brian Mawhinney said:

> A good deal of work will have to be done to achieve workable practical arrangements for seamless services for clients . . . It is essential that we break down any real or imagined barriers between health authorities and local authorities. Community care cannot be implemented successfully if people retain ideas of separate and unconnected responsibilities. (DoH, 1992).

Nowhere is this more true than in the field of learning difficulties.

Fragmentation versus seamlessness: the conceptual context

Fragmentation can take many forms. Hudson (1993a), for example, distinguishes between three types of fragmentation: resource, organisational and cultural.

Resource fragmentation

Resource fragmentation exists when responsibility for a particular domain of activity is divided between more than one budget holder. This has long been the position in relation to learning difficulties where, in 1986, 60 per cent of the combined health and personal social services budget was estimated to be locked into hospital care for a small and diminishing number of residents (Audit Commission, 1986). Taking a wider organisational perspective, the dilemma is compounded by the fact that community care funding comes from a number of budgets spread across different government departments: the hospital and community health services budget; the personal social services budget; housing and recreation from the Department of the Environment; education from the Department for Education, employment from the Department of Employment; and social security from the Department of Social Security. The resource fragmentation dilemma is exacerbated when no mechanism exists to significantly transfer budgets between cost centres to effect a shift in strategy – a position which characterises learning difficulties policy.

Organisational fragmentation

This refers to the inability of organisations with a shared interest in a domain of activity to develop a complementary or co-ordinated strategy. This goes beyond problems of budget transfers, to focus upon the dynamics of organisational life and the ways in which they may serve organisational rather than user interests. This is one important reason why many previous initiatives have floundered. The White Paper (DoH, 1989), for example, acknowledged that joint finance and joint consultative committees had been ineffective, while the Audit Commission (1989) reported difficulties with the dowry system and a 'lack of trust and common purpose' between health authorities and local authorities. One of the yardsticks by which to judge the effectiveness of the NHS and Community Care Act 1990 will be the extent to which this form of fragmentation has diminished.

Cultural fragmentation

Cultural fragmentation refers to the impact of distinct occupational socialisation processes which may create conflicting professional interests and stereotyping. The cultural fragmentation between medical, nursing and social care interests, for example, was starkly revealed in the aftermath of the Jay Report (1979), and has not been seriously addressed since that time. The legacy is such issues as the uncertain status of those with a Registered Nurse (Mental Handicap) qualification in a post-hospital world, and the unclear relationship between community learning difficulties nurses and social workers specialising in learning difficulties.

This brief account of the nature and influence of fragmentation suggests the need to be realistic about the attainability of a 'seamless service', and this tends to be the message from the theoretical literature on collaboration (Hudson, 1993b). Collaboration has no qualities of spontaneous growth or self-perpetuation, and in general both professionals and organisations will strive to maintain their autonomy.

From an agency's viewpoint, collaboration raises two main difficulties. First, the organisation loses some of its freedom to act independently. Second, it must invest scarce resources and energy in developing and maintaining relationships with other agencies when the returns on this investment are often unclear and intangible. Booth (1988) terms this the 'realistic stance' on collaboration and identifies the five following dimensions.

- Collaboration is a self-interested process in which organisations will participate only if it suits them.
- The spirit of collaboration cannot be invoked by an appeal to the public interest.
- Success of collaboration will be determined by the balance of incentives and constraints bearing on each of the main parties.
- Pursuit of narrow organisational interest is rational in terms of the agency's survival and security of its members.
- Organisations will generally seek to maximise autonomy and minimise dependency.

It is against this background that the White Paper and the subsequent policy and practice guidance emphasised improved collaboration as the key to the community care reforms. It is a challenge which has been laid down before, most notably in the 1971 White Paper (DHSS, 1971) which sought a redistribution of resources away from hospital services and towards more local patterns of care. There was only limited success in implementing this White Paper. Hardy et al. (1990) identified several reasons for this:

Definititional

The White Paper lacked both a definite commitment to change and an unambiguous set of principles to guide it. This in turn failed to address the absence of consensus both as to the needs of people with learning difficulties and the nature of appropriate forms of support.

Planning

The great majority of health and local authorities had failed to develop the degree of collaboration necessary to underpin a planned transition from hospital to community care. Any such attempts were then undermined by the rapid and unplanned growth of social security support to independent sector care homes and nursing homes.

Resources

The reduction in anticipated resources was dramatic. At the beginning of the period, central government had asked local authorities to plan on the assumption of 10 per cent growth per annum, but by 1976 this had been reduced to two per cent. The changes ushered in by the 1990 Act are similarly accompanied by spending constraints, and this is not the best climate in which to encourage collaborative activity.

More recent research into the resettlements of people with learning difficulties from long-stay hospitals to community settings suggests that these obstacles remain formidable. The 1990 Act and subsequent guidance directed that there should be joint health and social services assessment of the continuing care needs of people waiting to be discharged from hospital, but Collins (1992; 1993; and see Chapter 7) found these to be simply ignored. Most people who had left hospital had done so without the involvement of social services, and most people still waiting to leave had not been assessed by social services staff. Overall she found that the resettlement process and the course of hospital retraction was guided by the needs of hospitals and their staffs, rather than the needs of residents and, in particular, the following points are noted.

- Re-emergence of old hospitals as new self-governing trusts under the health care reforms, with a strategy of becoming monopoly providers in the community, just as they once monopolised hospital provision.
- A tendency to focus upon fitting people into existing provision, rather than organising provision to suit people's needs.

- Large organisations monopolising the resources available for learningdif-ficulties in their areas, thus preventing less traditional competitors from developing alternative support systems.
- Vital information about residents withheld from resettlement and community staff; residents' and relatives' anxieties about the unknown was deliberately fuelled.
- A number of hospitals planning their own continuation and abandoning the retraction and closure plans which were accepted before the attain-ment of trust status.
- Some resettlement officers admitting that they were forced to run 'escape committees' engaged in 'prising' people out of hospital.

All of this suggests that examples of good practice in health–social care relationships will be thin on the ground and will be surviving against the odds. Hardy *et al.* (1992), in their review of joint management schemes, come to just such a conclusion:

> Of those projects which appeared to have overcome the barriers, they were inherently fragile and vulnerable to organisational pressures that threatened their sustained development. They operate on the periphery of their parent bodies and may be viewed as either an administrative inconvenience or a threat to the professional or organisational status quo. They may rely too much on mutual trust and altruism, and may be over-reliant upon the personal networks of their original champions.

The critical paradox confronting the debate about a seamless service, then, is that accounts of failed attempts to secure collaboration are simply met with exhortations for better collaboration. Collaboration is simultaneously paraded as both the problem and the remedy. Few would disagree with the need for carefully thought out joint approaches to service development in the field of learning difficulties. Several features of current policy require this. They are: the accelerated rate of resettlement from hospital into the community; the associated require-ments for developing more appropriate patterns of community support; the introduction of assessment and care management which requires close co-operation between multidisciplinary teams; community care planning systems which need strong links across agency boundaries; and quality assurance which needs to encompass the activities of a wide range of professionals.

However, simultaneously with these imperatives for closer working, the health care and community care reforms have created a more complex and unpredictable environment within which to develop more positive relationships. The most notable of these have been the complexity of reorganisations within social services departments, the emergence of self-governing trust status for both long-stay hospitals and community health services, an unexpected extension of the purchasing remit of GP fundholders to cover community nursing and therapy services, and the introduction of contracting and a purchaser–provider split in health and social care. If Øvretveit (1993) is correct in arguing that in times of pressure, less time is spent informing, negotiating and consulting with others, then the collaborative agenda of the 1990s looks formidable indeed.

Vehicles for change?

Although the preceding analysis has served to warn against undue optimism, it should not be taken to imply that progress is impossible, but rather that it is more likely to be a case of moving slowly towards seamlessness rather than attaining it with effortless superiority. There may be four important vehicles for change: community learning difficulty teams; care management; primary health care teams; and joint commissioning.

Of the four the *raison d'etre* of community learning difficulty teams (CLDTs; the formerly named community mental handicap teams) has been:

> to confront head on those concerns . . . that care provision for people with a [learning difficulty] was fragmented, that services were inaccessible and that organisational and professional boundaries prevented continuity of care. (Brown and Wistow, 1990).

The idea of CLDTs was first promoted in the 1970s by the Development Team for the Mentally Handicapped (1978) and by the end of the 1980s most localities had some form of grouping. To that extent, the CLDT experience constitutes a useful test of the extent to which the system prior to the 1990 Act could develop an effective collaborative strategy.

Perhaps the most noticeable feature of CLDTs has been the variation in their size, membership and function. The survey of English CLDTs by Brown (1990) found two-thirds of them to have less than four members, which would imply a relatively limited multidisciplinary spread. The separate analysis of CLDTs in Wales (McGrath and Humphreys, 1988) described teams as being of four types: basic teams consisting solely of social workers and nurses (16 per cent); professionally oriented teams which included members of additional professions (29 per cent); service-oriented teams comprising social workers, nurses and service organisers (42 per cent); and integrated teams of social workers, nurses, other professionals and service organisers (13 per cent).

This range in size and membership is reflected in the variation in functions of CLDTs. Mansell (1990) cites the three following functions for CLDTs.

- A gatekeeping or co-ordinating role primarily concerned with direct 'routine family maintenance' which fills a gap in service provision.
- A service development role seeking to build up a range of residential and support services within the community, and which could involve little or no direct work with users.
- A direct service delivery role which is a logical extension of the service development role, where the CLDT becomes a managerial team appointing and employing basic grade direct care staff.

The balance of evidence would suggest that CLDTs have been only partially successful in securing collaborative working patterns, but that the achievements nevertheless are not inconsiderable. The English and Welsh CLDT surveys highlight the following positive results.

- Developing the recognition that planning must start from the needs of users and carers with a mechanism that allows them to participate in discussions.
- Helping to clarify the roles and responsibilities of different care professionals along with practical ways of fitting them together.
- Providing a vehicle for strengthening co-operation between health and social services authorities at field, management and planning levels.
- Offering an organisational framework for the growing number of health service staff working outside traditional hospital settings.
- Creating a mechanism for establishing a substantial, specialist fieldwork resource with a degree of ring-fenced protection.
- The very existence of multidisciplinary mechanisms is no small achievement given the pressures to retain separate identities and ways of working.

Notwithstanding these achievements, CLDTs have been far from an unblemished success. Three particular difficulties are the persistence of role ambiguity; problems in securing a co-ordinated response; and confusion over organisational accountability.

Role ambiguity

Given the lack of clarity about the original idea of CLDTs, it is unsurprising that many of them lacked operational policies: Brown's (1990) survey of the West Midlands found that only a quarter of them had been provided with a framework of operational objectives. The consequence has been that conflict and uncertainty, rather than consensus and rationality, have been the characteristics of policy making and policy implementation. This process of negotiation is not confined to the internal organisation of CLDTs, for they have also had to find a niche in the local service-providing environment.

Securing a co-ordinated response

It might be expected that one outcome of this complex role negotiation would be that CLDT members secured more co-ordinated patterns of working. The Welsh CLDT survey did indeed find that 'teams in general exhibited a high degree of commitment, mutual trust and support', but equally concluded: 'the various professions have different methods of working, value systems and priorities, and frequently show a lack of knowledge and understanding of other professions and a tendency to stereotype them' (McGrath and Humphreys, 1988). Both the English and Welsh surveys saw the relationship between social workers and community nurses as particularly difficult. Case owner-ship tended to be on an individual basis, with cases acquired through the separate networks with which they were associated. From then on, members worked with considerable independence from one another, despite appearing to perform broadly similar tasks.

Organisational accountability

Organisation is not a peripheral issue for CLDTs, but one which is central to their existence. The management structure within which the CLDT operates is a crucial factor in its effectiveness, and since multidisciplinary working also requires multi-agency working, the environment is complex. The Wales survey found CLDTs in difficulty where management support to the team was weak, with no over-arching system at middle management level to mirror the multi-agency nature of the teams. This tells us that the planning of multidisciplinary care packages on a 'bottom-up' basis requires clear lines of support in order to survive.

Although CLDTs may only have made limited progress in their search for co-ordinated patterns of working, it is arguable that they have made as much progress as the prevailing system of policy making encouraged. The danger in the 1990s is that the community care reforms may threaten to undermine that progress which *has* been made. Brown *et al.* (1992) identify several threats: genericism; the health–social care divide; care management; and organisational fragmentation.

Genericism

There is a concern that a specialist focus upon learning difficulties may not fit into the priorities being established for social services. The specialist expertise developed by CLDTs could be overlooked as social services departments become preoccupied with services for children and families, with learning difficulties becoming part of a more general category of 'adult services' or 'disabilities'.

Health–social care divide

The notion of a clear distinction between health care and social care has been promoted as part of the wider community care changes. Although offered as a means of clarification of respective responsibilities, it could easily create incentives to work separately. Brown *et al.* (1992) report that in some areas, health care purchasers have been seeking to fund only the distinct 'health element' of CLDT work, with community nurses working strictly to a list of 'health functions'. This runs counter to the efforts of CLDTs to work jointly across professional divisions and pool the resources of separate agencies.

Care management

Community learning difficulty teams may become marginalised as a separate care management system is developed, particularly in those localities in which care management is seen as solely a purchasing activity. Indeed, some would see care management as the 1990s response to the failure of 'old-fashioned' multidisciplinary working. Such an approach would be wasteful. In particular, care management has important parallels with successful individual programme planning (IPP) systems, and the IPP experience needs to be locked into care management development.

Organisational fragmentation

Community learning difficulty teams have sought to operate as both service delivery and service development agents, with an assumption that ground level information about need is vital to strategic level planning. This may be undermined by rigid versions of the purchaser–provider split, with needs assessment and planning seen as a purchaser activity, and multi-professional forums relegated to a separate provider role. The position of CLDTs and even joint care planning teams is unclear during these bouts of wholesale reorganisation.

The second vehicle for change is care management into which the government is putting considerable faith as a fresh means of attaining a co-ordinated approach to assessment and service delivery (Hudson, 1993c). The call for enhanced collaborative activity lies at the heart of several concerns that are critical to care management. These are: the recognition that boundaries between professionals, services and agencies militate against user-sensitive responses; the existence of some overlap and duplication of service coverage; and a feeling that services may be pulling in different directions.

It is still too early to make a judgement upon care management. The early projects funded by the Care in the Community initiative and evaluated by the Personal Social Services Research Unit at the University of Kent were optimistic in their findings, but more recent evaluations have been less sanguine. With learning difficulty, much interest has been generated by the evaluation of the Wakefield Care Management Project (Richardson and Higgins, 1990; 1991; 1992). On the particular issue of care management and collaboration, the Wakefield study threw up three problem areas.

The first was organisational and professional fragmentation. The project was established to facilitate the transfer of residents from hospital to the community, but it soon fell foul of the sorts of fragmentations discovered by Collins in her more recent study of resettlement. Care managers found difficulties in their relations with hospital staff who had a more traditional approach to residents, felt some prior ownership of them and saw the project as a threat to their security. Hospital consultants are key to the resettlement decision-making process, and they, too, tended to be sceptical about the project as well as resentful of the threat to their authority to determine client futures.

The second problem area identified was lack of interest on the part of the organisation. Whereas organisational and professional fragmentation destroys collaboration because of disputation over domain legitimacy, a lack of interest by the organisation destroys collaboration through simple neglect. The Wakefield Project found this to be particularly true of the local authority housing department, which was described as 'an embarrassment to the project'. The principal service required of the hospital leavers was housing, and the user-led nature of care management led to the expectation that users would move to individual houses and flats appropriate to their particular needs. In practice, the housing department simply did not respond other than to offer 'miscellaneous' properties – large or unusual properties of limited interest to families on the ordinary waiting list and traditionally seen as 'special needs' housing.

The third problem area was that of organisational inertia or the unwillingness or seeming inability of existing service providers to respond to change. Service development is an inherently political task and requires trying to interest those already working in a locality in developing new services and providing incentives to do so. The Wakefield Project seemed to be in a good position to do this, since it had funds waiting to be put to work, but found local agencies to be unresponsive. Richardson and Higgins (1990) argue that bureaucracies are simply geared to 'more of the same' and conclude that 'the real problem encountered was an organisational resistance to take on anything new'.

It would be wrong to place too much weight on the Wakefield experience, for the project was concerned with a particularly complex task and was operating some time before the DoH gave official backing to the care management process. However, it does suggest that it would be premature to view care management as the solution to the fragmentation dilemma. The realistic option would seem to be to continue experimenting with different models of care management in different places and with different objectives, and to tie this in with the positive developments which have arisen from local CLDT activity. Perhaps the most obvious delusion would be for social services agencies to immerse themselves in the procedural dimensions of care management without stopping to think about why care management is being used, which model seems most appropriate, and what outcomes it can be expected to be achieved.

The third important vehicle for change is the position of primary health care professionals, especially GPs, in a network of support for people with learning difficulties. This has been given little attention, but is an issue which is growing in significance. A part of this impetus is the extended purchasing remit which has arisen from Circular

EL(92)48 which widens the scope of the hospital and community health services element of the GP fundholding scheme (National Health Service Management Executive, 1992). Since April 1993, GP fund-holders have held an additional purchasing responsibility for health visiting, district nursing, dietetics, chiropody and community services for people with mental health problems and learning difficulties. Additionally, it seems unlikely that this extended role will be confined to fundholders in the future. The Audit Commission (1993), for example, has called for greater flexibility in local agreements to allow non-fundholding GPs to purchase some services on behalf of commissioning authorities through delegated budgets. Such a development would blur the distinction between fundholding and non-fundholding status and give impetus to the need for closer links with social care agencies.

In the guidance on the extended purchasing role, GPs are urged to liaise with social services departments and other members of the primary health care team 'to ensure appropriate and seamless care is delivered' – an injunction which is said to be particularly important during periods of transition, such as leaving hospital or residential care. However, Collins (1993) found that some GPs has misgivings about accepting former hospital residents with learning difficulties. Several reasons were given for this: they had little experience of this group; a fear of the expense they might create with, for example, high levels of obesity, hypertension, inactivity and medication; the absence of comprehensive medical notes; and the additional work required to bring both patient and notes up to the standard expected in the practice.

The issue of medical records was an important feature of Collins' findings in which it was noted that there was a reluctance on the part of some long-stay hospitals to release the medical records of resettled patients. In these circumstances, GPs may be expected to manage without any medical notes or with medical summaries which are incomplete and inaccurate; which pieces of notes are drawn from years of notes is, in large measure, quite discretionary. Collins argues that on return to the community, the fact that the institution has been a substitute for a GP is ignored. All of this suggests an urgent need to improve the physical health of long-stay NHS patients and facilitate the transfer of their care from hospital to community by developing primary care records to a format and standard compatible with those of patients registered with local GPs.

GPs, other members of primary health care teams and care managers will need to be closely involved when working on the same patch, but the relationships between them may be very different from the preference of the British Medical Association (1992) to simply add social workers to an extended primary health care team working to GP leadership. Indeed, there is a concern that the inclusion of community learning difficulty nurses within the fundholding empire could lead to the re-emergence of a medical model of learning difficulties. The Audit Commission (1992) argues for a radical locality model in which a single care manager holds a budget from health and local authorities and purchases both health and social care. This would require health care agencies to decentralise much of their purchasing and develop imaginative ways in which locality purchasing with SSD care managers might be developed. The new commissioning arrangements do seem to offer fresh opportunities for co-ordinating care, but it is still too early to make any judgement upon the pilot projects which are developing.

Joint commissioning is the fourth important vehicle for change and there are several imperatives which lie behind its growing popularity. These are:

- Minimising the potential instability created by the existence of multiple purchasers of health and social care.
- Allowing small purchasing authorities to develop purchasing expertise.
- Reaping economies of scale from savings in such items as staff costs, information technology support systems and office accommodation.
- Avoiding the possibility of a collusive relationship developing with a purchaser's 'own' providers.
- Combating problems of fragmentation at service delivery level.

In the health context, Ham and Heginbotham (1991) distinguish between three types of joint commissioning:

Informal joint purchasing

This is where authorities come together to share some of the work such as common service specifications and work on quality or contracts. In this model, authorities take opportunities for collaboration as they arise and these are sustained only as long as they prove useful to the participants.

Formal joint purchasing

This includes many of the same activities but is based upon a more explicit commitment to working together by the constituent authorities, and is more strategic than opportunistic.

Consortium

In a consortium, arrangements go further in terms of the degree of formality adopted. In effect, a consortium takes on all or most of the purchasing work of the authorities and acts like a common service agency. This is the strongest form of joint purchasing and may be a precursor to a formal merging of the authorities.

A number of localities have sought to develop joint commissioning arrangements for people with learning difficulties, but as with many aspects of the health and community care reforms, it is still too early to assess the effectiveness of such changes. However, the broader experience of inter-organisational work makes it possible to identify the following potential dilemmas facing joint commissioners.

Developing trust and understanding

Knapp *et al.* (1992) argue that the accumulated experience of 20 years of joint working suggests that it tends to work best when trust and confidence have been built up. However, it is not clear how such a relationship can be organisationally developed and sustained. At best it will probably take some considerable time to develop, implying that joint commissioning cannot be viewed as some short-cut panacea.

Linking different levels of purchasing

Both the health and social care reforms introduce purchasing at micro and macro levels – in the case of health through health authorities (macro) and GP Fundholders (micro), and in the case of social care through central commissioning units (macro) and care managers (micro). Linking these activities within single organisations will be difficult. Co-ordinating them across health and social care agencies constitutes a formidable task.

Pooling sovereignty

Essentially, the greater the degree of formal joint purchasing, the more organisational sovereignty will have to be pooled, and this may prove to be a political stumbling block. Clode (1992), for example, gives an account of the Lewisham Partnership, which is a joint commissioning project between Lewisham social services department and North Southwark Health Authority to cater for the needs of people with learning difficulties. He identifies two major problems in the development of the project – the construction of a joint budget and the political problem of deciding how that budget would be managed.

Overall, the general enthusiasm for joint commissioning can easily obscure practical difficulties: how much should each agency put into the pool? Who is to be held accountable for it? What are the limits of legality? Local authorities cannot purchase health care, but can pooled budgets be used to purchase it? Will joint commissioning undermine the local authority lead role in community care? Central government could do much to minimise the obstacles by clarifying the legal position and encouraging coterminosity. But ultimately it remains the case that joint commissioning is merely a means to an end, and if it does not produce more and better services for users than were available under separate budgets, then the whole enterprise will have had little point.

Overall, this chapter has not been optimistic about the ability to attain a seamless service between health and social services agencies. It has identified some of the problems encountered in past experiences and has cautioned against unrealistic expectations of current initiatives. However, boundaries need not be barriers and some progress may well be possible, but it is likely to be incremental and adapted to local circumstances. A realistic emphasis will be on the process itself rather than upon intangible results, with benefits accruing from such factors as mutual organisational learning; a clarification of differences; an upward spiral of trust; and a developing consensus about aims, principles and priorities. It would be too bland to seek to identify a checklist of pointers to good practice, but given a diversity of interests and values, the rational–altruistic model of collaboration has several prerequisites. These are that there should be at least some set of common goals; a system-wide view of needs and problems; some consensus about the nature of these needs and problems; agreement on how to tackle the problems; and agreement on the priority to be accorded to each potential claim.

Unless these fundamental prerequisites are addressed, the danger will be that much time and effort will be spent upon secondary issues of structure and accountability. The most important message has to be that joint working needs to be justified in terms of a better quality of life for users and carers.

References

Audit Commission (1986). *Making a Reality of Community Care.* HMSO, London.

Audit Commission (1989). *Developing Community Care for Adults with a Mental Handicap, Occasional Paper 9.* HMSO, London.

Audit Commission (1992). *Homeward Bound: A New Course for Community Care.* HMSO, London.

Audit Commission (1993). *Practices Make Perfect: The Role of the Family Health Services Authority.* HMSO, London.

Booth, T. (1988). *Developing Policy Research.* Gower, Aldershot.

British Medical Association (1992). *Priorities for Community Care.* BMA, London.

Brown, S. (1990). Finding a niche in the system: the case of the community mental handicap team. In *The Roles and Tasks of Community Mental Handicap Teams* (eds S. Brown and G. Wistow). Avebury, Aldershot.

Brown, S., Flynn, M. and Wistow, G. (1992). *Back to the Future: Joint Work for People with Difficulties.* National Development Team/Nuffield Institute, Manchester.

Brown, S. and Wistow, G. (1990) (eds) *The Roles and Tasks of Community Mental Handicap Teams.* Avebury, Aldershot.

Clode, D. (1992). Step by step. *Community Care,* 5 October.

Collins, J. (1992). *When the Eagles Fly: A Report on Resettlement of People with Learning Difficulties from Long-Stay Institutions.* Values into Action, London.

Collins, J. (1993). *The Resettlement Game: Policy and Procrastination in the Closure of Mental Handicap Hospitals.* Values into Action, London.

Department of Health (1989). *Caring for People: Community Care in the Next Decade and Beyond.* HMSO, London.

Department of Health (1992). Conference speeches delivered by Dr Brian Mawhinney. *Caring for People Newsletter,* No. 10.

Department of Health and Social Security (1971). *Better Services for the Mentally Handicapped.* HMSO, London.

Development Team for the Mentally Handicapped (1991). *First Report: 1976–1977.* HMSO, London.

Ham, C. and Heginbotham, C. (1991). *Purchasing Together,* King's Fund College, London.

Hardy, B., Wistow, G. and Rhodes, R.A.W. (1990). Policy networks and implementation of community care policy for people with a mental handicap. *Journal of Social Policy*, **19**, 141–168.

Hardy, B., Wistow, G. and Turrell, A. (1992). *Innovations in Community Care Management*, Gower, Aldershot.

Hudson, B. (1993a). Learning disability: is a co-ordinated service available? In *Community Care for People with Learning Difficulties, Report on CCETSW Conference Series*. Yorkshire Link Consortium.

Hudson, B. (1993b). Collaboration in social welfare: a framework for analysis. In *The Policy Process: A Reader* (ed. M. Hill). Harvester Wheatsheaf, London.

Hudson, B. (1993c). *The busy person's guide to care management. Community Care*/Joint Unit for Social Services Research, University of Sheffield.

Committee of Enquiry into Mental Handicap Nursing and Care, (Jay report) (1979). HMSO, London.

Knapp, M., Wistow, G. and Jones, M. (1992). Smart moves. *Health Service Journal*, 29 October.

Mansell, J. (1990). The natural history of the community mental handicap team. In *The Roles and Tasks of Community Mental Handicap Teams* (eds S. Brown and G. Wistow). Avebury, Aldershot.

McGrath, M. and Humphreys, S. (1988). *The All Wales Community Mental Handicap Team Survey*. University College of North Wales, Bangor.

National Health Service Management Executive (1992). *Guidance on the Extension of the Hospital and Community Health Services Elements of the GP Fundholding Scheme from 1 April 1993* [EL(92)48].

Øvretveit, J. (1993). *Coordinating Community Care: Multidisciplinary Teams and Care Management*. Open University Press, Buckingham.

Richardson, A. and Higgins, R. (1990). *Case Management in Practice: Reflections on the Wakefield Case Management Project, Working Paper No. 1*. Nuffield Institute, Leeds.

Richardson, A. and Higgins, R. (1991). *Doing Care Management: Learning from the Wakefield Case Management Project, Working Paper No. 4*. Nuffield Institute, Leeds.

Richardson, A. and Higgins, R. (1992). *The Limits of Case Management: Lessons from the Wakefield Case Management Project, Working Paper No. 5*. Nuffield Institute, Leeds.

Chapter 8

Putting people first?: Assessment and care management

Lynne Elwell, Helen Platts and Gillian Rees

This chapter looks at assessment and care management from the different points of view of three women: a service user, the mother of a woman with a learning difficulty and a service manager. It focusses on the introduction of care management into social services departments in response to the NHS and Community Care Act 1990 which required local authorities to establish, co-ordinate and monitor new assessment arrangements for access to community care services from April 1993. Our accounts show that although care management in its latest form is being presented as a coherent and consistent way of co-ordinating social care, basic tensions and contradictions underlie the new systems. In this chapter it is argued that only by being explicit about these issues, will real progress will be made in improving the services available to people with learning difficulties and their families.

At one level, care management can be seen as the positive and radical response by service agencies to an emerging role for them in supporting vulnerable people, including people with learning difficulties, away from institutional settings. 'Case management', as it was first called, was developed in the 1960s in North America as part of the general move away from segregating and congregating disadvantaged people in long-stay hospitals. This more individualised approach gained momentum in the UK throughout the 1970s and 1980s, when agencies started to define the complex task of supporting people in the community instead of in long-stay hospital and other residential and institutional settings. Case management was seen as a way of co-ordinating a range of services around the needs of one person, addressing the problems of lack of information about the different services available and the evident lack of organisation between services (NDT, 1991).

The political motivation for establishing care management as part of the recent community care reforms is based, in part, on similar concerns of giving people more autonomy and more control over their own lives. Care management fitted with the new right agenda of introducing consumerism into the public sector and making state bureaucracies more accountable to the end users of services. Reducing dependence by giving people more choice and more say in what services should be like appealed to policy makers and professionals alike. At the same time, there was political interest in reducing the costs of providing services. Care management was seen as a way of containing public expenditure by targeting services at those most in need of social care. Focussing on services for elderly people, the influential Griffiths report (1988) promoted care management as a process for allocating resources and developing low-cost, local supports to people in their own homes as an alternative to residential care. The shift in terminology from 'case management' to 'care management' by central policy makers in the second half of the 1980s, as well as reflecting the fact that service users were to be seen as equal partners rather than 'cases' (Hudson, 1993), made explicit the aim of using individualised planning as a way of accessing 'care', in other words 'services'.

The introduction of care management as a process for rationing services has led to concerns that the recent community care reforms may work against the interests of people with learning difficulties and their families. It is evident that identifying and meeting the needs of people already using services may not be compatible with the requirements of the White Paper *Caring for People* (DoH, 1989) that resources are targeted on those with the most complex needs (Beardshaw and Towell, 1990). Above all else, care management, set up under the new legislation to ensure that services are developed on the basis of good information about unmet need, still operates within local authority social services departments with limited funding where elected members make political rather than rational resourcing decisions. Alongside this political process, the new contracting arrangements introduced at the same time as care management may work against finding individual solutions. Although care management provides a system for obtaining information about individual consumer preferences and priorities in a systematic way, given that purchasing power is not vested directly with the end users of services, there is a danger that social services departments will respond to this information as before, by negotiating block contracts with service agencies. In so doing they are perpetuating the service-led model that care management, with its focus on the needs and wants of each person, originally sought to challenge.

Gillian Rees: Care management and what it means to someone who uses the services

Helen Platts put the following questions to Gillian Rees.

Helen Platts (services representative): What was it like when you had a social worker?

Gillian Rees (user): They got me into Selby [Houses, a housing project in South London]. It was good. They came to visit us. We talked about things – things that I wanted to talk about like Mum and Dad moving to Edinburgh. That was a couple of years ago.

HP: What did you like about having a social worker?

GR: Someone to talk to who wasn't at Oakfield [day centre] or Selby.

HP: What do you think about not having a social worker at the moment?

GR: I'd like one now. I'd talk about Mum and Dad moving. But I see Catherine [a psychologist] sometimes.

HP: If you had a social worker what would you like them to be like?

GR: Kind. Help out and do all different kinds of things. Talk to me about Mum and Dad moving. Talk to me about how I'll feel after they move. Ask me if I've got any brothers and sisters. That's all.

HP: If your Mum and Dad move away will it be important to have a social worker then?

GR: I don't know because I might get help from Oakfield and Selby.

HP: Do you know what care managers do?

GR: Do they go and see people who are on their own and things like that?

HP: Have you ever had an assessment?

GR: I don't think so.

HP: Have you ever had a review?

GR: Yes.

HP: What happens at the reviews?

GR: They ask how I'm getting on at Selby and how I'm getting on at Oakfield with work experience and things like that.

HP: How do you feel about reviews?

GR: They are normally good ones. I like them.

HP: What would be a bad review?

GR: If you'd been playing up and things like that all the time.

HP: What if you weren't happy with something at Selby or Oakfield?

GR: I'd say in a review.

HP: What would happen?

GR: They'd do something about it.

HP: Say you were moving away from your Mum and Dad's house for the first time. What are the important things to say?

GR: Tell them I want to move out of home. Tell them I want to live my own life. Tell them details about where I work. Give them my details. Then wait and see and ask them if there are any places I can move into.

HP: What really matters to you?

GR: Try and find a place like Selby.

HP: In what ways is Selby a good choice?

GR: Because you can live your own life. Can cook for yourself. Got your own key. Got your own bedroom key. They take you out on trips. You can have friends around. You meet different people.

HP: How would you feel if they didn't find what you wanted?

GR: Unhappy.

HP: What if it was a place where you couldn't cook for yourself, you didn't have your own key and you couldn't have friends round?

GR: I wouldn't take it.

HP: If social services said they were coming along to do an assessment how would you feel about it?

GR: Pleased.

HP: What would make it good? Say, if you start with a meeting?

GR: If I look smart – because you've got to look smart in meetings.

HP: What about other people in the meeting?

GR: They'll have to look smart as well because they're doing the interviewing.

HP: How should the meeting go?

GR: Tell them what I want.

HP: What about if a care manager comes along with a lot of forms?

GR: Sign them, if I agree with them.

HP: What if the care manager comes along with a lot of paperwork?

GR: Read through it.

HP: What if your Mum and Dad are there?

GR: They should have their say.

HP: Is this anything different from what you had with a social worker?

GR: No.

HP: What does community care mean to you?

GR: When people look after you when you are ill.

HP: What about living in the community? What does that mean?

GR: Talking about transport.

HP: Selby Houses is called community care. How do you feel about that?

GR: I like that because we all get on.

HP: Who else lives in the community?

GR: Everyone in Penge [the area in South London where Selby Houses are situated].

HP: What's community care about?

GR: When people come and see you. Being part of the community.

HP: What should people with learning difficulties get for support?

GR: Reading, writing, help with cooking.

HP: What does Selby give you?

GR: Help with shopping lists.

HP: What is care management?

GR: It's a manager. They look after people in the community.

HP: What does a care manager do?

GR: Stays in the office.

HP: How do they look after people?

GR: They go round and visit them.

HP: What good does that do?

GR: They talk to them. They have meetings.

HP: What happens there?

GR: They talk about things that the care manager is doing with the person.

HP: What sort of things might the care manager do with the person?

GR: Finding them a place. Going to a place to see if they've settled in.

Lynne Elwell: An experience of care management as the mother of a woman with a learning difficulty

There was a feeling of hope and change around before April 1993. Community care legislation that had been promised and then delayed for so long was at last coming into force.

We had hoped that at last we would have some power to make changes in our daughter's life that would enable her to enjoy and experience the things that our other children had taken for granted.

April came and went and no changes were apparent. In a discussion at our local carers meeting, we discovered that no one had been given any information and we were all aware of rumours that our local services had been moved out of town to another office. This was very worrying, especially for some of the older carers who were unhappy about having to leave messages on an answerphone. They felt that because of job reshuffles they would not be dealing with service providers who they knew and who knew their sons and daughters.

I had heard that I could make a request to have my daughter's needs reassessed and I decided to put this to the test. I telephoned our local office and was told to contact the main office. I asked who was responsible and whether there was a procedure for my daughter to have her needs reassessed. The reply to every question was 'I don't know'. Their only suggestion was to send a social worker to see me – the sixth in ten years. For a long time we have been seen as a 'nuisance' family because we asked questions that no one else would ask. For example, we objected to Nicola going on group outings from the day centre although we did explain what our objections were based on.

It was difficult arranging a time to meet the new social worker. I asked for an appointment after 4 o'clock so that Nicola could be there and because I go out to work. He said this would be difficult because he had a long drive home. When the social worker arrived, I asked him to explain the process of assessment to me. He said he was not sure. He had a six page form with him and suggested that we work through it. He also told me that he had not yet qualified as a social worker and had not had any training on assessments and anyway he was leaving the following week to take up a post in another part of the country. He said that he would take the completed form back to the office where a group of 'providers' would make decisions about it. It had been decided that the providers would do this because their background was in learning difficulty.

The form was made up of questions that did not seem to have much, if any relevance, to Nicola. It was like one of those questionnaires in a magazine where you tot up the numbers and they tell you how sexy you are. I asked him to leave the blank form with me so that we could take it to a meeting of Nicola's circle of support – the decisions were too important to be made in one short meeting. (A circle of support is a group of people who are invited to come together and meet regularly to offer support and advice to someone with a learning difficulty.) He refused to leave the form with me but I insisted and offered to take the blame for any problems caused. Throughout the two meetings we had with this social worker, it felt as if I was offering him more support than he was able to give me. So much so, that he thanked me for my help and said he had learned a lot from me. He said that the time he had spent with me was like being in a workshop and that he would find the things I had said to him helpful in his new job.

The members of Nicola's circle studied the assessment form and agreed that it was not relevant. They wrote to the director of social services saying how inappropriate the questions on the form were. Some time later we received a reply that did not address our concerns. The circle agreed at this point that we should fill in the form but carry on working in different ways to make changes in Nicola's life. Some weeks later Nicola received an acknowledgement that the form had been filled in and received.

A few months later I met, by chance, a senior social worker and asked what had happened to Nicola's form. She was surprised that we had expected a reply and said that as we had not asked for anything specific on the form they had assumed that we would not want a response. After being part of the individual planning process for a number of years without any outcome, it felt as if we had just taken part in another game, filling in forms so that the service providers feel as if they are doing something.

The general feeling coming from the service providers was that rather than April 1993 being a new start, they were totally confused. For the first time that I can remember the fears and confusion were being shared with carers.

We heard that a memo had been sent round to people doing assessments instructing them not to identify people's needs, because they could not be addressed. I contacted people I know and got all the information I could. I just read everything but none of it was specific and we all felt powerless. I still haven't a clue what the difference is between care management and social work. The word 'management' sounds as if it belongs to people higher up the scale, not those working directly with people. The way the assessment form was passed on to faceless people who do not know my daughter confirms this feeling. I know if I asked carers in their 70s or the younger ones, that they would feel the same way.

Earlier this year our youngest daughter started work. As Nicola has two brothers and two sisters, there had always been someone around if I could not get home in time for Nicola's arrival from the day centre.

Now I felt that this was my responsibility again and considered giving up work. I wondered just how long this parental responsibility was supposed to go on for and decided to share our latest problem with social services. They told me to look for someone who would be able to offer Nicola support and that they would find the money. I found two people who were happy to share the support and then social services told me this was not possible after all, because they could not get into employing these people. I feel that social services have not got the information to enable them to take innovative ideas on board. In the end we resolved it by taking on two support workers who are employed by a local residential home for elderly people. This is not an ideal solution but the two women happen to be wonderful and Nicola is happy.

Helen Platts: Care management from inside a social services department

January 1991 was an exciting time to be starting my new job. Care management was being introduced and the purchasing and provision of services was being separated, well ahead of the April 1993 deadline. This new way of organising social services offered hope to those of us who were working to change and improve local services for people with learning difficulties.

As a middle manager I was responsible for a range of services, most of which dated from the 1970s and early 1980s: a 25-bed hostel; a day centre for 90 people; a special care unit; a day centre for 45 people; and a group home service for ten people. We were being set up to operate at arms-length from the new care managers, whose job it was to assess the needs of all service users. Information from the assessments would be passed to the contracts manager who had been appointed to negotiate service level agreements for each part of the service. This meant that we as service providers would now be more accountable on the cost and quality of services.

I knew a number of people who benefited directly from the new care management arrangements. Jane moved back to the area from a registered care home 50 miles away to be nearer her family and to live more independently. With the support of her care manager, she had moved within the year from a group home into her own flat with her partner. For people attending the day, staff were able for the first time to challenge care managers to be specific about why they were making referrals. The emphasis was now on providing a service to the person with a learning difficulty, as well as meeting their carers' need for daytime care. When it came to designing a new service to replace the hostel, everybody living there was linked with a care manager who worked with them to make sure that their wants and needs were taken into account.

From our point of view as service providers, the new system called for real changes in the way we were working with service users. We wanted to create a culture of service delivery but this was difficult to achieve given the institutional nature of our services. Also, frontline staff were sceptical of yet another reorganisation and the change in management. Our commitment to taking complaints seriously and to taking disciplinary action in a few instances could be threatening to them. When some of them left, service users and their families expressed the view that the service was getting worse rather than better because of the high staff turnover and the delay in filling vacancies. Consulting with service users and their families about plans to replace the hostel and day centre was also a complicated process. Although we worked hard to involve them in discussions about the future, we had to face up to their lack of trust in us as social services' employees, founded partly on their fears that services were about to be cut.

This lack of trust also arose out of their anxieties about care management which from the start failed to live up to the expectations of some service users and their families. Well-established relationships with social workers had been broken off because of the reorganisation and even when the new care managers were in post, there were concerns that there were not enough of them to ensure that everyone who required a service could be assessed. Although locally care management assessments were carried out for all elderly people receiving a service, the system for people with learning difficulties was discredited because of the very small number of care managers for this client group. Carers were not sure what care management and the new eligibility criteria would mean in practice, but in the light of social services' stated intention of focussing on people with the most complex needs, they suspected that some of the 200 people with learning difficulties attending day centres locally would end up without a service.

Looking at the services we were taking over, it was clear that since they were first built, the hostel and day centre had not been able to change much to meet the requirements of the people who used them. In highlighting these shortcomings, we expected care management to lead senior managers and elected members to make strategic decisions about the location and design of new services to replace the hostel and day centre. In the event, care management, at least in the early stages, did not lead to any significant changes to local services for people with a learning difficulty. As yet care managers did not have control over their own budgets and inevitably, because of lack of training, lack of confidence and lack of time, they looked to existing services for off-the-shelf solutions. We did succeed in setting up a new supported employment service for 50 people, including some people with profound disabilities, but this was only possible because we, as service providers, secured funding from outside the local authority from the local Training and Enterprise Council, corporate sponsors and the European Social Fund.

It soon became clear that care managers and we as service providers had very little leverage to change the existing pattern of expenditure. In spite of the aspiration to purchase and provide services according to people's individual needs, we were all caught up in a political process in which the consent of elected members to major changes in services was required. In social services, other issues such as child protection, services for elderly people and budgetary problems were always treated as higher priorities. Two years after care management had been introduced, we were no nearer a decision to radically change the traditional, institutional services that we managed. As pragmatists, we now looked to the new alliance between social services and the local health service commissioners as a vehicle for bringing about strategic change in learning difficulty services. In looking at the health service commissioners who were purchasing services through block contracts and who had little or no investment in the new care management systems, we had moved to a position in which individual planning and assessment did not seem to be informing local decisions about services.

As a service provider I had learned that person-centred planning will always be constrained by the political, organisational and social environment into which it is introduced. I realised that care management alone cannot change the segregated and underfunded services which above all else reflect the low status accorded in our society to people with learning difficulties and their families. Care management has the potential to challenge the status quo but only if there are other changes in the way we, as professionals and citizens, work with and think about people with learning difficulties and their families.

Where do we go from here?

Given that care management is generally welcomed as an approach which focusses on people's individual needs and is also now written into the legislative framework for providing social care in England and Wales, it is important to learn from what has happened since the NHS and Community Care Act was implemented. A careful review of the experiences recounted above shows that even within the existing level of resources, there is a lot we can do to develop and improve the new care management systems to ensure that people with learning difficulties and their families benefit from this latest round of community care changes.

If we are to empower people through care management, it is important that the systems themselves make sense to the people for whom they have been set up. So far, the legislation has resulted in a version of care management that is primarily a bureaucratic and organisational response to the problem of targeting resources and containing public expenditure. This is demonstrated by the way that social services departments are introducing the changes. The emphasis has been on drawing up written procedures and setting up systems with the result that eligibility criteria, assessments and individual planning are based on forms and other official, written materials that make it difficult for service users and their families to share in the decision-making process.

From the outset, there is a need to involve people with learning difficulties and their families in setting up care management systems locally and in reviewing their effectiveness. Assessments and reviews have always featured in the lives of people with learning difficulties and the deficit model has prevailed. As Lynne Elwell explained in her account, it is important to take a holistic view, looking at the person's whole life, their aspirations and hopes for the future, rather than the functional–skills deficit model which still underpins many approaches to assessment. Gillian Rees, in describing her experience of reviews, indicates that to her it is still as if her behaviour is being reviewed rather than the effectiveness of the services she uses. Given that there is now a significant investment in setting up coherent approaches to assessment within social services departments, this is an opportunity to involve service users and carers themselves in designing an assessment process that makes sense to them.

Once the systems and procedures have been designed, it is important for care managers to use assessments flexibly and sensitively to ensure that a positive approach is adopted rather than focussing exclusively on a person's deficits. Care management has been recognised by purchasers and providers alike as an opportunity to move to a service delivery culture, giving people with learning difficulties and their families the chance to act as the quality controllers of the services provided to them (Pilgrim, 1990). Gillian Rees explained that reviews were a time when she could complain if things were not going well with the services she used, and Lynne Elwell expressed her view that care management should have enabled her to negotiate for the services needed by her daughter. If people like them are to start to have a say through care management, staff in service agencies need to support them with the new processes, in ways which take account of the possibility that they may not be used to feeding back criticism and may be concerned that services will be taken away from them if they do.

If people are to be empowered they need to understand the new jargon. A major criticism of the recent community care reforms is that the very language of care management, because it is abstract, prevents carers and families and especially people with learning difficulties from understanding these changes to the way that services are organised. The complexity of the ideas behind the reforms combined with a lack of detailed, practical information, leaves service users and their families and even social services staff confused about assessments, the purchaser/provider split and the difference between care management and social work. With their guide: *Oi! it's My Assessment*; People First, a group of self-advocates in London, have demonstrated that it is possible to explain how the NHS and Community Care will affect people with learning difficulties (People First, 1993). They succeed in explaining what the community care changes will mean in practice, using plain language and pictures. Every social services department needs to invest in providing good quality, straightforward information so that, at a local level, service users and their families can make sense of the changes that are happening around them.

Social Services staff, if they are to succeed in involving people with learning difficulties and their families, will need to be clear about how they are going to support them with the care management process itself. So far there has been very little discussion in service agencies about how to enable people with learning difficulties to participate in decision-making. This concern has been raised by People First:

> Right now there are no plans to help us learn to speak for ourselves or help us learn to make choices . . . to speak up for ourselves and make choices takes time and practice. (People First, 1993).

In this context, the importance of self-advocacy needs to be recognised. However uncomfortable, the role for social services and other service agencies in supporting self-advocates needs to be developed in ways which do not compromise their independence. Increasingly people with physical disabilities are critical of professionals and are asserting their right to be their own care managers. It is likely that as they develop their own confidence and their expertise in challenging service professionals, people with learning difficulties will call for similarly radical changes in the way that social care is organised for them.

The reorganisations which have arisen from the NHS and Community Care Act mean that discontinuity and loss continue to be recurring themes in the lives of many people with learning difficulties. Local authorities have framed the care management changes primarily as an administrative problem, because they faced the considerable challenge of taking over the management of residential care payments from the Department of Social Security on 1 April 1993. Consequently, organisational issues have taken precedence and priority has been given to restructuring and realigning staff. We need to recognise that the disruption and anxiety caused by these reorganisations has resulted in less rather than more continuity for service users and their families, in spite of the principle central to care management of ensuring continuity by having one co-ordinator of services for each person. Social services departments need to recognise the damage that has been done and to reassert the importance of continuity in relationships between staff and service users.

The emphasis should now be on developing flexible models of care management which help to sustain relationships by allowing for the contracting out of care management and assessment services to staff on the provider side where staff and service users already know each other well. This is particularly important for people with profound disabilities who often find it difficult to make their views understood. The recent preoccupation with organisational and administrative issues is reflected in the dearth of good information about service user experience of the care management process itself. Much of the recent research and writing about care management has focussed on process issues: managing change; developing joint strategies between social services and health; and ensuring effective multidisciplinary working. The time has now come to focus on what it is like for service users to be on the receiving end of care management services and to review in detail the extent to which the new systems are making a direct impact on their lives.

If care management is to succeed in promoting more individualised outcomes within the new systems for contracting for social care, social services staff need to develop creative ways of purchasing services for individuals and to move away from the block contracts which are in danger of perpetuating institutional services. We must develop creative ways of negotiating individual solutions with providers in a way that is consistent with the new contracting arrangements and also practical, given the large numbers of people receiving services. Voluntary agencies themselves need to be supported in developing less institutional services through the contracting process, while recognising that it is often low-paid, female employees who are disadvantaged by the move away from nationally negotiated terms and conditions to local agreements and casual contracts in the non-statutory sector (Brown and Smith, 1992).

At an organisational level, if care management is to succeed in promoting more individualised outcomes for service users, other cultural and organisational changes are needed in the way that service agencies operate (Stevenson and Parsloe, 1993). Care management is being introduced into large local authority social services departments which themselves can be criticised for being hierarchical, bureaucratic and disempowering to a whole range of people from service users to frontline staff (as reflected in the small number of women who reach senior management positions in these organisations). As Lynne Elwell explained, to many carers and people with learning difficulties the word 'management' is itself indicative of hierarchy and organisational structures which exclude service users. In spite of the new rhetoric about 'consumer choice' and 'customers', service users continue to have very little say or status in the service systems that purport to serve them. In particular, in many social services departments, the failure to really address equal opportunities issues at a practical level results in inadequate services and a lack of support for people with learning difficulties from ethnic minorities and their families.

To ensure that care management is introduced in a way that genuinely empowers people with learning difficulties and their families the following issues need to be addressed.

- Find out from people with learning difficulties and their families what a good assessment and care management service would look like for them.
- Give service users and their families clear information about what care management means in practice and how it will affect them, using plain language and pictures.
- Provide service users and their families with good information about the new eligibility criteria and be clear about their right of appeal and how they will be supported with this.
- Develop ways of supporting people with learning difficulties in making choices and having a say and recognise the importance of self-advocacy.
- Nurture existing relationships between service users and staff and see them as being important in the care management process. Resist reorganising.
- Involve people with learning difficulties and their families in commissioning and designing research which focusses on their experience of care management rather than on organisational and professional issues.
- Find ways of purchasing individualised services, as an alternative to block contracts.
- Find out from social services departments what they are doing to put equal opportunities policies into practice when it comes to delivering appropriate services for people with learning difficulties and their families from different ethnic backgrounds.

It remains to be seen whether the problems which have emerged with care management since April 1993 are transitional and whether care management, as defined by the recent community care legislation, has the potential to challenge the status quo. In spite of the early difficulties experienced by us, as a service user, a carer and service manager, we continue to have high expectations of care management. Our hope is that by listening to and responding to the people who directly exprience the services, care managers and other staff will be able to work with and improve the new systems to ensure that, at last, people with learning difficulties and their families have a say in what their services should be like.

References

Beardshaw, V. and Towell, D. (1990). *Assessment and Case Management: Implications for the Implementation of 'Caring for People'*. King's Fund Institute, London.

Brown, H. and Smith, H. (1992). Assertion, not assimilation: A feminist perspective on the normalisation principle. In *Normalisation: a Reader for the Nineties* (eds H. Brown and H. Smith). Tavistock/Routledge, London.

Department of Health White Paper (1989). *Caring for People: Community Care in the Next Decade and Beyond*. HMSO, London.

Griffiths, Sir R. (1988). *Community Care: Agenda for Action*. HMSO, London.

Hudson, B. (1993). *The Busy Person's Guide to Care Management*. Joint Unit for Social Services Research/*Community Care*, Sheffield.

National Development Team (1991). *The Andover Case Management Project*. National Development Team, London.

People First (1993). *Oi! It's My Assessment*. People First, London.

Pilgrim, D. (1990). British psychotherapy in context. In *Individual therapy: A Handbook* (ed. W. Dryden). Open University Press, Milton Keynes.

Stevenson, O. and Parsloe, P. (1993). *Community Care and Empowerment*. Joseph Rowntree Foundation/*Community Care*, York.

Chapter 9

Take it from us: Training by people who know what they are talking about

Liz Wright

Skills for People celebrated its tenth birthday in 1993. It is a small charity serving the north east of England and aims to promote self-advocacy amongst people with learning difficulties and physical disabilities – 'helping people to speak up for themselves, even when other people don't want to listen', as one planning team member put it. This is done in several main ways. The core of the work of Skills for People has always been the presentation of short courses aimed at helping people to speak up for themselves and have more say in their lives. The project also makes use of the skills of people with learning difficulties and physical disabilities to train staff working in the field, although the focus of the project's work is to work with people with disabilities and to resist the call to provide a great deal of training for professionals. Skills for People works to support the establishment of local self-advocacy groups by the offer of training or by providing advisors to work with new groups. In recent years Skills for People has been called on to help users of health and social services to express their views about services, either as part of a general move to increase user consultation, or, for example, to help people moving out of long-stay hospital to have more of a say in the running of places where they now live.

Skills for People is different from most other organisations because its work is largely planned and carried out by people who themselves have learning difficulties or physical disabilities. The organisation is made up of people with disabilities and non-disabled people who work alongside each other to share skills and give mutual support.

The project employs a small team of paid staff, but thrives on the work of the large number of committed volunteers (around 100 at the last count).

Central to the philosophy of the organisation is the belief that people who have disabilities should be enabled to speak up for themselves. Within Skills for People, every effort is made to ensure that this happens and the work of the project is planned according to the agenda of the disabled people within the organisation.

Management structure

People with disabilities are involved at every level within the organisation. Whether it is deciding work priorities for the year, running courses, leading workshops, ordering a buffet or checking out the accessibility of the toilets, the aim is to support them to be as actively involved as they wish.

The management structure aims to give people with disabilities a real say in the running of the project in the ways they choose. As well as a formal committee of trustees which meets quarterly, there is a programme committee whose job is to set the priorities for the project and to decide which pieces of work will be taken on. The committee receives monthly reports from all staff members and monitors the work of the project.

All courses are planned, presented and evaluated by teams of people, most of whom have learning difficulties or physical disabilities. Training for professionals is also presented by people with learning difficulties or physical disabilities. Most other work is carried out by people with disabilities in collaboration with staff who give support throughout the planning and presentation of work and provide facilitation in meetings.

Skills for People aims to cater for the special needs of everyone who plans or attends its courses or is involved in any other way. Video, role-play, games and small group discussions are used and transport, sign language interpreters and minutes on cassette tape are provided where necessary.

The methods used to help people play a real part in the work vary on each occasion and are determined by the needs and wishes of each individual member. For example, one planning team member might have difficulty in remembering, another may want somebody to help make sure his or her words are understood. Another might like to use photographs or drawings to get a point across. Of course, these are simple needs and easily met. Unfortunately, people with learning difficulties and physical difficulties say they have often been excluded because people have not listened to their basic needs.

Some simple factors help the process in most cases. We always write up what people say in their own words on a flip chart to make it clear that what they say is important. Minutes of meetings are produced in people's own words and as little jargon as possible is used is written and spoken language with people being asked which words they would prefer to use. People are involved in setting the agenda and the rules for a meeting and we listen, listen, listen. People are given plenty of time to say what they want, to find a way of getting their point across to others and to practise doing things until they feel confident. All these things sound simple and obvious, but at Skills for People we have been doing them and making mistakes and learning and trying again for ten years, and there is still lots of room for improvement. On a day-to-day basis there is little reliance on textbooks and theories; we have found that things go well when we ask ourselves basic questions such as 'What is most important to this person?'; 'What have we heard people say?'; 'Who is in control?' Things go wrong when we forget to ask the basics, or when we go too quickly, forgetting to go at the pace which involves people, or when we forget to take the time to listen.

The outcome of all this must be what was summed up by a programme committee member: 'At first it was hard to believe that Skills for People would really give me a say. Before I had felt that nobody really listened to me and I did not have a chance to say what I thought.'

Running and planning courses

The nature of the courses provided by Skills for People is determined by what people with learning difficulties and physical disabilities say they need. We are in contact with a large number of people, including those on our programme committee who decide what courses should be run. Local adult training centres and other services are visited to ask people what courses they would like to attend. The detailed content of each course is decided by the planning team. People who come as participants on our courses are asked if they would like to become members of planning teams for future courses. One planning team member said:

> This year has been really busy for me. I have been on lots of planning teams, planning courses and running them. I am about to plan my fourth 'Being your own boss' course, which is about helping people to have more control over their lives and to live more independently.

Our courses focus on helping people to have more control in their lives, to make themselves heard, to know their rights, to make their own decisions, to build relationships and gain in independence and confidence. Our courses have titles decided by the planning team such as 'Speaking up for Yourself', 'Being Your Own Boss', 'Building Relationships', 'Making Friends', 'Planning for Yourself', 'Speaking in Public'.

Each course is planned over many meetings, often as many as 15, for a course which might run for three or five days. In the words of a planning team member:

> Organising the courses was really hard work. We had lots to decide: Who was going to do what? Where the courses would be held? Organising the food. Designing the invitations and thinking about what we would talk about and do on the course.

As far as possible, the people on each planning team have personal experience relevant to the content of the course being planned. Planning is done carefully and slowly to ensure that each planning team member has a real say and plays an active part. For example, a course for people who 'speak without words' will be planned by some people who themselves speak without words. Similarly, a course for people moving out of long-stay hospital will have on its planning team some people who have themselves been resident in long-stay hospitals. Being a member of a planning team helps people to gain in confidence and build on their own skills. A staff member works with each planning team, taking care that everyone is actively involved in the planning process and is enabled to make their own decisions. The staff member facilitates the process, helping communication, offering suggestions and ways of getting messages across, and gives advice about the structure of the course. Someone will write up (or perhaps draw) what everyone says and then minutes (in writing or on cassette tape) are produced after each meeting.

Planning needs to be taken slowly. The process is different each time, but it may be that we begin by thinking about the course, what it is to be about and a lot about the role and tasks of a planning team. We then explore the subject matter of the course and begin by finding out what the subject of the course means in each of our lives: What experiences have members of the planning team had? What lessons have they learned? What do they want to learn? What do they think other people need to know? We piece together the content of a course based on the views and personal experiences of those planning it.

The planning team might then think about the presentation of their ideas. Planning team members will often know of favourite rounds or ice-breakers, games or exercises which they have found helpful. It will then test these, along with any new ideas. Often the personal experiences of planning team members are woven into the course as personal accounts, as role plays or as case studies.

A long time is spent practising and working out who will do what on the course. Care is taken to make sure people are supported and take on what they feel able to do. Some people might want simply to welcome people, or to introduce the ice-breakers. Other members of the planning team will be happy to play role play situations and so on. Everything is practised. We need to be imaginative about helping people to speak, to remember, to understand.

Planning team members are actively involved in the practical organisation of the course. They might visit the venue to make sure it is accessible. They will order the buffet and draw up rotas for making tea and coffee.

When a course finally happens, the planning team faces many challenges. One of the most difficult things it must do is to be flexible to meet the needs of course participants. Some planning teams have decided to hold pre-course meetings with participants so that they can be sure that the course they are planning fits the particular needs of the people who will attend. The courses allow plenty of time for socialising and meeting people, because this is what people have told us is important to them.

After each course, planning team members evaluate their work and celebrate by having a meal together.

Training schemes

Skills for People concentrates on helping people to speak up for themselves. We do devote some time to working with professionals and staff who work with people who have physical disabilities or learning difficulties. We consider it vital that staff training includes sessions led by disabled people. We have contributed to various staff training programmes including Diploma in Social Work courses and courses aimed at staff working with people with disabilities such as nurses, social workers, residential care staff or managers.

The training is usually related to self-advocacy and might address such things as labelling, stigma, rights, self-advocacy, relationships, our homes, where we work, and how Skills for People works. It can be a very fulfilling experience for trainers, as one explained:

> 'I never thought I would ever talk to people like that. Along with other volunteers, I have been talking to them about our lives, our rights and how they might make things better for the people they work with. Staff need to know what people are thinking.'

The methods used by Skills for People volunteers and staff to present this training are much the same as those used in any other Skills for People courses. The training will be planned and presented by people with learning difficulties or physical disabilities supported, as necessary, by staff and other volunteers. Training is based on the personal experience and views of the trainers. Planning a session often begins by taking it in turns to relay our experiences about the issue. These personal accounts will often form the basis of a training session supported by other training materials. The aim of a session will be to get over to staff messages thought to be important by the people with disabilities who are presenting the session, and to try to get staff to take more steps to address these issues in their own work. The sessions will use interactive exercises and rely on simple jargon-free language.

The role of the Skills for People staff members or other supporters will depend on the needs of the trainers. They will often help the trainer to draw out lessons which staff could learn from their experiences. They provide guidance about the process of training, the need for confidentiality and so on. They may provide practical help; for instance, in writing, using interview techniques to aid memory, explaining jargon, challenging course participants and the like. They will aim to help the trainer to present his or her material in an interesting, useful way and feel ownership of their own ideas as well as understand their role as trainer. The nature and level of support is explicitly defined by the trainers with learning difficulties and physical disabilities.

The training sessions often use directly the personal experiences of the trainers; for example these might be recounted and used as a basis for looking at how the person has experienced discrimination, or as a basis for problem solving. Other materials such as videos or checklists will be used to generalise from the particular. Trainers, like others elsewhere, have found it useful to ask participants to consider their own lives and aspirations as a basis from which to consider the lives of the people they work with – be they called clients, residents, patients. Participants are asked to give concrete examples from their own work about how they might help empower those they work with.

The sessions are usually vibrant, relevant and helpful to participants. The issues addressed are complex and dealt with in depth. The subject matter is often difficult and loaded with emotion. Participants are challenged to think imaginatively about their own practice and yet the value of the work they do is not undermined; the very real difficulties faced by staff are acknowledged and strategies for overcoming them are identified. There has been good feedback and requests for more training.

The personal way in which most trainers choose to present their material, using their own experiences and that of their friends and colleagues, appears to have a great impact on people receiving the training. The down-to-earth examination of day-to-day practice throws up huge ethical and professional questions, whilst offering some practical solutions. It has not been possible to gauge the longer term effects of training, which must have limitations since it takes place over such a short period of time, often for just one session or one day.

The philosophy and nature of the work at Skills for People has remained the same over its ten years of existence and it continues to be seen as innovative. Many of the volunteers have now been with the organisation for many years and have attended and planned a great number of courses. The project continues to face the same challenges in its work. It requires constant self-evaluation to make sure that people within the organisation and the people who attend its courses are allowed to speak up for themselves and have a real and important say in its work. We must continue to think of new and imaginative ways to involve people. Many of the people we work with can be suggestible and we try to ensure that we do not 'put words into people's mouths'. It is important that people come up with their own ideas about the way they want to be treated.

It is easy to underestimate the ability of people with learning difficulties and physical disabilities and this happens many times. Often staff members believe that the people they work with will not be able to take part. The staff at Skills for People will regularly find that people who attend or plan the courses have unexpected abilities, skills, insight and understanding. These abilities can be overlooked by people without disabilities acting on preconceived ideas.

Enormous patience is required to ensure the full involvement of people who have often come to feel that they have very little of value to say and very little power. The work can seem painfully slow to people who want to see end results, that is, the course, the decision. But the process is as important as the end result and the time taken pays off, ensuring that the courses and the decisions do really belong to the people who make them and not to those paid to support them.

Chapter 10

Contracting for change: Making contracts work for people with learning difficulties

Hilary Brown and Paul Cambridge

> It is unlikely that contracts will change or eradicate . . . historical problems . . . Instead it might be better to see them as a new language to describe old problems (Ward, 1990).

Contracts and their limitations

In this chapter we want to look at the problems as well as the possibilities inherent in the new contract culture because we believe the best way of making contracts work for people with learning difficulties is to be very clear about their weaknesses as well as their strengths. Trading and exchanging people and services is nothing new: joint working and joint finance, coupled with financial transfers and agreements with voluntary agencies had been developing a quasi-market in care for well over a decade, but now the arrangements have become more overtly commercial. What used to be framed as an agreement or partnership between funders and providers of care is now couched in legal terms and the parties might include companies, both commerical and not-for-profit, whose goal is profit as well as professional or organisational gain.

At best, contracts set a framework which enable service agencies to tailor finite resources to the needs of individuals, thereby supporting people with learning difficulties and their families, in accordance with their wishes and circumstances. At worst, fragmented contracting allows commissioners to abdicate responsibility for providing high quality services or sustaining networks of service providers and local expertise. What we see in the new arrangements is an attempt to replace management functions, which were located within single hierarchies, with agreements reached across agency boundaries. In some instances this has simplified lines of accountability, but in others, important functions have fallen between different agencies and specific knowledge and expertise has been lost or dispersed. Often there are reduced opportunities for economies of scale and the development of specialist services, and fractures in user involvement, accountability, information and communication.

But do people with learning difficulties have increased power and choice within the new system, and does competition lead to higher standards or set up pressures which lead to cost-cutting and fragmentation? Fundamentally, a philosophy of consumer choice represents a shift from civil rights to consumer rights and inevitably brings with it inequity in access to goods and services: only those who have money to buy can exercise their rights to buy, while less powerful groups of consumers do not have access to the same options nor do they exercise the same degree of leverage over what is available.

Are consumers really powerful?

Once funded there are still a number of fallacies in the argument that being a consumer is more powerful than merely being a receiver of public service. It is supposed that individual consumers influence products or services by virtue of choosing where to spend their money and that when individual decisions are accumulated 'good' suppliers survive at the expense of bad ones. Also, it is posited that consumers have the power to complain about unsatisfactory conditions or products and to return goods which do not fulfil their expectations. Increased choice allows the user either to 'shop around' for 'off-the-peg' services or opt for 'commissioning' tailor-made packages which suit their individual needs and circumstances. In theory they have an impact on what is on offer by knowing what they want.

Undoubtedly, there are circumstances when consumers do exercise such influence but even with money, there are times when individuals are at the mercy of, rather than powerful in relation to, those who supply them with goods and services. It is because the individual consumer is vulnerable in the market place that regulations and independent bodies exist to mediate in these situations, that there are sources of independent information, evaluations and guarantees. In the field of care, when the consumer is actually being served *because* of their vulnerability these checks and balances take on an added urgency.

Churchill (1992) contrasts the notion of consumers and 'end users' in the computer field, where they can often become hapless victims of a technology which they do not understand, to the fancy-free fodder of car adverts, characterised by the industry as 'user-choosers'. It is an illuminating dichotomy: end-users are not powerless because they are unable to take their business elsewhere but because they do not have enough knowledge of what is possible and how to get the best out of the system. In other words, they do not have the expertise to accurately interpret their needs or to know what is best for them. Some people with learning difficulties and their carers may also be in this position, for example someone who has difficult behaviours may not be in a position to know what is appropriate in terms of programming or interventions. They cannot act for themselves in the role of powerful consumers even where monies are devolved to them directly. Indeed, individual brokerage tends to cut across the employment of profession-ally trained care workers (Brown, 1992, personal communication) and make it unlikely that people who have complex needs will be able to access 'state of the art' solutions.

Setting up the market

Who does the buying?

It can be seen that it is not necessarily the person with a learning difficulty or their family who are in a position to strike a good deal or to exercise sanctions. As Churchill (1992) asserts: 'There is the all-important question as to who the contract is between'. He goes on to point out the danger 'that bilateral contracts will become the norm and that . . . any element of consumer influence must be grafted on to a supplier–purchaser relationship which essentially excludes the person receiving the service.'

Commissioning bodies are authorised to operate in this respect *on behalf of* people with learning difficulties, not merely to purchase but to activate and actively structure the options available in the marketplace. To do so they need 'top–down' information about demography, that is, projections as to the number of people they will need to serve, but also 'bottom–up' information from individual assessments about the particular, and often changing needs of people using services and how they want these to be met.

How are providers developed, identified and selected?

Aggregate commissioning arrangements between the major players do not, in themselves, diversify the pool of services from which they can purchase. An important strategic decision is to strike a balance between purchasers of services acting proactively, to ensure that a range of services is available and to develop new service models, and a more *laissez-faire* approach which leaves the market to develop according to its own logic. Recently, a particular example of this has been the planning of services for people with learning difficulties who have been sexually abused. It is no good being a responsive service and allocating money for specialised counselling to an individual in the aftermath of a crisis, if no such service or expertise exists. Pump-priming appropriate initiatives is a necessary first step.

Flynn and Common (1990) describe the following ways commissioners can operate in respect to providers in the market.

- Opt for open tendering, that is, leaving providers to come to them.
- Invite providers to apply to be put on an approved or 'select' list.
- Negotiate with a single supplier, or with a range of suppliers.
- Actively encourage and develop new organisations to meet specific needs or provide services to an identified group.

They conclude: 'the approach chosen affects choice for the consumer. Formal contracts with one provider inhibit choice while informal, open-ended arrangements . . . promote choice'.

Does it save money?

Cost-effectiveness and efficiency are stated aims of the government's community care reforms, but there is little evidence that these are either more compatible with, or more achievable through, contracts as opposed to more participative devices.

Wistow *et al.* (1993) examined the social care market from the perspective of economic theory to determine whether it is structured and operating in accord with markets in general. They identified weaknesses in the structure of supply, with insufficient competition between providers undermining quality, choice and price improvements. They also noted that providers in specialised markets can create monopolies (an example might be challenging behaviour services) which could find them in a position to 'name their price'.

As Wistow *et al.* (1993) point out, while costs seem to be contained within the contracting process:

> There are costs which arise from operating a market system. The fundamental issue is whether authorities can avoid incurring a level of transaction costs in agreeing and monitoring contracts which exceeds the efficiency savings from commissioning lower cost providers to deliver services. In addition other costs arise from inspection, accreditation and other regulatory mechanisms.

Insofar as a mixed market does offer cheaper services, these have been bought at the expense of the conditions of service of the workforce. Badly paid staff, with few rights and job insecurity, are not the best advocates for other relatively powerless people. Concern about the position of workers in newly privatised industries has led to an increased awareness of the position of the 'whistleblower'. There is clearly a risk that the market will produce perverse incentives to good practice, cost more to operate and produce less.

What if the service does not measure up?

If the contract is the defining element in the setting up of a service agreement, it also has to govern circumstances in which this might be terminated. The consumer analogy clearly works on the basis that by withdrawing custom, individuals influence the quality of services which survive. Similarly, in the field of social care, it is supposed that formal complaints procedures will empower service users:

> By giving residents the ability to complain about poor services in a way which could bring positive results (nothing empties a home faster than bad publicity) it is hoped that dissatisfied customers or their representatives can exercise power and counter poor standards of care service. (Churchill, 1992).

In fact, the problems in closing a home militate against the natural forces of the market place operating to improve quality, indeed, discontinuity in service provision is a major breach of quality for both people with learning difficulties and their carers. Unless alternative services are standing by for consumers ejected from unsatisfactory services, commissioners cannot assume that the market place is offering any inducement to quality.

At a systemic level commissioners cannot afford for individual services to be penalised or shut down in an unplanned way as these outcomes disrupt comprehensive service planning at a local level.

What is specified in contracts?

It can be seen that the contract does not exist in isolation, but as a component within a wider commissioning process which includes the key tasks of agreeing a mission statement, assessing the population needs, identification of potential service providers, service specification, contract agreement, performance review taking account of user's and carer's views, contract renewal or termination and information feedback to inform a continuing sequence of evaluation and service development (Knapp and Wistow, 1992). These other functions determine the environment in which contracting operates.

There are many variations in the way contracts have been drawn up and in what they specify. Flynn and Common (1990), in the official guidance which accompanied the community care legislation, developed a model to differentiate what is actually specified in the contracting process, that is whether what is spelt out is the resources given to the user (inputs), the way care is offered (process), what is achieved by way of output (such as how many trips out into the community) or outcomes which describe what is achieved on behalf of the person in terms of their quality of life and integration into the community. They reported that they had 'observed a wide range of contracts, from informal exchanges of letters attached to grant payments to very detailed specification of inputs, services, pay scales and what to do with spilt body fluids'.

Recent trends, particularly with the spread of quality audit, tend towards the belief that it is possible to specify and price everything. But as Flynn and Common (1990) observe:

> The main influence on the contract seems to be the amount of trust between the supplier and the authority and the pressure on the process from outsiders such as accountants and auditors. Some authorities assume that very detailed specification leads to strong control.

In fact, the opposite may be true as the monitoring process may encourage services to become secretive about any difficulties they encounter in operating on a day-to-day basis. Running a quality service involves taking risks, being open about complaints or allegations of individual mistreatment, collecting objective data about the lives of people using the service and monitoring progress. By overspecification, the purchaser can unwittingly encourage the provider to look for loopholes.

In addition to varying what is specified, and at what level of detail, there is the tension between authority wide block commissioning and local and individualised commissioning. Block contracts depend on aggregate information and central budgets while local or individual contracts are based on devolved accountability and budgets. These have sometimes been called strategic and tactical commissioning, respectively (Knapp and Wistow, 1992). Evaluations of pilot care management projects suggest that devolution leads to more cost-effective services and improved client outcomes in services for elderly people (Davies and Challis, 1986; Challis and Davies, 1986) but there have been limited attempts to replicate such arrangements in learning difficulty services (Cambridge, 1992).

What models of contracting have been tried?

The tension referred to above has led to a dichotomy between one-off placement contracts for individuals and block purchasing of services whether or not individual placements are taken up. The Association of Metropolitan Authorities (AMA, 1993) strongly recommends that a standardised procedure be adopted which consists of three stages:

- A pre-placement agreement in which terms and agreement over conditions for potential placements is set out prior to the placement of named individuals. Adherence to the detailed service specification can become a part of this agreement.
- A detailed service specification outlining the type of services required for people with learning difficulties.
- An individual service contract outlining the particular care arrangements needed for each individual and the resources attached to this specific placement.

The advantages, it suggests, of authorities adhering to uniform practice in the contracting process, are twofold: first, reduction in time and cost especially for purchasing authorities who frequently deal with out-of-authority placements or providers who deal with several pur-chasers and second, that involvement of users and their advocates can be safeguarded. The report adds: 'it is also hoped that standardisation will minimise tension between purchasers and providers and thereby assist in the building of partnerships between the two parties'.

Setting up a pool of approved providers who are able to provide a comprehensive range of services makes placement decisions more efficient and avoids having to start from scratch each time. A minimum standard would be registration under the Registered Homes Act 1984, but the specification allows a further layer of scrutiny and discussion. Moreover, where gaps in services are noted or anticipated a tendering process can be instigated.

The AMA standard pre-placement agreement guarantees the following safeguards: residents' rights to dispose of their own money; the obligation to provide specified statistical information and co-operate with monitoring exercises; and an agreed framework for financial transactions to be made between purchaser and provider.

The service specification elaborates this framework and allows the commissioner to set particular standards in relation to the client group, to the employment of staff (for example, adherence to equal opportunities policies) and to any other policies or codes of good practice (such as sexuality guidelines or guidance on responding to difficult behaviour). It also allows the commissioner to set the tone by setting out a statement of values and principles. This then lays the groundwork for an agreement about meeting the specific needs of individuals.

We have identified ten important elements to be included in service specifications and individual contracts.

The service specification should set out the following:

- Philosophy and mission.
- Aims and objectives of the service as a whole.
- The daily routine, social and physical environment.
- Policies, guidelines and procedures.
- Protocols for managing vacancies or withdrawal of services and/or clients.
- Management arrangements.
- Staff deployment patterns.
- Staff recruitment and the mix of skills and competence required.
- Staff development and training.
- Planned investment and targets.

Individual service contracts should specify:

- Individual's aspirations and needs in relation to their participation and integration into the community and development of their competence.

- How to meet these goals.
- Nature of staff intervention required.
- User preferences and views.
- Level and nature of personal care required and how this should be offered.
- Communication needs and/or additional sensory handicaps which need to be taken into account.
- Additional professional input required by this person and how this is to be accessed and paid for.
- Any difficulties, for example, escalation of challenging behaviour or deteriorating health which would legitimate the negotiation of further resources.
- How the person's money is to be handled.
- Support needed to maintain their social network and family relationships.

There are critical areas in which the two types of contract interact and these need to be addressed by protocol and procedures. An example is in the handling of empty places when it needs to be agreed whether the purchaser or provider will bear the increased burden of costs.

Principles of principled contracting

Despite the inherent problems in contracting as a mechanism for planning comprehensively for, and maintaining standards in, services for people with learning difficulties, there are ways in which the process can be harnessed to support the rights and interests of those who use services and their carers. We have identified six elements to principled contracting:

- Specifying radical models.
- Building in a commitment to equal opportunities outcomes.
- Setting up information systems and accountability.
- Keeping 'bricks and mortar' in the public domain.
- Setting up counter-controls such as user-advocacy, independent case management, open systems, access to professional advocacy and intervention.
- Commissioners maintaining the strategic initiative in developing an array of service options.

Specifying radical models

A primary purpose of the contracting process is to define the characteristics and parameters of the service to be offered. It has been clear for several decades that models of care which are predicated on the basis of institutionalised and segregated establishments serve only to isolate and contain people with learning difficulties. Increased levels of difficult behaviour (see Querishi and Alborz, 1992) may ensue from these conditions alongside decreased levels of participation and social skills. Research has clearly linked smaller scale, more ordinary accommodation, with better outcomes for people but also with higher costs (Cambridge *et al.*, 1994).

For better outcomes to be possible, the service has to demonstrate that it has the capacity to organise the daily activities of staff and their shift patterns, to ensure that household tasks are done with the person and not for them, that risk-taking is the subject of negotiation and scrutiny, that individual strategies are developed to assist those with severe disabilities or sensory handicaps to become involved in everyday activities and that all people with learning difficulties are supported in making positive contacts in their local communities.

Existing contracts, for example, that suggested as a model by the Association of Residential Care, (Churchill, 1992), set out the separate elements of the service to be provided such as hotel service, residential care, day care, holidays and leisure, education and training, employment, medical and paramedical, admission and review procedures, variations, arrangements for terminating, quality assurance and financial arrangements. Such contracts tend to specify what rather than how. Unless positive models are stipulated, that is, those which detail the amount and nature of the support to be offered, the emphasis on static features will drown out more important issues about staff interaction and purpose. Of course, buildings need to be clean and attractive, but if the people who live in them have no involvement in the day-to-day running of their own homes, their lives will be essentially as empty as they were in hospitals.

Advertising and the proliferation of smaller providers demonstrates how such commitments can be lost. Services are packaged as 'hotels', 'farms' and all sorts of unlikely formulations. One service for people with challenging behaviours was able to specify that it would provide a 'continental breakfast' but not to demonstrate that it had any understanding of why people might have challenging behaviours or what sorts of interventions would be used to manage these.

Commitment to equal opportunities outcomes

This emphasis on active support highlights the key role staff have in facilitating the involvement of people with learning difficulties in household and community activities and in acting as mediators to gain access to generic community services such as primary health care, legal representation and so on. For them to fulfil such a responsibility requires continuity and skill. A model of care which stresses 'house work' as opposed to personal ties and development is, therefore, inappropriate: the staff member is not easily replaceable because they are not delivering a 'routinised' package which can be easily replicated but are part of a complex web of social contacts and interaction. Encouraging staff to stay means offering planned progression and not relying on a pool of low paid and badly protected workers.

There are particular equal opportunities issues in the way services are delivered to users who risk their own cultural ties being broken when they enter services. People with learning difficulties who use English as a second language should not have to adapt to workers who do not know their language or customs, nor should carers have their own needs and support networks misrepresented. Developing an appropriate service for users necessitates building a workforce which can work as a team and represent all views. Security of employment, rights and training are crucial components of work force stability. Measures of continuity, skills development and of sound personnel practice should be included in contracts and monitored by commissioners. Contractors who are not fair employers are not in a position to be fair providers of care since the provision of care requires openness and negotiation. Moreover, poorly paid and underprotected workers cannot act as advocates or key workers if their hands (and tongues) are tied.

Setting up information systems and accountability

Many contracts specify ambitious goals but stop short of devising any means to see whether these are met. While it is usual to focus on the measurement of outcomes, we believe that in the case of long-term care it is important to monitor both input and outcomes. Monitoring of input is required to ensure that people with learning difficulties receive goods and services which are being paid for on their behalf. Inspection and monitoring must, therefore, be sufficient to detect poor heating, food, staff cover, as well as to monitor the outcomes of teaching programmes, social contacts in the community and engagement levels. At the individual level this should include monitoring daily or weekly activity plans and at the service level, staff meetings and the exchange of information and records.

Varied methods should be used to collect data, balancing prearranged and spot visits, exit interviews, consumer satisfaction surveys involving both users and carers, monitoring of individual care plans and the achievement of goals drawn up as part of the planning process. People with learning difficulties constitute a very small proportion of the people on whose behalf commissioners purchase services. This level of detailed monitoring may not be sought in other services where what is offered and delivered is less complex. In judging the efficacy of a surgical operation it will be clear exactly what should be done and what happens if something goes wrong, but in the provision of long-term care, staff interaction *is* the intervention not merely the means to an end. Moreover, the client group concerned are among those who are least likely to be able to make a complaint or formulate a request for more respectful, or different kinds of, support.

At the time of writing knowledge about long-term care is held within provider units but this must soon be transferred to commissioners if they are to exercise sufficient authority to ensure that public accountability for the quality of the services and the use of public resources can be assured.

Keeping 'bricks and mortar' in the public domain

We believe that wherever purchasers have a choice they should contract with agencies who will ensure that buildings and assets currently being bought for individuals with learning difficulties are kept in the public domain and are therefore ultimately going to contribute to a pool of resources for people with learning difficulties who require services in the future. Purchasing services from housing associations meets this requirement, as it encourages public housing authorities to provide ordinary housing which meets the needs of people with a range of disabilities. Purchasing from a private provider may, on the other hand, see public money used for the purchase of buildings which revert to private assets if the service is no longer deemed necessary or satisfactory.

There are related issues with reference to training and accreditation since public funding is being used to buy skilled intervention as well as buildings. A motivated and skilled workforce is something which will continue to be required. It is untenable for non-accountable providers to purloin trained staff from the public sector provider units, whose unit costs are thereby deemed to be higher and less productive. Development should be built into each and every contract and where providers fail to commit a proportion of their receipts to accreditable staff training the commissioner should withhold a cost relating to this element of the contract and invest directly in training for this client group.

Ethical commissioning should take account of these potential conflicts of interest between stakeholders. Private providers explicitly use the contract as a commercial device but there are hidden beneficiaries in other sectors as well. Not-for-profit status masks a complex interplay of personal and organisational interests. Management buy-outs, units floating-off to become trusts or consortia, and other arms-length arrangements, create opportunities for personal gain based on what is essentially insider information. New executive and managerial structures are required by these quasi-independent providers, representing transactional costs to users, funders and tax-payers. New, well-paid jobs have been established for managers while care staff wages have been held down and the workforce is becoming increasingly polarised. In drawing up new contracts commissioners should bridge the gap between personal gain and public service.

Setting up counter-controls

User involvement, independent care management, open systems, access to independent professional advice and advocacy are all vital if people with learning difficulties are to be given power to make the ideology of consumerism a reality. User consultation does not happen on its own and in smaller agencies may not happen at all, unless it is stipulated that people with learning difficulties must have access to self-advocacy groups or to people in a position to act as independent advocates for them. At a conference involving users of service in Kent and East Sussex, held by the South East Thames Regional Health Authority's Institute of Public Health, users asked commissioners only to contract with agencies which could demonstrate that they were taking user involvement seriously.

Contracting separately for different elements of the service is also important as it will ensure that agencies are offering services independently of each other and would be in a position to blow the whistle if they have evidence of another agency failing to offer an adequate standard of care. They may also pick up if a service is under stress, if deadlines fail to be met, reports are promised and not written and so on. Goffman (1961), in his seminal description of institutions, identified the management of all spheres of a person's life under one roof and by one authority as the essential feature of institutionalisation. In one service where allegations of physical abuse had previously been raised by a day care worker in an independent day service, the contract had been renegotiated on the basis of the residential service providing daycare itself, with the unlooked-for side effect of isolating some very vulnerable clients. Building in checks and balances is the only way of protecting vulnerable people.

Commissioners maintaining the strategic initiative in developing an array of service options

Throughout this discussion it is clear that a market operating for people with learning difficulties must be a managed one. The only way for people with learning difficulties to have access to a comprehensive range of services is if commissioners maintain control of and strategically manage the development of a range of service options, rather than allow themselves to be influenced by ready-made products. Would-be providers should be given adequate information and support to enter the market place and to tender for the right to provide a well defined service to an identified group of clients. Resources must be protected so that other more vocal groups do not attract a larger share at the expense of people with learning difficulties, and monitored to ensure that they are delivered as specified.

If the management function is to be effected through the contracting process then commissioners have to retain more control over smaller than larger agencies, maintaining some direction over how they relate to other parts of the whole system and managing economies of scale between several smaller providers. The relationship *between* agencies in the market place has to be attended to in the contracting process. For example, if the commissioners were to fund a peripatetic team whose role was to build up the competency of the district's services to provide care for people with learning difficulties who display, or are at risk of developing, challenging behaviour, the contract with other providers would need to specify what authority should be attached to the team's interventions. Individual provider units would need to know if they are obliged to accept training or be bound by the service plans drawn up by the team. The team may need sanctions it can apply if programmes are not followed or if proper records are not kept. Unless the relationships between agencies are specified in contractual terms, a commissioning agency could be in the position of purchasing services which effectively cancel each other out and specialist input to the most needy people could be watered down.

Despite its somewhat evangelical introduction, the contract culture is no panacea to the problems of providing social care and has been imposed at a crucial juncture in the development of community-based services, when idealism had run into the sand and it was being realised that skilled intervention was necessary to make ordinary life a reality. Many concerns about the nature and quality of direct care have yet to be solved and now have to be translated into, and articulated through, the new language, images and icons of the market. Using the new language to create solid contracts and robust relationships between the different parties involved in specifying, funding and delivering services, must be the current goal. To achieve this, contracts have to be made on the basis that people with learning difficulties are not powerful consumers: it is the function of the contracting process to build up their power base by negotiating high standards on their behalf and applying the sanctions of the market place if they are not delivered.

References

Association of Metropolitan Authorities (1993). *Guidance on Contracting on Residential and Nursing Home Care for Adults.* Association of Metropolitan Authorities.

Brown, R. (1992), personal communication.

Cambridge, P. (1992). 'Case management in community services: Organisational responses', *British Journal of Social Work*, **22**, 495–517.

Cambridge, P. *et al.* (1994). *Five Years On: Community Care for People with Learning Disabilities.* Personal Social Services Research Unit/Ashgate, Aldershot.

Challis, D. and Davies, B. (1986). *Case Management in Community Care.* Gower, Aldershot.

Churchill, J. (1992). Contracts or partnerships. In: *Standards and Mental Handicap*, (eds T. Thompson and P. Mathias) 74–93, Balliere Tindall, London.

Davies, B. and Challis, D. (1986). *Matching Resources to Needs in Community Care.* Gower, Aldershot.

Flynn, N. and Common, R. (1990). *Contracts for Community Care, Caring for People Implementation Document.* HMSO, London.

Goffman, I. (1961). *Asylums.* Penguin, Harmonsworth.

Knapp, M. and Wistow, G. (1992). *Joint Commissioning for Community Care*. Personal Social Services Research Unit/Nuffield Institute Paper, University of Kent, Canterbury.

Querishi, H. and Alborz, A. (1992). Epidemiology of challenging behaviour. *Mental Handicap Research*, **31**, 147–162.

Ward (1990). Community Care – Implications of Changes for Black Communities. In *Equality By Agreement?* Report of a day conference on contracting issues and progress with black community groups and organisations. National Council of Voluntary Organisations, London.

Wistow, G. *et al.* (1993). *Social Care Markets: Progress and Prospects*. Nuffield Institute for Health/Personal Social Services Research Unit, University of Kent, Canterbury.

Chapter 11

From the bottom up: Ensuring quality with service users

Peter Allen

Inclusion of people with learning difficulties in evaluating quality is one of the few ways we have of judging whether or not services are meeting the needs of individuals. 'Agencies cannot be truly responsive to the needs of families and consumers if they are unwilling or unable to solicit their input . . .' (Kennedy, 1990).

If this assertion is accurate we must question why we are now in a position where inclusion poses such major challenges and why existing systems and structures typically make this goal seem like defying gravity.

The four definitions of quality identified by Bradley (1990), are characteristic or property of a thing or service; aspiration consistent with high level of achivement; subjective notion where different people will express varying opinions about the quality of the same thing; and value which equates to the outcome or benefit of a service. This brief illustration of different ways in which the term can be used or applied begins to illustrate the depth of exploration which will be needed when venturing on the new journeys which must result in better outcomes for people who use services.

This chapter asks readers to undertake their own quality audit, explores some of the ways which attempt to include people with learning difficulties, and describes some of the changes we should be anticipating in our approach to including people with learning difficulties in looking at quality.

The NHS and Community Care Act places a much more specific emphasis on the need to involve and include the users of services by providing clearer information, establishing procedures for consultation, publicising ways in which people can make complaints about services and also ensuring that mechanisms exist to monitor dissatisfaction. The goal of attempting closer participation is to be applauded; however, those involved in service planning and provision know the reality is much harder to achieve.

Closer and focussed relationships have been prescribed between local and health authorities and voluntary organisations. In services for people with learning difficulties this has reopened discussions about who the consumer is. Is it the family, the person with learning difficulties or both. It has been recognised that there is a need to involve people with learning difficulties in making decisions about plans for their own lives, but despite the growth of self-advocacy and many services saying they subscribe to individual planning, the structures and systems for achieving such an objective on a broad scale are far from clear.

At a time when we are all struggling with new ideas such as the joint commissioning of services, and wrestling with ideals which should result in more individualised approaches, we are still working with many of the cumbersome committee structures which have served us so poorly in the past.

It is important to separate activities which aim to develop and change services from those necessary to monitor, regulate and address quality.

Strategic development and community care planning

Planning structures will vary from place to place, but are likely to have some similarities to the following points.

- Will generally include people who are relatively experienced at attending meetings.
- Contain people claiming expert clinical or operational knowledge.
- Will have relatively limited experience at including people with learning difficulties as equal partners.

This is a situation which needs to change if users are going to be included in quality initiatives, because they must have ways of directly influencing the future.

Community care plans will typically be written documents, and provide information barely accessible to either the general population or to people with learning difficulties. There is an irony in that the people to whom the information should be directed are, therefore, excluded from the content. Surely this is an example of *un*equal opportunity.

Monitoring quality and standards

There are only few examples of methods and strategies to monitor, and therefore safeguard the quality of services for people with learning difficulties which deviate from the traditional professionally lead techniques:

> Professional theory contributes much to the standard-setting process, including standards having to do with the development of individual plans, staffing standards and staffing credentials, reporting requirements and so forth (Bradley, 1990).

We have to look much harder to find explicit statements about a quality assurance programme that genuinely asks people with learning difficulties what *they* think or feel, and undertakes to act as a consequence: '. . . service providers cannot fully assess the impact of their programmes unless they actively involve families and consumers in monitoring and evaluation' (Lehr and Lehr, 1990).

The proliferation of standards and requirements, for example, through the Registered Homes Act and its amendments and the care and service specifications resulting from the implementation of the NHS and Community Care Act, is not surprising; they aim to protect individuals and may be the basis for funding renewal. This growth seems to parallel the US experience with community systems serving more people in a variety of settings. What we need is an appropriate balance between systems which protect and regulate, and those which are more likely to bring about informed and appropriate change through user involvement.

A quality audit?

A brief look at our local practices will soon identify the strengths and weaknesses of existing systems and structures. As far as *people* are concerned: what are the existing ways in which you listen to people and learn from their experiences? Who does this listening and how? What happens to these stories? What is the right of redress if nothing happens?

What about *structures*? Are there planning groups which look at the service, finance, community care planning and long-term issues? Do people with learning difficulties know these exist? How are people with learning difficulties involved in them? (For example, fully, not at all, as a sub-group, by intention but not in reality.) When people attend are they supported and how? Are transcripts, visual representations or tapes of the proceedings or decisions made available?

What kind of *monitoring systems* exist? Are there systems to monitor quality in the full range of service provision? How are people with learning difficulties included in this process? Is monitoring mainly restricted to registered homes? Who asks people with learning difficulties what they think about services? Are there independent citizen or self-advocacy groups which have a real voice? How do these link in? Are the results of monitoring activities only available to the organisations or to the users as well?

For *training and support* the following questions need to be addressed: do professionals go to disability awareness training? Is there training and support available for people with learning difficulties who wish to attend meetings? Are there open workshops on quality assurance? Do professionals have the necessary communication skills?

It is tempting to suggest that the answers to these questions could form the basis to improving quality as a quality assurance initiative in readers' own services.

Quality action groups

This section traces the development of a quality action group and is based on a series of conversations held between the remaining members of the group before it stopped meeting. The quality action group was focussed at a resource centre for adults with learning difficulties in East London. The following looks at its achievements and the potential conflicts between what the group set out to do and the pressures of running such a group at a time of change and financial constraint.

The resource centre operated by trying to find activities, mainly in the community, which were suitable for people with learning difficulties who previously lived in hospitals. The quality action group was set up because a psychologist working in the borough was invited to take part in field testing of the *Quality in Action* pack (Ritchie and Ash, 1990), and because managers were expected to address quality in their services more and more.

The group met monthly about 30 times with breaks each summer. It originally involved users of the centre, representatives from the local college, a volunteer worker at the centre, a support worker, the deputy manager at the centre (who acted as the group leader) and the psychologist (who acted as the group's co-ordinator).

The first few meetings concentrated on members getting to know each other, learning to work together (sometimes in quite different ways) and building up group trust. For all of us, working in a diverse group, in quite different ways, this was intriguing and challenging.

It seemed something of a luxury to be able to spend plenty of time on introductions. Photographs were taken of group members and time spent talking in pairs and as a group. In one exercise, stories were drawn of our lives, including any events which were felt to be important. Connections and differences were identified between the lives of different members of the group but the talking, the process of getting to know each other, was the important part. This introductory work helped to raise common themes. The exercises also helped to obscure the boundaries of different roles, to blur the distinctions between service users and service providers. Spending time learning to work together helped to emphasise equal status as group members.

This was a really enjoyable time, sometimes hard work had to be done on reconciling having fun in the group with the more usual view of meetings as rather drab and tiresome, and sometimes not very productive. Meetings often relied heavily on discussion; this was not the best way to involve everyone in the group, or to make the most of our varied talents and different experiences. The more lively meetings involved using different models of communication such as drawing, Makaton, photographs, and so on. Some group members had to concentrate on not hiding behind jargon or using long words; it was a challenge to make things clear. The group began to talk and think about the service that the centre offered. It began to think about quality.

Members of the group felt that the term 'quality' had been taken over and jargonised. Quality control, quality assurance, total quality man-agement: these terms complicated the idea of quality. In reality everyone understands what quality is; if something has quality it feels right, it's stylish, well-made, or really effective, or luxurious. It is like the 'shoemaker's rule'; you don't need to be a shoemaker to know if a pair of shoes fit and feel really comfortable. Time was spent trying to demystify the word; to think of tangible things which were examples of quality.

The group made posters about a 'quality service' using pictures from magazines, diagrams, drawings and words, working in new, non-traditional ways. Collages had images of lovely food, beautiful houses and people involved in many different activities. Sometimes the vision of quality in magazines and the media was very far from the experiences of people with learning difficulties in the group.

These posters included words such as 'choice', 'privacy', 'friends', 'work', 'hobbies' and so on, and became reference points. Lots of things to do with quality are not just being luxuries or money but are to do with personal choice, having your own space, having good relationships, freedom to come and go as you please, entertainment, variety, health and so on. Some of the abstract things became more meaningful when related to something *real* like choosing what activity to do on a Monday morning, or choosing to have a lie-in, or to go out late.

Making a collage to demystify quality also helped the professionals in the group to recognise that it is service users who are the experts at describing and defining what a quality service should offer them. Again the pace of doing things was slower and surer, amidst the snap-snap decision making going on around us.

Collages were a good way of trying to look at the centre as a whole, but the group wanted to look at individual aspects of the service which needed improvement. The list made included more work experience for service users; more opportunities for people to learn to travel on their own; better taxis; more activities to choose from; more meetings for service users, more information and consultation; more customers for the centre café; and a better phone system, with someone to answer the phone.

The group tried out different ways of assessing these things, measuring how good or bad something was, using pictures, Makaton signs for good and bad, smiling or unhappy faces and diagrams. We had a thermometer with a coloured stem; up to the top if something was very good, or just a little way up if something was bad.

As the group became more established, its profile was raised, with contributions to the centre newsletter. The collages were displayed in the centre's foyer and taped minutes of meetings circulated. More service users were asked to join the group. Notably the group was involved more in centre activities. Requests came from management that the quality action group become more involved in, for example, the annual service review.

Six months after our group started, members went to a national workshop in Bristol for groups field testing quality in action materials. This was exciting and encouraging, sharing ideas and successes as well as setbacks and disappointments. There was talk about how groups got started, ways of involving everyone and feedback on the materials used from the draft pack.

A year after the group started, it held an open morning to which many people in the borough were invited, including all service users, staff at the centre and relevant managers. There was a display of the pictures made and materials from the *Quality in Action* pack (Milner *et al.*, 1992). Large sheets of paper explained why the quality action group was important for members individually. Group members gave short talks and mingled with as many people as possible. The open morning and the conference were good opportunities to look back at what had been covered thus far, to concentrate on achievements and work done, rather than setbacks.

There was another meeting of quality action groups who had field tested materials early in 1992, an opportunity to share experience – good and bad – with other groups. Some were going strong and had notable achievements to their credit. Sadly other groups had folded, withered, or lost momentum. Our group experienced more changes in membership. There was a problem of divided loyalties. How do you involve managers of services as equal members of the group? How do you *not* turn to them automatically with the problem? How can professionals 'de-role', think of themselves as part of a resource, hold on to a vision and not simply answer problems by saying 'because of money, or staff, or time, or this, or that, we can't change the problem'?

Although there were achievements, perhaps the big issues were beyond the group's control. This was brought home to the group when there was a major reorganisation of the space at the centre – something that would affect the quality of service – yet the group was not appropriately consulted. And if it had been, would it have been possible to do anything? This was clearly a huge issue and, perhaps, if it had been taken on the group would have set itself up to fail.

The group made a positive decision to finish meeting, but as a final action wrote up and circulated its achievements, providing information and raising questions for those undertaking similar work. These were: how can quality action groups be helped to go from strength to strength; carry through difficult times; survive changes in membership and people leaving? How can they claim space on busy timetables? How can group members maintain their enthusiasm? How can a group function as an entity greater than the sum of its parts or ensure that its ideas and suggestions are truly influential?

We came up with a number of ideas which may prove helpful. First, the group needs to be empowered. It is not enough that managers simply see the *existence* of a quality group as evidence that quality is really on their agenda. They must agree to respond fully to quality action group suggestions with explanations if ideas are not taken on. There need to be links built at different levels so that the group can have access to management and decision-making groups, committees, or whatever. The group could perhaps be given decision-making control over certain areas of the service, or management could present problems or difficulties to the group who would then be used as a resource. Second, it needs to be clear and agreed that people are fully committed to the group so that the issue of divided loyalties does not slip in. Group members need to feel able to superimpose the group's agenda over their own. It does not work to have someone in the group to whom the group automatically turns with a problem. A manager in a group needs to be there simply for ideas; someone else has to take on the response role.

Group members need to be able to suspend all cynicism in the group, think laterally and creatively. Nothing is a bigger barrier to creativity than people rubbishing ideas or silently implying 'there'll never be the money for that'. The group can then perhaps come up with creative alternatives rather than judgemental responses.

Involvement in joint planning and community care

There are now many more attempts to involve people with learning difficulties in the development of services, particularly since the NHS and Community Care Act. My own local experiences are probably not all that different from those of others involved in services. At the joint planning level the right decisions were made to include consumers in the planning process, and ensure the development of appropriate consultation. But in practice there were inevitably difficulties establishing such structures. Traditional wisdom suggested setting up a number of subgroups which would focus on a number of identified problems, namely, respite care, transition from child to adulthood and day services. The list went on and included service user involvement. The idea that a separate group could be established by a professional, working in the service, to address issues around service user involvement is inherently flawed. Yes, we did meet as a group on a number of occasions, but were struck by the inequality of information available to us. Many users had only a scant idea of what services were available, who controlled access to them and how it might be possible to bring about change let alone how they might be more involved.

It was time to recognise that this was the problem which needed priority consideration. While addressing the need to make more accessible information available to people, we also began to dismantle the subgroup and started working with People First (London) in order to identify a more vibrant approach to user involvement.

This new approach has resulted in the following number of initiatives listed, which we believe will lead to more relevant inclusion of people with learning difficulties in contributing toward the quality of services.

- Consultation on the community care plan was facilitated by People First, independently of service providers. Comments were presented back to the joint planning group.
- People First also acted as consultants over the assessment process used locally, and attempted to make sure it was one which they felt was relevant to their needs. As a result of this work they published 'Oi! It's My Assessment' (1992).
- Joint finance was identified for a three year period with the goal of more fully including people with learning difficulties in the whole community care process. Even though it is too early to anticipate the results of this work, it is possible to consider some of the anticipated benefits.
- The process is independent of existing groups and structures.
- People First hope to be undertaking similar work with other boroughs, and will, therefore, be able to bring broader experience to the consultancy.
- Local groups will be set up, and facilitated by People First. Included in this will be a focus on a small number of people yet to return from hospital to the borough.
- Funding is being made available for a period of three years, which increases the likelihood that work can develop at an appropriate pace.
- The long-term aim is to get people with learning difficulties fully involved in the planning and consultation process, but under conditions which are acceptable to them.
- The work is being monitored by senior officers in health and social services, who are looking at this as being a possible model for other user groups.

Whilst the focus of this work is community care planning, this itself is an all-embracing and essential part of our local quality initiative. It should lead to an increase in the quality of the service provided because it will become more accountable to users of local services and the questions we are asked will become more and more relevant.

To be successful in our attempts to ensure quality with people who use services we will need to bring about a number of significant changes in attitude and service approaches.

A more comprehensive approach to quality is likely to comprise a number of inter-related systems, which should include people with learning difficulties in a variety of ways. It will be a challenge to each of us to examine how it might be possible to do this in such a diverse range of areas such as: regulation; standard setting; documentation; training people to carry out service evaluation; using checklists or forms in an attempt to measure the performance of a service; policies, procedures and their application; being clearer about the anticipated end results of an intervention or delivery of service (that is, the effects the benefits, rather than just what is done); and encouraging evaluation teams to learn from and listen to users.

Are the quality audit tools we use developed independently from the people who use the range of services? If so, how can we ensure that that is changed?

Supporting user-lead initiatives and attempting to include people with learning difficulties will, it is hoped, result in our regaining their confidence and working toward joint and shared goals. There will be tensions, but these may be harnessed for their creative potential. Listening is a relatively easy, low-cost activity which can make considerable difference to our understanding, confidence and competence. It may also mean greater respect from users for our more enlightened approach!

Greater inclusion means that we need to consider a number of issues.

- What will it mean to empower service users involved in groups and teams? Where will meetings be held, under what terms and conditions and who is seen to own the meeting?
- People will be bringing forward their own views and opinions. As professionals we often hide behind the belief that we only bring a professional or organisational stance, and that this is divorced from any personal feelings, attitudes or values which we may hold, but this is not so.
- Inclusion must be viewed as a positive, relevant activity, which is consistent with well-functioning services, rather than an irritant, or inconvenient or difficult 'bolt on'.
- The pace, style and nature of the ways in which we work may need to be changed. Regular working groups, lengthy meetings, committee style approaches and dependence on words may become less significant and

possibly inappropriate. The use and development of graphic forms (Sibbet, 1981; 1993) to share ideas will become highly relevant and liberating.

- We have to learn to check what we intend to do in services and how. Whenever possible this should be *before* we act. We have to enter into a real dialogue, and be prepared to change.
- Patronising stances must be avoided with people who use our services, and we must understand the impact that we and others can have on lives.
- Evaluation, even when well intentioned, will have an impact on people using services. Kennedy (1990), in a letter to his senator, described a government official who visited his home, who could 'stare a hole through me . . .'
- It is important to decipher the grand statements we make and the language we use: while the ideas we use may be laudable, we must appreciate that they are not self-implementing and need checking at a practical level.
- Information must be made much more available and accessible.

Quality, involvement of users in service development and monitoring, empowerment, advocacy – these are too important to become cliches or buzz words. It really matters that we, in our privileged positions of power, influence, interest and authority, constantly strive to improve the quality of services in partnership with the people who use our services. It is likely to be a long but worthwhile journey, but we will know when we have arrived, it will be like achieving weightlessness!

References

Bradley, V. (1990). Conceptual issues in quality assurance. In *Quality Assurance for Individuals with Developmental Disabilities* (eds V.J. Bradley and H.A. Bersani). Paul H. Brookes, Baltimore.

Kennedy, M. (1990). What quality assurance means to me: expectations of consumers. In *Quality Assurance for Individuals with Developmental Disabilities* (eds. V.J. Bradley and H.A. Bersani). Paul H. Brookes, Baltimore.

Lehr, S. and Lehr, R. (1990). Getting what you want: expectations of families. In *Quality Assurance for Individuals with Developmental Disabilities* (eds V.J. Bradley and H.A. Bersani). Paul H. Brooks, Baltimore.

Milner, L., Ash, A. and Ritchie, P. (1992). *Quality in Action: A Resource Pack for Improving Services for People with Learning Difficulties*. Pavilion Publishing, Brighton.

People First (1992). *Oi! It's My Assessment*. People First, London.

Ritchie, P. and Ash, A. (1990). Quality in action: improving services through quality action groups. In *Better Lives, Changing Services For People With Learning Disabilities* (ed. T. Booth). *Community Care*/University of Sheffield.

Sibbet, D. (1993). *Graphic Guide To Facilitation, Principles/Practices*. Graphic Guides Inc., San Francisco.

Sibbet, D. (1981). *I See What You Mean: A Workbook/Guide to Group Graphics*. Graphic Guides Inc., San Francisco.

Chapter 12

Partnership in practice: User participation in services for people with learning difficulties

Andrea Whittaker

People First, the self-advocacy organisation run by people with learning difficulties, celebrated its tenth anniversary in 1994. During those ten years it has changed from a single group of individuals from various parts of London to a nationally known organisation tackling major issues affecting the lives of people with learning difficulties and advocating successfully for changes in their services. Those ten years have also seen major changes in services and the way we think about them. User involvement has become accepted, at least in principle, and some areas are making good progress. However, many areas are still at the starting gates.

This chapter gives examples, mainly from People First, of how people with learning difficulties are influencing the direction of services, and gives some pointers as to what needs to happen if user involvement is to become such an essential factor in planning, developing and monitoring services that it would be unthinkable for any service purchasers or providers to expect to deliver quality services without it.

How do users get involved?

In their book, *Achieving User Participation*, Fiedler and Twitchin (1992) outline a continuum of user participation which is helpful as a framework when considering the major areas of involvement. The first step on this pathway is information, followed by consultation, then participation and finally delegated control. All four steps are important

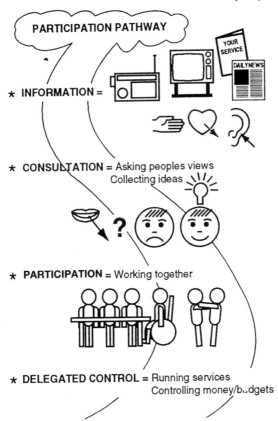

Fig 12.1 Participation Pathway

but as the last one – delegated control – is still not much more than a dream in relation to services for people with learning difficulties; we will concentrate here on the first three where it is possible to point to progress.

Information

Surely we have enough information already? We are swamped with masses of information produced from a variety of sources. But in spite of laudable efforts by plain English campaigners for example, much written material still remains incomprehensible to many ordinary people and quite unusable by people with learning difficulties. So a basic first step is to produce information in a way which people with learning difficulties can understand and use. We must think in terms of clear, simple language and develop effective use of signs, symbols and pictures.

'No jargon'. This is a constant cry of People First and other people with learning difficulties. We need to strip the language down to its bare essentials. Do we really need many of the complications of our language structure in order to get a message across? People First has taken a lead in producing publications which are truly accessible to people with learning difficulties, one of the best being *Oi! It's My Assessment* (People First, 1992) which explains clearly, with many pictures, the meaning and process of the whole community care assessment procedure. Brian Stocker, People First's community care worker says:

> The aim of my work on community care is to help people to understand what community care is. Part of this is about making documents easy for people to understand. For example, when documents come into the People First office or papers which we need to use when we go to meetings about community care, we have to translate these into easy words . . . We are working on a leaflet about community care – explaining about group homes, hostels, living independently in the community. I am working on this with Kelly who draws the pictures. Kelly helps me to write things down as well as putting in the pictures. This leaflet will help us to answer queries when people phone in asking about community care.

Good use is being made of symbol and picture systems like Makaton and Rebus but this tends to be done by individual enthusiasts for their own local use, resulting in scattered pockets of good practice and no doubt a considerable amount of overlap (King's Fund Centre, 1991; 1993a; 1993b). There is a great need to generalise this work so that it can be used in a much more comprehensive way across the country but this is not easy. Many people with learning difficulties, particularly those with profound disabilities, are helped best by having a very personalised symbol or picture language which they can relate to, but which will only be understood in their local area. Also devising the picture language is just the first step. It needs to be combined with understanding of the symbols and training in their use.

In Somerset, a county-wide system developed by the health authority's speech and language therapy department, incorporates local signs and symbols which people with learning difficulties have devised for their own personal use along with other symbols which are understood county-wide. This is combined with an intensive staff and user training programme with the aim of producing a total communication package which really works.

In Bristol, the Phoenix Trust funded Connect to produce accessible materials for people with learning difficulties, including a resettlement survey questionnaire using symbols and pictures as well as words. As well as 'translating' official documents they publish *Buzz*, a magazine produced by and for service users.

Funding from the NHS Management Executive has enabled the setting up of a pilot project to develop materials and methods to improve access to health information and health care services for people with learning difficulties. This project is based in Oxford Regional Health Authority and is working with local people with learning difficulties but its results should be applicable nationwide.

Consultation

The idea of asking people with learning difficulties for their views has been established for a very long time but good practice in consultation is still the exception rather than the rule. As various reports of the first round of consultation on community care plans have shown, while many people had good intentions, true consultation was rarely achieved. If people with learning difficulties are to be effectively consulted, we need to rethink our current methods of working. Too often consultation just means attempting to respond to a draft document within an impossibly short timescale. This rarely works well with any groups consulted and many people with learning difficulties will find it particularly difficult. The system needs to be turned on its head.

We need to start with the service users: go to them and ask how they would like to be consulted. They need to be respected as equal partners and what they say valued. This means actively developing listening skills beyond what might have been previously needed. It means planning further ahead to allow longer lead-in times for consultation. Better still, developing continuing ways of collecting peoples' views so that we don't rely so much on deadlines. In fact, it means slowing the system down. This will be frustrating to some, but areas which are serious about involving users and value their contribution, will recognise that in the end, better service delivery will be achieved.

A number of People First members are involved in quality action groups (see Chapter 11) where service users meet regularly with staff, relatives, professionals, advocates and members of the local community to look at the quality of their service. Working this way has resulted not only in small-scale achievements like changing a lunch menu, but also larger scale, more dramatic outcomes like moving house (Millner, 1991).

Mid-Downs Health Authority asked People First to set up and run a group for people with learning difficulties to learn about health services and how to make them better. Lloyd Page who has been facilitating the group says: 'We talk about how important it is for us to get good information about our health. We meet with people who work in health services – like doctors and nurses. We visit places like doctors surgeries. The group meets fortnightly and has now been running for over a year. There are plans to set up additional groups in the south west Thames area'.

Getting more out of meetings

Love them or hate them, meetings in some form or another are still the most commonly used way of achieving consultation. Involving people with learning difficulties in meetings again means being prepared to rethink the usual ways of doing things (Whittaker, 1990). Making meetings more effective for people with learning difficulties will almost certainly mean they will be more effective for everyone else as well.

So much has been written about meetings that there is a risk of restating the obvious, but the following checklist may be helpful.

- Are your venues wheelchair accessible, informal in atmosphere, and local?
- Are you prepared to hold meetings in the evenings or at weekends if necessary?
- Do you provide transport?
- Do you have flexible meeting procedures, for example, some parts of the meeting in small groups, language breaks, tea or coffee in the middle instead of just at the end?
- Do you provide independent support for the people with learning difficulties to prepare for the meetings?
- Do you provide summaries of the minutes or dictate the minutes on to tape?

People First is now represented on many influential committees such as the National Association of Health Authorities and Trusts, Central

Council for Education and Training in Social Work, a team at the Open University, producing a new course on learning difficulties, and the Department of Health's Users and Carers National Committee. Etherington (1993) speaks of her experience on one of these committees: 'It has been going for a year. Important issues we talk about are: getting rid of the term "mentally handicapped"; people coming out of hospitals and living in the community. For the first few months it was difficult. They spoke to me after the meeting. Now it is easier. It is generally good and people listen to me. If we don't understand any words, we tell them. Some jargon has been changed'.

Participation

It is now possible to point to an increasing number of examples where involvement has gone beyond the information and consultation stage to working together with users to change services. While there is undoubtedly still a considerable amount of tokenistic involvement, there are also more examples which show real partnership and positive action. Users are being involved as members of planning and policy groups within the traditional service structure and new ways of working with users are being explored. Clwyd in Wales was one of the early good examples of participation within the conventional system and the way this developed is well-documented (Hosker and Roberts, 1991; Murray, 1991). In Clwyd, users are involved at all levels including county planning teams. Norfolk social services has taken steps to overcome the problem of tokenism by ensuring that equal numbers of service users, parents and professionals are members of their learning difficulties reference group which is a part of their overall consultative structure.

In south west Surrey (Leat, 1992) the development of a structure to enable managers and users to work together began with consultation meetings with users to see how they would like to organise this. First of all, people had the opportunity of speaking up for themselves in their individual planning meetings and at their own house meetings. From these, representatives attend a residents' committee once a month and service issues brought up at these meetings were then taken to a quarterly meeting with managers. One result of this collaboration was that users gained more control over their own spending money and they then began work on producing a user-friendly complaints procedure.

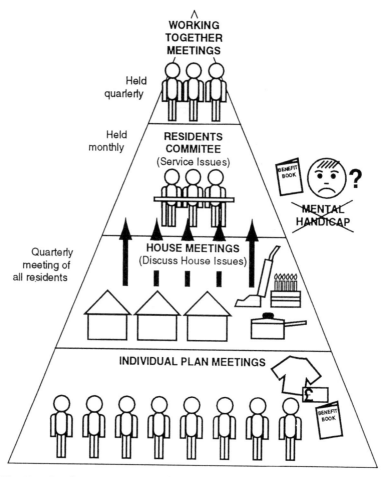

Fig 12.2 South West Surrey Heath Authority

Training together

For some years now, People First has been fostering the principle of users and staff training together and has developed considerable expertise in this area. People First members devise and run the workshops and one of the conditions is that staff and users attend together as participants. A Department of Health grant enabled People First to run three such courses, in different parts of the country, which aimed to achieve the following.

- Train staff to help users speak up for themselves.
- Help users to say what they expect from their services and understand what is possible.
- Help staff understand what the users want and users to understand what the staff do.
- Show staff what it feels like to be a service user.
- Show staff how they can actively include self-advocacy in all areas of the service.

The importance of this way of working is emphasised by the People First trainers: 'We organise the days so that there are some sessions where everybody is together and some sessions where users and staff work on their own. We can train staff to know how it feels to be a service user – staff should 'be in our shoes' to know how it feels. These workshops help staff to realise that they should share power with the users.'

Training together with users almost always has a deep effect on staff. One can see how their attitudes change towards the people with whom they work. They see people's abilities more and thus they show greater respect. They talk about positive changes in people, even during the comparatively short time of a two-day workshop. Also, the majority of staff have never been trained by people with learning difficulties before. Training together encourages a sense of partnership, working together and equality.

Perhaps the most pioneering area of user involvement is user-led evaluation of services. In 1990, People First carried out an evaluation of residential services for the London Borough of Hillingdon, looking at the lives of seven people living in two houses in the borough. People First members devised the questionnaires, carried out the interviews and wrote the report. It was the first time that people with learning difficulties had been given responsibility for such a task (Whittaker *et al.*, 1990). More recently, they have published a report of a much bigger evaluation covering two boroughs which has focussed particularly on the experiences of people moving from hospital to the community (People First, undated). Both pieces of work have proved that people with learning difficulties, given the right training and support, can offer a view of services which is unique because of their own personal experiences and is therefore different from anything which a professional researcher can undertake. There are many facets of involving users in evaluation and monitoring which need further exploration and development but these pioneering projects are pointing the way to further possibilities of working in partnership with users.

Recognising good user involvement

An organisation that is practising good user involvement will show this clearly on both an organisational and individual level. First, everyone, at all the levels of the organisation, must be committed to the idea. This means that clear statements of intent are not only written into policies but put into practice. Working in partnership with users will be demonstrated by employing people with learning difficulties. Users will be involved as trainers, not just for a one-off demonstration exercise, but as a regular and integral part of the on-going staff training programme.

On an individual basis, there will be a policy of enabling staff at all levels to get to know service users and this requirement will be written into job descriptions. Senior managers will keep in touch with users, not just at the annual Christmas party but on a regular basis, by, for example, taking their turn at answering calls on an open phone line to the public and working alongside service users on various committees and planning groups. Money will be made available to user groups. Purchasers will insist on clear plans for user involvement before contracts are agreed. As People First members say: 'Working with staff to change services is about people recognising our abilities and working with us as partners. It is about giving us choices. It is important to get our voice heard, to let the world know what we are all about and to get our messages across to purchasers and providers'.

Acknowledgements

My thanks to Alice Etherington, Lloyd Page and Brian Stocker for helping me to plan this chapter and for sharing their own experiences of user involvement.

References

Etherington, A. *et al.* (1993). *Self-Advocacy Awareness and User Participation*, (unpubl.) People First, London.
Fielder, B. and Twichin, D. (1992). *Achieving Participation*, Living Options Project Paper No 3. King's Fund Centre, London.

Hosker, P. and Roberts, D. (1990). Having a voice in service planning and development. In *Supporting Self-Advocacy*, (ed. A. Whittaker) King's Fund Centre, London.

King's Fund Centre (1991). Involving service users in appointing staff and using pictorial methods to enable people to communicate more effectively. *Information Exchange on User Participation and Self-Advocacy*, Issue No 1, November.

King's Fund Centre (1993a). Involving users on management committees and consulting users about community care plans. *Information Exchange on User Participation and Self-Advocacy*, Issue No 5, May.

King's Fund Centre (1993b). Involving people who have multiple disabilities. *Information Exchange on User Participation and Self-Advocacy*, Issue No 6, November.

Leat, M. (1992). Working together. *Information Exchange on Self-Advocacy and User Participation*, Issue No 3. King's Fund Centre, London.

Milner, L. (1991). Collective Action. *Lias*, Autumn.

Murray, N. (1991). In the driving seat. *Social Work Today*, 10 October.

People First (1992). *Oi! It's My Assessment – A Guide to All You Ever Wanted to Know about Community Care, your Assessment and your Care Manager*. People First, London.

People First (undated). *Outside but not Inside . . . Yet*. People First, London.

Whittaker, A. (1990). Involving People with Learning Difficulties in Meetings. In *Power to the People*, (ed. L. Wyn). King's Fund Centre, London.

Whittaker, A., Gardner, S. and Kershaw, J. (1990). *Service Evaluation by People with Learning Difficulties*. King's Fund Centre, London.

Chapter 13

The right to complain: Making complaints procedures for people with learning difficulties

Ken Simons

> None of the legislation currently in force confers clear entitlements, nor does it specify what level of service should be available, or what outcomes should be achieved. There is no national consensus about what should be provided to whom and under what circumstances, or even according to which principles. (Doyle and Harding, 1992).

The development of complaints procedures is a central plank in the government's attempt to reshape public services. Linked with the development of various charters, the idea is that every actual or potential user of a publicly funded service should have a clear idea of what to expect from that service, and should it fail to deliver the appropriate goods, the individual should have access to a straightforward and accessible means of seeking redress.

However, as Doyle and Harding (1992) point out, agencies like social services departments have a lot of discretion about the way they work. In the absence of substantive rights to services, Doyle and Harding argue that procedural rights become even more important. The right to be treated fairly, to be heard, and to have access to a means of redress feature prominently in their list of such rights; there have to be ways for users and their families to challenge the system.

This chapter draws on two separate research projects, both supported by the Joseph Rowntree Foundation. The Bristol Advocacy Project (Simons, 1993a; 1993b) was a study which explored the views of people involved in both self-advocacy and citizen advocacy. Although not specifically about complaints procedures, it looked in some detail at the experiences of both adults with learning difficulties and advocates who had attempted to question what was happening in services.

In contrast, the project entitled *I'm Not Complaining But...* (Simons, 1995) is concerned specifically with the workings of complaints procedures in social services departments. The main focus of this study is complaints involving (directly or indirectly) adults with learning difficulties. This research is not completed, so any findings described here have to be seen as tentative impressions.

Although this chapter concentrates on social services departments, many of the issues apply equally well to complaints procedures in the NHS and the independent sector. It begins by looking at some of the barriers to complaining experienced by users and carers, before examining concerns about the way the procedures are currently working. Finally, ways of encouraging and supporting potential complainants are discussed.

Barriers to complaining

Most studies of complaining (more or less whatever the context) have found evidence of dissatisfaction that does not get translated into recorded complaints; what Kemp *et al.* (1992) rather colourfully call the 'dark figure'. Reluctance to use the procedures appears to be greatest when the potential complainant is relatively less powerful, more vulnerable or less articulate, and is forced by circumstances to have a continuing relationship with those about whom he or she wishes to complain. It is perhaps scarcely surprising therefore that relatively few people with learning difficulties and their carers appear to be making complaints. As a group they are markedly under-represented in all the statistics available from social service departments. Understanding the reason for this reluctance to complain is crucial in designing a system that is genuinely accessible. The following points relate to the barriers to complaining perceived by users and carers taking part in the two research studies.

- Users are only too aware of what has happened in the past to people who are seen to be 'challenging': 'I don't complain. I don't want no trouble' (user).
- Citizen advocates interviewed said that at some stage their partner with

---

Social services complaints procedures

The practice guidance on complaints procedures is contained in *The Right To Complain* (SSI, 1991). Briefly, there are meant to be three stages:

- *Problem solving.* Where possible complaints should be resolved 'locally' (that is dealt with the point at which people complain, by frontline staff or their immediate managers).
- *Formal registration.* Where the complaint cannot be resolved at stage 1, or if the matter is of sufficient seriousness to miss out stage 1, then it should be formally registered and investigated. This investigation should, as a minimum, be carried out by someone who does not have line-management responsibility for the services being complained about.
- *Review stage.* If the complainant is still not satisfied with the outcome of the investigation and the department's subsequent response, they have the right to seek a review of the investigation. This is carried out by a panel of three people, at least one of whom (the chair) must be an independent person from outside the department.

The procedures should be accessible and widely advertised. Staff are meant to be clear about their role in relation to the procedures. All departments are meant to have a designated officer whose job is to co-ordinate the procedures and ensure that the department provides a prompt and 'considered' response to criticism.

---

learning difficulties had been reluctant to let them pursue an issue: 'He sometimes worries he will get into hot water. "They'll think I've been stirring it up" ' (advocate).

- These fears are not confined to the people with learning difficulties; the advocates themselves often had similar concerns, as did carers: 'You've got to be careful about tackling things head on. It does Emma no good' (advocate); 'They might take it out on her' (carer).
- All too often these worries have been heightened by what are perceived (and as one sometimes suspects, intended) as implicit threats from staff: 'You realise we are not obliged to care for your son' (comment reported by carer).
- These worries are not limited to fears or retribution. Users and carers have little sense of being in control and, for them, making a complaint has the potential for starting a process that might have unpredictable consequences: 'You don't know what might happen' (user).
- Many have learnt over many years that the best way to survive is to keep their heads down: 'You've got to be careful what you say.'

Most users and carers are forced by circumstances to rely on services for support. They tend to work hard to build up relationships with some staff. Some users, in particular, are worried that a complaint could get valued staff into trouble. Any complaint is seen to reflect badly on staff: 'I don't complain, staff are good here.'

Many users and carers can point to some aspects of the service that they appreciate. As far as they are concerned, complaining represents a risk; there is always the danger that a professional will decide that your day centre or your home 'no longer meets your needs' and will whisk you away somewhere else (or provide no service at all). Better to tolerate a few imperfections than lose everything!

Rightly or wrongly, both users and carers interpret many of the 'messages' coming from services in ways that undermine any encouragement to complain.

Both users and carers have absorbed the idea that times are hard and budgets squeezed, and they have lowered their expectations accordingly: 'They have got no money, haven't they?' (user).

In their reluctance to blame professionals, many carers accept that services are short staffed, that this is more or less inevitable and is not something about which they can complain. Similarly, many carers with adult children (or in some cases brothers and sisters) with learning difficulties living at home are frustrated by the lack of opportunities for the latter to leave home and live somewhere with some appropriate support. Many have stories about being told by managers that social services can only help in a crisis. One comment reported by a carer was: 'We can only do something if they are likely to be on the street.' While this may unfortunately be no more than a statement of reality, the message it gives is that services are so stretched that complaining is pointless.

Many users and carers have taken part in consultation exercises, without any obvious impact on the policies or practice of the departments in question. Indeed their experiences of consultation were often unsatisfactory. For example, one carer described how she had attended a public meeting and had finally screwed up the courage to ask a question about the local problems with short-term care. A councillor 'just dismissed' her concerns and moved straight on to the next topic without giving her the chance to question what he had said. Why, her carers group wanted to know, would using the complaints procedure be any different?

Some users and carers have negative associations with the word 'complaining'. They see it in terms of appearing ungrateful and not being polite. In the past, these feelings have often been reinforced by services; complaining was rarely presented in a positive light, or as an assertion of a *right*.

For other carers and users the lack of a truly independent element in the complaints procedures means they are simply not convinced that justice will be done, particularly where their relationship with the services has been poor in the past: As Lindsay (1991) says: 'To be credible and effective, complaints procedures need to be genuinely independent.' Or, in the words of a carer: 'It's all just chums investigating chums, isn't it?'

Although some authorities have used external investigators for a few serious complaints, the complaints procedure is effectively a form of self-policing. Some dissatisfied complainants may be able to take their case to the local government ombudsman (if there is evidence of 'maladministration', that is, if the authority has broken its own procedures or has acted in a way that is inherently unreasonable). They may also be able to seek a judicial review in the High Court if they believe they have been the victim of a misinterpretation of the law. Indeed, recently there have been several important instances where complainants have successfully challenged social services departments over the interpretation of the law (see, for example, Eaton, 1993; George, 1993). However, as far as most complainants are concerned, there is no independent appeal.

Complaining about the NHS is a notoriously complicated task (Consumers Association, 1993), with a complex array of procedures relating to the different parts of the service. The problems facing a user of services of the independent sector can also be pretty bewildering; depending on whether or not the local authority is acting as a purchaser of the service for that individual, they may or may not have access to the social services complaints procedures. In some authorities, complaints relating to the independent sector are seen as the preserve of the inspection unit. In others they are handled like any other complaint. Most difficult of all are complaints about services which span organisational boundaries. Even if the service is seamless, the complaints procedures will not be.

In Avon, services have gone some way to addressing this muddle by developing a co-ordinated response. Rather than deflecting misplaced complaints, the local NHS provider, the social services department, and some of the local voluntary organisations have all agreed to help people complaining make their voice heard in the right quarter.

Concerns about procedures

Having overcome the barriers that might have inhibited them, how do the people who have made complaints feel about the experience? This is one of the issues being addressed by the research on complaints procedures. It is too early to report the final results here, but the omens are not good. Most authorities seemed to view a complaint not taken further as a complaint 'satisfactorily resolved'. However, there is little reason for such complacency. The Social Services Inspectorate (SSI, 1993) has done a detailed inspection of complaints procedures in five social services departments, and as part of this exercise they carried out a postal survey of people who had complained. Over 65 per cent of those who replied were dissatisfied with the experience. In addition, there is evidence that the proportion of complaints that are upheld varies wildly between authorities. All this suggests that the procedures do not always work as intended. Already a number of areas of concern are emerging.

Many people complain not because they want to get compensation or have staff disciplined, but because they do not want other people to have to go through the same experience (Consumers Association, 1993). Many will therefore be complaining on the assumption that the agency will be learning the lessons from their particular circumstances. The guidance on complaints procedures (SSI, 1991) makes a similar assumption; agencies ought to see complaints procedures as part of a range of quality assurance mechanisms. Those responsible for the procedures should be identifying and disseminating the general lessons from the complaints that are made.

However, the SSI inspection (1993) found that in this area, the performance of the social services departments studied was 'disappointing'. The recording was poor, there was little systematic evaluation of the available data and there were few attempts to monitor the impact of the procedures on policy or practice.

An early assessment of annual reports produced by social services departments carried out as part of the research project on complaints confirms this picture. A few departments do provide comprehensive descriptions of how the procedures have worked, and clearly identify changes that have taken place in response to complaints. Some provide a detailed breakdown of who complained, and to what effect. A small number have carried out surveys of complainants to gauge the extent to which they are satisfied and to evaluate the performance of the procedures. However, these are very much a minority. Most are content to simply provide aggregated data on formal complaints, broken down by area, departmental division, or client group. Such crude statistics provide little scope for drawing conclusions about what needs to change. Additionally, the information gathered and the way it is presented tends to reflect the individual authority; it is almost impossible to compare the performances of different social services departments on the information available.

There are inherent dangers in formal 'high level' complaints procedures. According to the Family and Community Dispute Research Centre (Hill *et al.*, 1991) they tend to lead to an emphasis on the way decisions are made (do they conform to procedures?), rather than the substantive issues (are we doing justice to this complainant?); what the researchers refer to as 'ombudsman-proofing' decision making. Such an approach biases decision making in ways that can act against the interests of service users. More formal procedures also tend to involve more red tape, and they cost more. The emphasis on the informal problem solving in the guidance on complaints procedures (SSI, 1991) would appear to be well placed.

This problem-solving approach is meant to be most apparent in the first stage of the procedure prior to formal registration complaint, when every effort should be made to solve problems locally. However, there is remarkably little evidence to show that this part of the procedures is working as was intended. The vast majority of authorities have little or no information about what is happening at a local level. This is apparent from the annual reports produced by social services departments, it is the case with the social services departments taking part in *I'm Not Complaining But . . .* , and it was also true of the five authorities included in the SSI inspection (1993). The SSI comment that some managers showed a 'marked reluctance to record issues as complaints until all other possibilities were exhausted', while others simply failed to record complaints that were appropriately dealt with.

A procedure that puts a lot of emphasis on local resolution will not necessarily act as a good alarm system. For example, the inquiry into the case of Frank Beck (the Leicestershire child care worker who was found to have been sexually abusing children in his care for a decade) found that local managers had received 30 official complaints about

Beck's activities, but that they were not properly investigated (Marchant, 1993). There is a danger that the informal stage of the procedure may be used to contain problems by staff who are themselves part of the problem, and that the emphasis sometimes placed upon complaining to local staff first may inhibit vulnerable users from voicing their fears, unless they know both about their right to make a formal complaint and how to access the wider system.

The experience of the citizen advocates interviewed as part of the Bristol Advocacy Project found that frontline staff often reacted very defensively and aggressively to criticism (Simons, 1993b) and that conflict frequently became very personalised. However, some also found that the intervention of a manager acting in an impartial way sometimes helped to resolve at least some of this conflict. The meetings arranged by managers seemed to provide a forum where staff and advocates could discuss the principles involved rather than getting bogged down in the muddy detail of 'who said what to whom'. Not that these meetings necessarily met all the advocates' concerns, but they did seem to offer a model of problem solving in action.

Yet this approach seemed to be relatively rare. Even in the first stage of the procedures, there seemed to be more emphasis on investigating whether or not a complaint was justified, rather than exploring other more constructive avenues.

Some potential complainants have found complaints procedures interpreted in very narrow terms. John Keep of the Royal Association for Disability and Rehabilitation has come across examples of individuals who have been told that they can only use the procedure if their complaint is about 'maladministration' (personal communication, 1993), while others (NCC, 1992) have found social services departments claiming that 'political decisions' (that is policy decisions made by councillors) fall outside the remit of complaints procedures.

Ths issue cropped up in the SSI (1993) inspection of complaints procedures. They found confusion about the precise role of review panels (the final stage of the procedures); were they to consider the 'justice' of the situation, or do they have the more limited role of simply judging whether or not the complaints procedure had been properly applied? The SSI report gives the example of a department where panel members were told they should not challenge 'professional' decisions.

These attempts to limit the role of complaints procedures runs contrary to both the spirit and, in many cases, the letter of the guidance on the procedures. To exclude any areas of practice or decision making from the procedures is to effectively insulate them from criticism; a highly dangerous course of action.

Promoting complaints

For the system to be effective there has to be both encouragement for people to try complaining and support for them when they do. This section looks at some of the ways that this might be done.

According to the Department of Health (1991), social service departments are meant to ensure their complaints procedures are accessible and widely publicised. People with learning difficulties are an obvious group on whom to target information in more accessible forms, yet most authorities were slow to start producing material specifically designed for this group of users. The situation is changing slowly, and an increasing number of leaflets are being produced with Makaton symbols or graphics; some authorities now provide information on audio tape, and a few have produced videos.

However, making complaints procedures accessible means more than just telling people that the procedures are there. There has been a tendency for much of the information produced to concentrate on the technical aspects of the procedures (for example, what will happen at which stage) rather than attempting to address people's fears and concerns. Given the fears many users and carers have about complaining, there is a clear need for reassurance that complaining is OK, that people will not get into trouble because they have complained, that their views will be taken seriously, and that nothing will happen as a consequence of the complaint without them being consulted.

For information to have an impact on users, it must actively engage them and be meaningful to them. A few authorities have tackled this imaginatively by getting local theatre groups involving people with learning difficulties to explore what complaining means. One of the best ways of ensuring that material is accessible to users is to involve them in its production. A good example of this strategy is the *Residents' Rights* pack (Allen and Scales, 1990), a video for people with learning difficulties that explores (among other things) the right for users to complain about the behaviour of staff. Adults with learning difficulties are themselves starting to produce effective material. For example, a Gateshead self-advocacy group has made a video on complaints.

It is easy to be cynical about charters, but by letting people know what rights they have and what they can reasonably expect from a service, they may provide an important set of yardsticks against which users can judge the performance of the service. The problem has been that most local service charters are at best cautious affairs, and do not really address the concerns of users and carers.

Based on the experiences of people involved in citizen advocacy, Simons (1993b) lists some suggestions for a local charter; for example, ensuring that the elements of the Disabled Persons' Act 1986 that were not implemented by the government (including the right to appoint and have contact with an independent advocate) are enshrined as *local* policy. By specifying the general rights that users and carers have, as well as making it clear what the service will not do (for example, preventing contact with friends and family as punishment or as a way of controlling behaviour), a charter can help remind staff what is (and what is not) expected of them and can protect the organisation against unwittingly infringing people's rights, as well as providing a clear framework to help those who want to complain when things go wrong. The act of producing such a charter may also force services to decide exactly what they are offering. For example, can users change their social worker, key worker or care manager if they do not get on?

When the members of the Somerset Self-Advocacy Network were consulted about the development of complaints procedures in the county, they made it clear that some people would need help to complain, and that while staff would sometimes be able to do this, there would also be times when it was important to have support from someone who did not work for the council. The local citizen advocacy organisation was suggested as one source of support. A citizen advocate is an unpaid private citizen who is independent of local services, who is matched on a one-to-one basis with someone who is vulnerable or isolated. The value of having someone who is known and trusted, who can provide both moral and practical support, and who is there to be on the side of the person complaining, cannot be underestimated. Traditionally, citizen advocacy organisations have tried mainly to find people who would act as long-term advocates. However, several have now also set out to to recruit and train short-term complaints advocates (Simons, 1993b).

Citizen advocacy organisations are not the only source of independent support. The SSI (1991) mentions a whole range of organisations that have been asked by social services departments to provide independent advocates for people who want to complain. These include the Samaritans, Citizen Advice Bureaux, Age Concern, Mind and The Children's Society. A complaints leaflet for one London borough includes no less than 20 telephone numbers of organisations who might be able to offer help, including some specifically aimed at particular minority ethnic groups.

Another important source of support for people complaining has come from people with learning difficulties themselves. Some self-advocacy groups have put considerable energy into discussing both complaints procedures and the things that have upset users. These groups can provide a safe and supportive environment where people can talk about their experiences, particularly if the group is able to meet in a venue outside the main service. A service user said: 'I felt comfortable there!' For example, as a result of a group meeting in an adult education setting a number of users were able to make a complaint about the way they were treated in their hostel. This complaint was successful and staff were suspended as a consequence.

It is also important not to underestimate the importance of very informal sources of support, like friends, family and other users. Potential complainants have usually discussed the problem with others long before they get to make a formal complaint. This helps them crystallise the issues (Hill *et al.*, 1991). The extent these supporters are encouraging or discouraging can also be an important determinant of whether the person goes on to complain. Regular direct contact between the people responsible for the procedures and users and carer groups is one way of trying to engage potential supporters.

For user groups and advocacy organisations to be effective, they need resources. Finding ways to provide funding in ways that do not undermine their independence (for example through joint finance monies) has to be seen as a priority.

Complaints procedures are particularly important for groups who have tended to miss out on services, or for whom services have been inappropriate. For example, people from black and ethnic minority groups have often been badly served, and it is vital to ensure that complaints procedures are accessible to and usable by them as a tool to challenge discrimination. Equal opportunities ought to be a key issue for complaints procedures. Take the case of Geoff Smith. He is black, and has recently experienced a lot of racial abuse from other service users at his day centre. He finally complained about the lack of action from staff. He initially got support from two white complaints advocates. They were full of indignation about the way Geoff had been treated, but in the end Geoff decided that he wanted support from someone who was also black. Without contacts in the black community the local co-ordinator of the advocacy scheme was unable to find someone, and in the end, as a compromise, a black member of staff from another area was asked if she would help Geoff.

Finding supporters for people from the same culture or community can be crucial, particularly where, like Geoff, people are facing overt discrimination. This means establishing links with all of the local communities and ensuring that they are involved in developing support mechanisms. For example one citizen advocacy organisation in Leeds has appointed a black co-ordinator, co-opted black people onto the management committee, and set out to recruit black and ethnic minority advocates (Baxter *et al.*, 1990).

Most authorities do not seem to have moved beyond having basic leaflets translated into various languages, although some have acknowledged that this is an area that needs further developments. In a few instances, further steps have been taken; for example, establishing a budget to pay for interpreters.

In-house complaints chasers

A few authorities have established individuals or groups whose role it is to monitor and follow up complaints. Some are quite separate from those who are responsible for managing and implementing the complaints procedures. For example, Bedfordshire has appointed a county-wide ombudsperson (not to be confused with local government ombudsmen who have a national remit). On a rather different tack, Leeds social services department has appointed a children's rights officer (with some additional funding from Save the Children). This officer is responsible for investigating some specific complaints (offering at least a degree of independence), but also is charged with identifying issues of strategic concern in relation to services for children. Being insiders, complaints chasers have the advantage of knowing how the system works. However, they should never be seen as substitutes for effective independent support.

Complaints procedures that are developed and run by professionals in isolation are less likely to be accessible to users and carers than those where the latter are directly involved. The SSI (1993) is keen to see much greater consultation of front line staff, users and carers over the way procedures work, in the hope that this will generate feelings of 'ownership and confidence'. Nevertheless, its inspection found that the authorities involved had 'some way to go'.

There is enormous scope for involving people with learning difficulties and their families in any review of complaints procedures, yet there is little evidence that this is happening on any scale. A small number of authorities have started to co-opt users and carers into steering groups overseeing the development of the procedures, but these are the exception, rather than the rule.

Ultimately, the responsibility for ensuring that internal complaints procedures of an organisation work lies with the staff who work in it, from top to bottom. The importance of the way that staff behave is underlined by the finding from the SSI inspection (SSI, 1993) that people complaining were much more likely to have learnt of the existence of the procedures from professionals than from information leaflets. Staff need to be equipped with the knowledge, skills and confidence to carry out the following tasks effectively.

- Ensure that users and carers know about, and understand their rights.
- Identify when users and carers are unhappy, and to offer the procedures as a way of tackling the situation.
- Provide effective support to people who want to complain (including ensuring that they have access to independent advice and advocacy).
- Deal positively with 'informal' complaints (including appropriate recording).
- Behave appropriately in the context of formal investigations.
- Challenge bad practice by their peers.
- Identify the wider lessons from complaints.

These issues can be partly tackled by effective staff training. But they are also related to the way that organisations view complaints procedures. They have to be seen as a high priority. Resources have to be committed to making them work, and there has to be support both for staff who are helping individuals complain, and for those who are the subject of complaints. Above all, the organisation has to show its workforce that it takes complaints seriously.

The requirement that social services departments should have a complaints procedure covering all their operations was an important step in the right direction, but it was very much just a first step. Despite the commitment of many complaints officers, too many of their fellow professionals have yet to see complaints as a high priority. Most authorities have only set out a narrow range of initiatives in this area, and some seem stuck firmly in a 'no complaints equals no problems' complacency. The absence of complaints can rarely (if ever) be interpreted as a sign of good services. A responsive system should actively seek the views of users and carers, should encourage people to complain if they are at all unhappy, should ensure that there is a range of support for those who do complain, and should learn the wider lessons from all the complaints that are made.

Complaints procedures can be made to work for people with learning difficulties. With the right support and encouragement, some users and carers have been able to take on the system. However, the procedures are not a magic wand. In themselves they are not sufficient to carry the burden of expectation placed upon them; there have to be other complementary mechanisms to ensure that vulnerable people are both encouraged to speak up, and are heard by decision makers.

> The spirit in which complaints procedures are implemented will largely determine their effectiveness . . . They are most likely to ensure quality and protect individuals when they stem from a recognition of user's needs and rights. (DoH, 1991).

References

Allen, P. and Scales, C. (1990). *Resident's Rights: Helping People With Learning Difficulties Understand Their Housing Rights*. Pavilion Publishing, Brighton.

Baxter, C., Poonia, K., Ward, L. and Nadirshaw, Z. (1990). *Double Discrimination*. King's Fund Centre/ Commission for Racial Equality, London.

Consumers Association (1993). Complaining to the NHS. *Which?*, April, 11–15.

Department of Health (1991). *Community Care in the Next Decade and Beyond: Policy Guidance*. HMSO, London.

Doyle, N. and Harding, T. (1992). Community care: applying procedural fairness. In *The Welfare of Citizens*, (ed. A. Coote). Institute for Public Policy Research, London.

Eaton, L. (1993). Needs versus wants. *Community Care*, 22 April, 6.

George, M. (1993). Legal storm brewing. *Community Care*, 29 April, 18–19.

Hill, M., Walker, J., Cracknell, S., McCarthy, P., Simpson, R. and Corlyon, J. (1991). *Citizen's Grievances about Local Authority Services: A Report to The ESRC*. Family and Community Dispute Rsearch Centre, Newcastle Upon Tyne.

Kemp, C., Maguire, M., Minkes, J. and Morgan, R. (1992). *Complaints Against Central Government Departments*, School of Administrative Studies, University of Wales, Cardiff.

Lindsay, J. (1991). Complaints procedures and limitations in the light of the 'Pindown' enquiry. *The Journal of Social Welfare and Family Law*, 6, 433–441.

Marchant, C. (1993). A catalogue of complaint. *Community Care*, 18 February, 7.

National Consumer Council (1992). *Getting Heard and Getting Things Changed: The Report of A Conference On Complaints Procedures For Users of Social Services Departments*. National Consumer Council, London.

Simons, K. (1993a). *Sticking Up For Yourself: Self-Advocacy and People With Learning Difficulties*. Joseph Rowntree Foundation/*Community Care*, York.

Simons, K. (1993b). *Citizen Advocacy: The Inside View*. Bristol: The Norah Fry Research Centre, University of Bristol.

Simons, K. (1995) *I'm Not Complaining But. . . . Complaints Procedures In Social Services Departments*, Joseph Rowntree Foundation/*Community Care*, York.

Social Services Inspectorate (1991). *The Right to Complain*. HMSO, London.

Social Services Inspectorate (1993). *The Inspection of the Complaints Procedures in Local Authority Social Services Departments*. HMSO, London.

Part Three

Changing Issues

Chapter 14

Confronting colour blindness: Developing better services for people with learning difficulties from Black and ethnic minority communities

Carol Baxter

> The message to all those who choose to care for others is that, unless their actions are guided by a sense of importance of every human being, their competence and professionalism will remain questionable. (Nirza, 1986).

The fact that the UK is a multiracial society is now well established. According to the 1991 census 5.9 per cent of the total British population identified themselves as being a member of a minority ethnic group. In some cities the proportion of people from ethnic minority communities is close to 50 per cent (OPCS, 1993). People with learning difficulties come from all sections of society and from different racial and ethnic backgrounds. Most service providers in health and social welfare agencies pride themselves on the fact that they treat everyone the same and that they do not differentiate on the basis of colour or ethnic group. Services, however, have tended to develop an inflexible structure of their own and many aspects are specifically geared to the needs of the dominant white majority population. This type of structure has contributed to an inadequate response to the needs of people from black and ethnic minority communities, many of whom will have experiences, priorities and expectations which differ from those of the white majority population.

Over the last ten years this 'colour blind' approach has begun to be challenged. It is now accepted by many that providing the same services in the face of differing needs is not the same as providing equitable services. There are also legal and statutory requirements. Public agencies do not have complete discretion as to whether to take account of the cultural implications of how they offer care and support. They are bound by the Race Relations Act 1976 (Home Office, 1977) which outlines a responsibility to ensure that neither direct or indirect discrimination is taking place. Race equality is also implied in the Patients' and Citizens' Charter and other professional statements about rights and quality of life. This can however easily get lost in day-to-day practice and processes. There are therefore some essential steps which will need to be taken to ensure any theory of racial equality is translated into reality. It is not difficult to gain superficial support for ideas of fairness; race equality in service provision has become a good thing to which all right-thinking people subscribe. Unfortunately, that is sometimes as far as it goes. So commonplace is the idea that many service providers are expected to know and understand all about the issues involved without the benefit of any exploration of the practical implications. This chapter will identify how racial discrimination operates in services for people with learning difficulties and present some guidelines for the development of services which are appropriate and sensitive to this section of the population.

An essential starting point is to identify the ways in which racism exists and is prepetuated within services. It is not difficult to appreciate that white people in the UK enjoy more privileges and have more opportunities and power than black people. Their colour confers rights that are often denied to black people. Black people are more likely to live in run-down inner city areas and in substandard housing, to be found in semi-skilled jobs, to be disproportionately affected by unemployment and are economically worse off than their white counterparts (Brown, 1984). There is also evidence that black people have poorer health and less access to appropriate health care (McNaught, 1985) and consistently receive less than their entitlement in benefits or services (Gohil, 1987). These inequalities have their roots in racism. Racism is the legacy of historical and contemporary power relations between the UK and the rest of the world which has created a situation of imbalance in which ethnic minorities are seen as subordinate by the dominant white majority for whom relations are marked with notions of inferiority and alienness (Alexander, 1987).

But what has racism got to do with providing better services? Racism is reflected in all institutions, including health and social welfare agencies – both in the behaviour of individuals as well as in institutional practice. Although there will be incidents of individual racist behaviour, individuals are often not consciously aware of how racism shapes the way in which they respond to those for whom it is their responsibility to provide services. Most people in the caring professions would not deliberately withhold care or treat people differently on the basis of their colour. It is institutional discrimination which is the more common and damning form of racism. This is where things are done in a way which assumes that all clients are from the same racial, cultural and linguistic background as the rest of the white majority population. For example, despite the fact that not all families speak English as a first language, services are on the whole provided in English. Link-workers and interpreters are not routinely employed within services.

Stereotyping is another way in which racism is perpetuated in services. Negative stereotyped views are still prevalent in our society and black and ethnic minority people continue to be seen and evaluated in this way. People responsible for making decisions about services can often base their decisions on racist assumptions and stereotyping. For example, fostering and adoption agencies have until recently been resistant to recruiting black parents on the racist assumption that their childbearing practices were inferior to that of whites and that black families were not interested in fostering children. The popular myth that black families prefer to 'look after their own' and do not want to use services has recently been exploded: the truth is that many black people have a greater need for support than their white peers.

It has been argued that skin colour is the greatest single factor that governs society's attitudes to members of minority groups. Hence people whose skin is visibly different from the white majority population are particularly vulnerable to racial discrimination (Pumphrey and Verma, 1990). Racism is a dynamic and complex force in society which takes many forms, most of which are covert and inherently part of the way in which services are planned and delivered. Black people with learning difficulties experience different types of oppression concurrently – there being clear parallels between the way in which society views and treats black people and the way people with learning difficulties are perceived and responded to (Baxter *et al.*, 1990). This creates more challenges for services in meeting their needs. Race equality in service provision requires that services challenge racial discrimination, understand the experiences of those who suffer it and develop ways of responding to black and ethnic minority people which values their culture.

Over the last four years the planning, management and delivery of health and social services has experienced considerable change in their structural, organisational and ideological approaches. Within this climate of reform, however, might these changes in reality further work

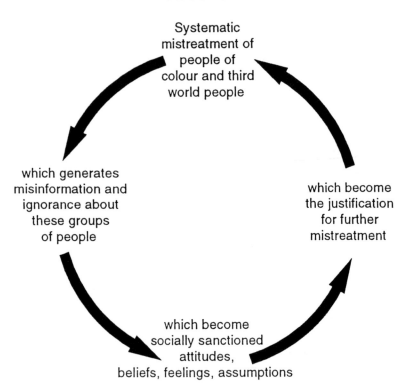

RACISM

Systematic mistreatment of people of colour and third world people

which become the justification for further mistreatment

which become socially sanctioned attitudes, beliefs, feelings, assumptions

which generates misinformation and ignorance about these groups of people

Racism is one consequence of a self-perpetuating imbalance in economic, political and social power.

Racism hurts all of us, whether or not we are members of the targetted group.

Fig 14.1 Racism (adapted from Ricky Sherouer-Marcuse, *Unlearning Racism Workshops*, 6501 Dana, Oakland, CA94609)

against black users of services? Four areas within services for people with learning difficulties warrant close examination: community care, normalisation, assessment and individual care planning.

Community care

The community care White Paper, *Caring for People* (1989) states:

> Minority communities may have different concepts of community care and it is important that service providers are sensitive to these variations. Good community care will take account of the circumstances of minority communities and will be planned in consultation with them.

This is however a very minimal statement as there is no specific guidance on how this might be achieved. The new framework for delivering community care services to people with learning difficulties has required a change in assessment procedures and policies and in the management of individual cases. While these changes in themselves may be welcome their impact on service users from black and ethnic minority communities leaves much to be desired. The implicit assumption is that black and ethnic minority people have access to and are using services in the community. While voluntary organisations are now playing an increasing role in providing services in the community, experience, however, has shown that mainstream organisations do not cater adequately for the needs of black people (Dungate, 1984). Such services are still largely based on the needs of the majority of people who are white. The few black voluntary organisations which exist are grossly underfunded and too under-resourced to take on this role. There will, therefore, be an increased burden on black families. Meanwhile, the values underpinning service delivery contrive to reflect the norms of the white majority population so that black and ethnic minority people with learning difficulties and their facilities often fail to get the community care support they need.

Normalisation

Normalisation and the service assessment tools with which it is associated provide a critical analysis of services which have been of considerable benefit to people with learning difficulties. Normalisation promotes the social value of people with learning difficulties. People are encouraged to see their fellow citizens with learning difficulties in a more valued way. Service providers are urged to enable them to experience an everyday life which is as close as possible to that experienced by the rest of society. Cultural values are key factors in the implementation of service actions which are proposed by normalisation. However, racism as an integral part of the culture of the dominant white society is not explored and normalisation thus fails to help services to recognise and address the effects of racism on the users and providers of services. Since those who plan and manage services are largely white, there is concern that the normalisation principles are not being interpreted in ways which are appropriate or beneficial to black people with learning difficulties. An exercise carried out by a community learning difficulty team in Harlesden for example, demonstrated that what white staff would value for themselves would, in many cases, conflict with what black service users valued. (Baxter *et al.*, 1990) while normalisation largely ignores issues of race, racism and culture, a racial equality approach to assessing a black person's needs would see a focus on their racial identity as desirable and constructive (Ferns, 1992)

Assessment

Assessment tools used in the UK fall prey to the 'colour blind approach'. They are often based on white British norms which bear little relationship to the everyday life of black people. Many standard test procedures and equipment involve images based on white middle-class lifestyle and experiences. For example, a test still widely used has a picture of a couple involved in a Western style wedding ceremony. Hindu, Sikh and Muslim wedding ceremonies bear no resemblance to this and many Asian children may have difficulty in recognising the image. Another concern regarding the assessment of black and ethnic minority children is the fact that interpreters are not routinely used in these procedures even when this involves children for whom English is a second language. Consequently, such children are being disproportionately placed in schools and units for children with severe learning difficulties. In Tower Hamlets, Bangladeshi parents felt that if their children were assessed in Bengali instead of assessed in English, they would have achieved a more positive result (Chaudhury, 1986).

Individual care planning

Accordingly, individual care planning is another area of concern. In the processes involved, the focus is on the individual; the aim being to

Table 14.1 Race and mental handicap workshop: Normalisation exercise

| | Positive | | | | Negative | Sample |
	1	2	3	4	5	
Living independently	10					Afro-Caribbean
			5		5	Asian
	7		3			White
Being good at sewing	2		4	4		Afro-Caribbean
			5		5	Asian
	2		6		2	White
Having a boyfriend/girlfriend	2	4	4			Afro-Caribbean
					10	Asian
	5		1		4	White
Eating with your fingers	2		4	4		Afro-Caribbean
	8	2				Asian
					10	White
Being black*	10					Afro-Caribbean
	10					Asian
	2	2	3		3	White
Being severely mentally handicapped					10	Afro-Caribbean
				2	8	Asian
					10	White
Remaining closely linked to your family in adult life	10					Afro-Caribbean
	10					Asian
			4	5	1	White
Going to pubs/discos	2	2	2		4	Afro-Caribbean
				2	8	Asian
	5	2	3			White
Wearing a sari			4		6	Afro-Caribbean
	8	2				Asian
	1		6	1	2	White
Being extrovert	2	2	4	2		Afro-Caribbean
			5	2	3	Asian
	5	2	2		1	White
Drinking alcohol	2		4	4		Afro-Caribbean
				2	8	Asian
	3	2	4		1	White

The exercise was completed by 30 people: 10 Afro-Caribbean, 10 Asian and 10 of white British and Irish origin who lived in Harlesden, London Borough of Brent, in Autumn 1985.

*For Afro-Caribbean and Asian samples, self; for white sample, of a friend.

Source: Baxter et al. (1990).

enable service providers to recognise and meet individual needs. However, in black communities the family and community may take precedence over the individuality which is encouraged more in white British society. The former requires skills in working with families which currently do not receive the required emphasis in the training of professionals. Furthermore the goals of training for independence which are identified in individual care planning – such as the teaching of skills to enable the individual to live on his or her own may conflict with the values in some families where there is a tradition of an extended family network.

Furthermore, complex and highly bureaucratic assessment and review procedures are not always easy to understand. This will be particularly confusing for those parents who are not familiar with how the system works or whose mother tongue is not English. A study by Contact a Family (1989) showed that often parents were expected to provide their own interpreters who might be relatives or friends who were themselves not familiar with professional terminology and procedures. Unfamiliarity with professional jargon may have negative consequences for black families; for example, parents believing that special education meant better quality than that offered in the ordinary schools (Chaudhury, 1988).

Role and position of black staff

Black staff, especially those from backgrounds similar to service users, are vital in providing good services to a multiracial clientele. Experience has shown that employing staff who share the same social experience of the black and ethnic minority people they serve and who can communicate with them in their own languages can result in a dramatic increase in the take-up of services by potential clients who are non-English speaking. A survey carried out by the Social Services Inspectorate of the Department of Health in Kirklees illustrates this very clearly. The survey covered three areas: Batley, Fartown and Dewsbury. In Batley, where there was a team with Asian staff, an estimated 17 per cent of the total clients referred were Asian, compared with 11 per cent of the Batley population. In Dewsbury, with a similar proportion of the population who were Asians, but no Asian workers, only three per cent of the total clients referred were Asian. (Dearnley *et al.*, 1986).

There are however a number of concerns about the role and position of black and ethnic minority staff (Baxter *et al.*, 1990). The particular perspectives, experiences and skills of such staff are often undervalued; the initiatives and approaches they develop can be viewed as unprofessional by their colleagues or managers. Ahmed (1988) points out that:

> These criticisms have ranged from the accusation of 'over-identification with clients' to 'oppressing of the individual with family and community expectations' and 'hindering the liberation of the individual'.

Many black and ethnic minority staff become labelled as 'the race expert', thus relieving white staff of their responsibilities in this area. This also has the effect of restricting full use of their professional skills and consequently limiting their career prospects.

Developing better services

In seeking to improve services so that they reflect the needs of the whole community, including black and ethnic minority service users, there are a number of key areas of priority: challenging racism; appropriate consultation; access to more appropriate residential and personal care.

Challenging racism

First and foremost it is essential that services address the issue of racism whether it be personal or institutional. The consequence of racist behaviour (conscious or unconscious) should be identified and challenged where it exists. Those responsible for the planning and delivery of services need to address the following questions.

- Is the way they relate to black service users influenced by unhelpful racist stereotypes?
- What measures have been taken to learn about and understand the nature of racism and how it affects practice in the workplace?
- Are racist jokes or slurs from clients or colleagues challenged?
- What types of policies are there to ensure that where clients' rights are violated, appropriate action is taken?
- Are black clients given assistance to minimise destructive self-criticism and focus on their positive self-worth?
- Are clients addressed by their preferred name? Attempts should be made to accurately pronounce and record clients' names. These should not be changed to more English-sounding ones.

Tackling racism should not be seen as going beyond the call of duty. It is enshrined in the professional requirement to treat service users with respect and dignity. Doing so will be in keeping with the recommended good practice of making underlying values explicit and in exposing myths and stereotypes within services. Neither should it be seen as a personal threat but as a means of working towards developing higher professional standards in future practice. A service which recognises and challenges racism will remove the image of agencies as instruments of state control and win the trust of the black community.

Consultation

It is essential to ensure that the full range of wants and needs of potential service users and their families are ascertained. A priority must, therefore, be to develop consultation mechanisms which do not ignore the views of black and ethnic minority communities. There will need to be a greater emphasis and confidence in working with, listening to and accepting the views of a wider range of people – balancing needs of the individual with those of the family and the long-term relationships between them. Black and ethnic minority groups and individuals with some knowledge and interest in particular areas of service provision should be specifically targeted. They will also need to be approached about community care plans *before* these are drawn up. Ways of consulting the community should be flexible enough to ensure that people are communicated to in their preferred language and that options for women and men meeting separately are made available if required. The following checklist will be instrumental in establishing good practice.

- What is the ethnic mix of your local population? This is now readily available through the 1991 census data.
- What are the local community languages spoken?
- How comprehensive and up-to-date are lists of local black and ethnic minority organisations?
- What attempts have been made to ensure people understand how the system of consultation works?
- Are publicity materials written in a user-friendly manner and translated into appropriate community languages?
- Has the information been disseminated and distributed widely and appropriately with a good lead-in-time to be useful to consumers?
- In publicising meetings and plans, is the local ethnic press and radio used?
- Are there opportunities for people to set their own agenda for meetings?

- Is the attitude of the chairperson to black and ethnic minority people, to consultation and to user involvement positive?
- What attempts are made to elicit the views of individuals who do not belong to groups or organisations or who do not attend meetings?
- Are funds made available to reimburse people who become involved in participation activities such as acting as advisors, consultants or as members of formal working groups?
- What mechanisms are in place for finding out from individuals and groups whether they found the process useful?

Residential and personal care

Attention also needs to be paid to these services used by the most vulnerable people, that is, those who need assistance in their daily lives through residential care. One area of great concern to black and ethnic minority families is whether staff are competent in providing for the physical care, hygiene and grooming needs of their relatives.

Personal hygiene is very important to a person's feeling of well-being and it is important that workers should be able to give appropriate attention to these areas. The preferred routines adopted at home should be followed, for example, showers and bidets being made available for those who prefer to wash in running water rather than baths.

Hair and skin care is still an area of gross neglect for black clients. Grooming of the client should be carried out to reflect cultural preference. This can be learnt from relatives. Support workers and care assistants will also need to appreciate that some people require their skin and hair to be moisturised, especially after procedures which deplete hair and skin moisture, for example, swimming or a bath. Where such procedures are neglected, this could lead to damage.

Religious and cultural requirements for modesty may mean that support workers of the same sex may be preferred when carrying out intimate forms of care.

Black service users will also need assistance in maintaining and developing their religious and cultural identity. There are basic standards to which service providers should consistently work:

- Clients should have the opportunity to have personal possessions which reflect their culture.
- Appropriate and preferred dress is important in helping service users to maintain personal appearance. For example, a support worker should be able to help Asian girls to wrap their saris or a young man to wrap his turban if this is their wish and that of their family.

- Service users should be encouraged and assisted to join organisations or attend events in their own communities. A support worker should be able to be involved with service users if this is necessary.
- Celebrating events such as Diwali, Chanukkah and Christmas will be an important part of many people's lives. Very little adjustment to services is needed to achieve this.
- Wall-hangings, toys for children (such as dolls), books, television programmes and other artefacts should reflect a multiracial society. Videos from most ethnic minority communities are now widely available and would be helpful. Golliwogs and books and other artefacts which portray negative images of black people should be removed.
- The service user's religious beliefs (if any) should be established and respected. Assistance to make available places for those who may wish to practice their religion should be given. Mosques, Afro-Caribbean churches and Sikh gudwaras and temples are welcoming to anyone who wishes to support members of their communities.
- Catering arrangements should ensure the availability of a choice and range of foods to suit individual preferences. This should include those normally eaten at home. For example, vegetarian, halal and kosher meals should be available if required.
- Service users should be encouraged to speak in their first language and be assisted in finding situations where this is possible.
- Play and learning expriences and other daily routines for adults should be of sufficient variety to promote positive identification with their own racial and cultural background.

Ways forward for purchasers and providers

There are clear tensions between a moral stance that emphasises rights and entitlements and an organisational and managerial approach concerned with efficient delivery of services in a climate of restricted resources. There is, however, no necessary conflict between the two, rather the reverse, since cost effectiveness requires that money should be spent on services that people want rather than those they do not. Today greater efficiency and effectiveness are essential in any evaluation of services. The absence of a race equality perspective may well mean that scarce resources are being applied inappropriately and thus wasted.

There are a number of practical suggestions which, if implemented, would enhance the quality of community services to people from black and ethnic minority communities. Nadirshaw (1993) summarises what purchasers and providers need to do:

- Acknowledge and validate the role of black and minority ethnic voluntary

organisations who offer a more holistic service and enable such organisations to negotiate a contract.

- Consult black and ethnic minority users, carers and service providers by
  organising groups for the discussion of planning and resource issues.
- Provide information about services to black and ethnic minority communities and plan future service provision from the norms and values of
  black and ethnic minority users.
- See that the criteria for assessment are specified by people with appropriate training, awareness, understanding and knowledge of the needs of
  black and ethnic minority people with learning difficulties.
- Be responsible for providing specialist training in assessment tools and
  techniques which do not label or strengthen stereotypical and prejudiced
  views about learning difficulties in black and ethnic minority communities.
- Acknowledge diverse and differing needs as an essential prerequisite for
  providing different community care services as opposed to the same
  approach adopted for the white indigenous population.
- Make specific recommendations for recruiting black and ethnic minority
  staff and incorporating equal opportunity policies.
- Recognise the need for and implement anti-racist and anti-discriminatory
  strategies for providing services. Provide anti-racist training for all staff
  responsible for designing and delivering care packages.
- Clarify statutory duties and legal responsibilities that service planners,
  care managers, providers and co-ordinators have for providing appropriate relevant, accessible and adequate services to black and ethnic minority
  people with learning difficulties.
- Make it mandatory for statutory agencies to assess in their local profiles
  the demographic statistics of black and ethnic minority communities and
  the way in which they access present service.
- Create a system that genuinely centres on black and minority ethnic
  groups' needs and preferences – and those of their carers – ensuring that
  available resources are targeted to those most in need and used effectively.
- Recommend participation by black and ethnic minority people with
  learning difficulties and their carers in the active monitoring and reviewing
  required for effective provision and delivery of community care services.

To adopt these measures would be to move toward services that meet
the current imperatives of cost effectiveness and efficiency, while
ensuring the dignity and well being of all citizens whatever their racial
or cultural background.

Acknowledgements

Some of the material in this chapter is based on information which first
appeared in *Double Discrimination. Issues and Services for People*

with Learning Difficulties from Black and Ethnic Minority Communities (see Baxter *et al.* in references). This publication was based on a research study project carried out from the Norah Fry Research Centre, University of Bristol, established in response to concern about the lack of information on good services for people with learning difficulties who came from those communities.

References

Ahmed, B. (1988). Community social work: Sharing the experience of ethnic groups. *Social Work Today*, 14 July, p. 13.

Alexander, P. (1987). *Racism, Resistance and Revolution*. Bookmarks, London.

Brown, C. (1984). *Black and White Britain. The Third PSI Survey*. Gower, Aldershot.

Baxter, C. (1987). Parallels between the social role perception of people with learning difficulties and black and ethnic minority people. In *Making Connections. Reflecting the Lives of People with Learning Difficulties* (eds A. Brechin and J. Walley). Hodder and Stoughton, London.

Baxter, C., Nadirshaw, Z., Poonia, K., and Ward, L. (1990). *Double Discrimination. Issues and Services for People with Learning Difficulties from Black and Ethnic Minority Communities*, King's Fund Centre/Commission for Racial Equality, London.

Chaudhury, A. (1988). How special is special? *Issue*, Spring.

Contact a Family (1989). *Reaching Black Families? A Study of Contact a Family in Lewisham and the Relevance of Services for Black Families who have Children with Learning Difficulties*, Contact a Family, London.

Dearnley, J. and Milner, I. (1986). *Ethnic Minority Development (Kirklees MDC)*. Social Services Inspectorate, Department of Health, London.

Dungate, M. (1984). *A Multicultural Society. The Role of National Voluntary Organizations*. Bedford Square Press, London.

Ferns, P. (1992). Promoting race equality through normalization. In *Normalization: A Reader for the 90s* (eds H. Brown and H. Smith) Routledge, London.

Gohil, V. (1987). DHSS service delivery to ethnic minority claimants. *Leicester Rights Bulletin*, June/July, No. 32.

Home Office (1977). *Racial Discrimination. A Guide to the Race Relations Act 1976*. Home Office, London.

Department of Health (1989). *Caring for People. Community Care in the Next Decade*, HMSO, London.

McNaught, A. (1985). *Race and Health Care in the United Kingdom. Occasional Paper 2*. Health Education Council, London.

Nadirshaw, Z. (1992). *Implications in the Assessment and Care Management of Black and Ethnic Minority People with Learning Difficulties and Their Carers. Occasional Paper No 2*. Boroughs Disability Resource Team, London.

Nzira, V. (1986). Race: The ingredients of good practice. In *The Residential Opportunity? The Wagner Report and After* (ed. T. Philpot) Reed Business Publishing/*Community Care*, Wallington.

Office of Population, Census and Surveys (1993). *Census Data 1991*. OPCS, London.

Pumphrey, P.D. and Verma, G.K. (editors) (1990). *Race Relations in Urban Education*. Falmer Press, Basingstoke.

Chapter 15

A woman's place?: Issues of gender

Dorothy Atkinson and Jan Walmsley

> There is a double jeopardy involved in being a woman and having a disability. Women with disabilities experience all the barriers that women in our society normally experience; in addition they endure the problems that people with disabilities face in their daily lives (Hutchinson *et al.*, 1992).

These are the views of three Canadian women with learning difficulties, expressed with the support of their adviser Peggy Hutchinson. We use this as the starting point of our chapter for two reasons: we are not only interested in *what* they say about their experiences as women with learning difficulties but also in *how* those views came to be aired. This chapter is based around the airing of women's views and indeed it could not have been written without the changes in recent years which have made it possible for women's voices to be heard.

The importance of listening to people with learning difficulties has been acknowledged relatively recently (Williams and Schoulz, 1982). The increasing readiness to listen has led to the beginnings of person-centred research where the lives and experiences of people with learning difficulties have been sought by researchers. We include ourselves in this process and draw, where we can, on our own work (Jan Walmsley's work on caring and Dorothy Atkinson's oral history work). There is, however, little research which directly features the lives of people with learning difficulties and there is even less documented about the specific experiences of *women*. We are introducing, therefore, a gender perspective to some of our own, and other people's research, in order to build a picture of how life was in the past for women, and how it is now.

The research cited here was not specifically designed to explore 'a woman's place' but, by bringing together personal accounts by women from several sources, it can at least begin the process of discovery. Wherever possible links are made with ideas developing both in the learning difficulties literature and more widely in feminist writing.

It is only in very recent years that the experiences of women with learning difficulties have begun to be differentiated from those of men. The traditional practice has been to generalise about 'people' with learning difficulties (Walmsley, 1993a) and focus on men's issues rather than those of women. Even the principle of normalisation, which has done much to highlight and counteract the devaluation of people – or men – with learning difficulties, has itself reinforced traditional sex roles which serve to maintain a woman's place as being in the home or in low paid work (Brown and Smith, 1992).

The danger of not addressing women's issues directly is that the policies and practices generated by normalisation may replicate the gender divisions of the wider world. This point is made by Williams, who suggests that although it may become easier for women to marry, and thus gain a measure of independence and status, nevertheless they may then enter 'a set of unequal personal relations in which they find themselves responsible for caring, cleaning, cooking and budgeting, or even subjected to violence and abuse' (Williams, 1992). While the dangers of women being confined to the private and domestic sphere have been highlighted (Brown and Smith, 1992), the recognition of the part played by women with learning difficulties as carers rather than, or as well as, people who are cared for, has been an important one (Williams, 1992; Walmsley, 1993b).

The recognition that women with learning difficulties share some of the experiences of women more generally in British society also points to some interesting contradictions, particularly in relation to caring. Feminist scholars have argued that the duties women assume as carers for children, older relatives and disabled offspring are often exploitative and exclude them from participation in society as citizens (Lister, 1990). On the other hand, being in a position to offer care to others can also be seen as something many women value as an expression of female identity (Graham, 1983). Although caring can be a means by which (non-disabled) women enter the public world these opportunities do not necessarily transfer to women with learning difficulties. Indeed, they may well find that informal and domestic caring at home effectively traps them in the private sphere (Williams, 1992).

What do women with learning difficulties themselves say about their 'place' in the world? We draw together a number of personal accounts by women, taken from recent research, which begin to tell us about their lives. As none of this research was designed to find out specifically about women's experiences (that task remains to be done) we are adding that gender dimension. We take an historical view, as well as a contemporary one, because we want to look at the continuities, and the differences, between women's experiences then and now. The current interest in biographical research has given us, and other researchers, a *means* to find out about people's past and present lives. In this chapter we focus on two important areas of women's life; relationships and work.

We start with relationships because this is where differences between women and men have been noted:

> Men, it seemed, were more at ease with the chronological life-story approach which chronicled the main changes in their lives and how they felt about them; whereas women's stories often seemed to be about people who mattered and their relationships with them, rather than a systematic account of life events. (Atkinson and Williams, 1990).

This gender difference in the presentation of personal testimonies is not confined to women and men with learning difficulties as it is a trend noted more generally by oral historians (Thompson, 1988).

Relationships

The switch, in recent years, from institutionalisation and segregation to a policy of community care has had a major impact on the relationships described by women with learning difficulties. At first sight this seems entirely beneficial though the reality, as we see below, is quite complicated.

The institutional era was characterised by the loss of, or rejection by, families at the time of admission and by strict separation of the sexes within the institutions. Although the explicit policy, in the early days of the development of the colonies, was the *protection* of people with learning difficulties the practice, in relation to women was to prevent sexual relationships which might result in the birth of unwanted and possibly defective children. Thomson (1992) shows that the Mental Deficiency Act 1913 targeted girls as a sexual problem, and that once they were institutionalised they often stayed for life. The Act led to the separation of many thousands of people from their families in an attempt to curb what was seen as a threat to society, particularly by women with learning difficulties who were widely regarded as over-fertile, promiscuous and the likely bearer of defective offspring:

> Feeble-minded women are almost invariably immoral and, if at large, usually become carriers of disease, or give birth to children who are as defective as themselves. The feeble-minded women who marries is twice as prolific as the normal woman. (Fernald, 1912).

Separation from families could come in childhood as well as in later life but, whenever it came, the effect was devastating. In the words of Margaret (quoted in Atkinson, 1993): 'When I was a little girl, I was put away. I was 14 and a half. I went to Cell Barnes to live because they said I was backward.'

Jackie (quoted in Atkinson and Williams, 1990) said: 'I got a mam but she's abandoned me. Put me in the courts. My dad and mam split up. It's all in the record book.'

While Doreen suffered the loss of a child: 'I moved to Northgate, I was 20. I had a bairn . . . a baby. He died.' (Quoted in Atkinson and Williams, 1990). Elizabeth's comments (quoted in Potts and Fido, 1991) were: 'I didn't go home 'cos they knew I was in trouble – they knew what had come. When I did go home, she [mother] said, "If you are having a child," she says, "I won't have neither the child nor you near me doorstep".'

One purpose of the long-stay institutions was to regulate contact between the sexes, thereby preventing the development of sexual relations between women and men (Potts and Fido, 1991). This strict segregation of the sexes is described by Elizabeth, Margaret and Grace, older women who remember how these practices had impinged on them (quoted in Potts and Fido, 1991):

> I just say, 'What's up with this place?' when I first came and you couldn't talk to any o' lads. 'Oh God!' I said to one o' lasses, 'Is this how you've been brought up – without talkin' t' lads?' (Elizabeth)

> We never used to talk to men in them days. Daren't even speak to them when we used to go to school. Don't know why. The girls were on one side and the boys were on the other side. We daren't even talk to them. Daren't even look at them! (Margaret).

> All the girls used to have to sit on one side. You couldn't go near the boys. They were watching you. You were even watched when you went to dances or anywhere. (Grace).

Although these experiences were common it is important not to become pessimistic about the restricted lives led by women with learning difficulties and see them only as victims of an unjust system. To do so would be to ignore ways in which women themselves describe their lives. Despite the oppressive regimes of the colonies there is some evidence that people resisted the harsh regulations. Some women, for example, found ways to be with men, as Isobel told Jan Walmsley in a research interview (1991): 'I had me dress on, me and Brian used to go round the walls kissing and cuddling. Bloody sister comes round. You go up your ward, you go in there she says. Used to kiss and cuddle round the corner. Good, it was.'

Other women like Grace found their own ways around an otherwise inflexible institution: 'I did cabbage you see. And love letters were sent through cabbages; used to fold them up. They used to cut 'em in half, cabbages, and stick it together again. And when boys came in with their pot of tea in the morning there used to always be a letter underneath'. (quoted in Potts and Fido, 1991).

Sometimes it was possible for women to get their own back on staff as Isobel informed Jan Walmsley in an interview: 'She's terrible, sister, one day I went in the canteen, long time ago, stopped all me money for me work in the laundry, told me brother, he told Dr Fleming [medical superintendent], he rang up and Dr Fleming told me, he said, "don't worry about it Isobel, don't worry about it." So I got me money back and she got the sack.'

Even though people were moved around from ward to ward, as part of a deliberate institutional policy of separation (Potts and Fido, 1991), close friendships still developed in which women helped one another. Margaret, one of Potts and Fido's oral history group, helped the interviewer to understand her friend Brenda's speech by acting as her interpreter, an ability based on long years of living together. The practice of encouraging 'high grade' patients to care for 'low grades' may represent exploitation; it also gave some women an opportunity to form close relationships and contribute to the welfare of other people. In the words of Anna, when interviewed by Jan Walmsley: 'I used to be there at seven, dress 'em, some of 'em can't dress themself. I used to dress one of them, always the same one, yeh. I didn't mind doing it, no. I was down there before breakfast, then I came back have me breakfast, then I went back to him.' In the following extract (quoted from Potts and Fido, 1991), Grace talks about her sister's child: 'She only put her in the colony because she knew I were there and she knew that I should look after her. She were only 21 when she died. I used to go up every night to see her – put her to bed.'

These accounts remind us that even in such outwardly unpropitious circumstances women can still retain a sense of themselves as more than just victims. They are capable of resistance because, it seems, they possess a personal identity which is at variance with the label others have placed on them.

While admission to hospital, and complete separation from home and family are largely things of the past, it is possible that a different sort of segregated living is emerging through prolonged periods of living with ageing parents, or through life in hostels and group homes which in some ways emulate the nuclear family (Brown and Smith, 1992). Although sexual relationships and marriage are more likely for women with learning difficulties than they were, the division of labour in the home itself may reflect traditional sex roles and, in practice, motherhood often remains an unachievable goal (Williams, 1992). We will look, in turn, at the effects on their relationships of women's reported experiences of segregated living; traditional division of labour in the home; and the prevention or management of motherhood.

What opportunities are there for developing relationships in segregated settings, even where those settings are not long-stay institutions? The following accounts from women suggest that the nature and quality of relationships can be restricted through prolonged enclosure, not only within the family, but also in schools, hostels and group homes. (Quoted in Atkinson and Williams, 1990).

> I don't know how much money I've got. Mum does it for me. (Christine).

> When I was at school we always used to have to go in lines – like the army does. When the classes were finished we had to line up in two's. We got up at seven o'clock and made our own beds. The dormitories weren't brilliant. The food was mainly salads. Some of the girls were spiteful. (Susan).

> I went into St Lawrence's Hospital when I was small. It was horrible in there. Horrible grub and tatty clothes. Viv got me out of there and I went into a group home. It was horrible. I didn't like it at all because there were too many rows. (Carol).

Some women have moved from segregated settings to their own homes in the community, sharing with a partner or husband. Their experiences, as captured by Flynn (1989), often reflect the traditional division of labour between husbands and wives:

> He gives me the housekeeping money . . . he takes me out. If I haven't got any money left, he'll take me out for a packet of ciggies or a drink . . . He

used to help me with the shopping a lot, because I got cataracts on me eyes, I can't see. (Mrs Heaton).

I do the cooking in the kitchen and the washing . . . and cleaning and all that. (Mrs Sewell).

I spoils him . . . I bought him a new suit and then I gives him money for spending money, then I buy him cigs . . . then if he's short I gives him money. (Miss Greaves).

Motherhood for women with learning difficulties still tends to be discouraged. Where it occurs, it is strictly regulated. The following personal accounts by women (quoted in Atkinson and Williams, 1990) reflect both the external forces at work, and the internal, learnt, prohibitions which women carry with them.

Staff can have children. People like us need help. (Women's group member).

Babies are a lot of hard work. People like us might not be able to look after one. Babies wake up at night and cry. (Women's group member).

People like us don't have babies. No one in the centre does apart from staff. Some people have their stomachs taken out. (Women's group member).

We had a big meeting about us getting married. They said: 'Would epileptics like you want to get married?' We said we'd give it a go. Things have turned out very good. I know we won't have children but we still love each other. (Sue).

I have a kid aged $5\frac{1}{2}$ and I am a single parent. Social workers and headmaster, teacher, police and doctor all together talk about you and your child when they think there might be a family problem. They have a case conference and talk about you and your child. (Angie, quoted in Craft, 1993).

Although there are continuities between past and present, there are real differences too. One major difference is the opportunity to speak, and be listened to, but there are also more possibilities now at least for some women to be involved and active in a range of relationships. Friendship, for example, is celebrated (Richardson and Ritchie, 1989; Atkinson and Williams, 1990), and some of the leading lights in the advocacy movement are now women.

Work

Work is also important as it is a means by which we gain a sense of who we are, and how we are seen and see ourselves. Paid work carries with it at least the possibility of some degree of independence and autonomy – important issues particularly for women who have had few choices in their lives. Work for women with learning difficulties, however, in the present as well as in the past, tends to be low paid or unpaid, and is often domestic 'work' at home. This chapter looks at women's personal accounts of their working lives.

Finding real jobs is the aspiration of many women, and men, with learning difficulties. It was one of six major issues discussed at the Third International People First Conference in Canada in 1993: 'Delegates were united in calling for real jobs with proper wages.' (Booth and Booth, 1993). In many respects both women and men face similar difficulties in obtaining and keeping work which will give them financial autonomy and self-respect. Jobs are hard to come by, and the work that is available to people with learning difficulties is often low paid and low status. It is our purpose here to acknowledge that while these are problems shared by both women and men, there are particular issues for women.

It is easy to overlook the degree to which people with learning difficulties were expected to work in the past, particularly in the colonies (described by Thomson, 1992, as 'patient exploiting work regimes'). Indeed, it was officially recognised that their continuing viability depended upon the labour of patients:

> there is no objection to the creation of a class of paid patients who would be given definite responsibility and a regular wage but who would not rank as staff, and who would not be left in sole control of patients. (Letter dated 1935, quoted in Thomson 1992).

The extent to which patients were employed within the colonies can be demonstrated by reference to the annual reports made by the Board of Control on institutions. For example, in 1943 87 per cent of the patients at Bromham Hospital, Bedfordshire were employed on the day of the inspectors' visit.

There was a clear division of labour based on gender; 41 men were engaged on farm and garden work, and 14 on ward work. Of the women, 22 were employed in the laundry, five in the kitchens, 14 in the sewing room and nine on domestic work. The inspectors stated that women did not work outside, whilst some men were employed on local farms (Board of Control annual report on Bromham Hospital, 1943). These statistics are borne out by people's own memories. Irene, for example, remembers: 'In t'olden days I worked on a villa. Scrubbing on your hands and knees. I worked at night, till seven o'clock at night.' (quoted in Potts and Fido, 1991). Margaret's memories were similar (quoted from Atkinson, 1993): 'The sister on the ward didn't like me and I didn't like her. I was there 20 years and I was always scrubbing.' While Edna (quoted in Atkinson, 1993) remembers: 'I was at Leavesden Hospital. I used to polish and work at the nurses home.' Similar assumptions about the appropriateness of gender roles informed the development of adult training centres in the 1960s. Bramingham ATC, Luton, was founded in 1966. In reporting on its opening the Luton Society for Mentally Handicapped Children's 1967 annual report describes: 'the carpentry shop where boys are introduced to tools and given an awareness of danger'; 'the domestic training room where the curriculum [sic] states that groups of girls shall cook themselves a meal, wash clothes and do simple mending and ironing, shopping and budgeting'. If any adults who went to Bramingham were to find real jobs it is clear that their gender was expected to be a major determinant of the type of employment.

Contemporary oral evidence offers corroboration that women with learning difficulties find themselves at work within the private sphere of the home:

> When I was younger I lived with my mum. I used to scrub the floors – there were no hoovers in them days. I used to do all the cleaning outside my mum's house, on my hands and knees. You know, you used to scrub in them days. I got housemaids knee for it, using a scrubbing brush and soap. (Edna, quoted in Atkinson, 1993).

> It would be better if I did not have so much work to do at the hostel, because I wouldn't get so worn out. In ten years time I will be 42. I hope things will have changed. I would like to live in a flat with my boyfriend. We would be sharing the housework. (Member of women's group, quoted in Atkinson and Williams, 1990).

> Mum used to go to R Lodge [day hospital] and I used to come here every day. I looked after her you know when I came back from here. Bit of a bind but I had to do it. (Gwen, research interview with Wamsley, 1989).

We have been selective here, choosing quotations where women emphasise the burdens of domestic and caring work in the home. It is equally possible to demonstrate that women derive satisfaction from having a useful role to perform.

> My mum's done a lot for me, I always think I'm the worst one of the lot, but I'm not. I'm a great help to my mum with the cooking and the washing up. (Linda).

During the Easter holidays I was doing the housework for the whole two weeks, doing the shopping and cleaning, and it was good. It wasn't boring. It was something to do. (Anne Marie).

I like to do my housework. Sometimes Billy helps. I cook in my own slow cooker. I got it as a wedding present from the staff at the hospital . . . cook mince and chicken. Do shopping on Thursday mornings. (Jackie, quoted in Atkinson and Williams, 1990).

I help in the group home when there's only one member of staff on duty, help wash up, they say 'course you can'. Look after Kevin and Maggie when staff are busy. (Deirdre, research interview with Jan Wamsley, 1991).

These accounts help us to understand that the contradictions which beset many women in their work at home, as domestics and carers, also apply to some women with learning difficulties. Although caring is one way for women to find a place in society (Graham, 1983), it is often unpaid or underpaid, unnoticed, and relatively lacking in status. It is important to acknowledge that women with learning difficulties, like other women, vary in their response to such work. Our quotations show that some women felt oppressed and burdened by their domestic work, whilst others derived satisfaction from being able to look after themselves and people they are close to. The work may be the same, but the meanings individual women attach to it are different.

Women with learning difficulties, we contend, face particular pressures to conform to traditional gender roles in which they undertake domestic and caring work in the private sphere of the home. It is hard to be certain of this in the absence of much research which explores gender issues though Noonan Walsh's study of men and women in Ireland (1988) and Lonsdale's research into disabled women (1990) tends to substantiate our position.

Conclusion: a research agenda

There are two agendas emerging in relation to women's issues. On the one hand, there is now a climate in which the discussion of 'a woman's place' is increasingly recognised as important and valuable, and good practices are being developed in working with women with learning difficulties. On the other hand, while there is little research which directly addresses and reflects women's lives and experiences, the means for doing so are emerging through the growth of participative and reflective research methodologies. It is our hope that the two agendas can come together, so that practitioners can find the space and encouragement to write about their work with women, and qualitative researchers will use their methods to find out from women themselves about their lives and experiences. We hope this chapter will be a step in that developing process.

In terms of the practice agenda, there is a growing recognition that women with learning difficulties may not automatically share the interests of men with the same label. Turk and Brown's research (1992) into sexual abuse shows that women are more vulnerable than men, and that some abusers are men with learning difficulties. There is a growing recognition of the vulnerability of women service users to abuse in the development of policies on sexuality (Booth and Booth, 1992). Such policies can embrace more than just a recognition of women's vulnerability; they can also acknowledge that women have a right to choose leisure activities and voluntary or paid work which contravene sex stereotypes, with whatever support they need in exercising these choices.

Secondly, the idea of 'meaningful association' (Brown and Smith, 1992), which encourages women with learning difficulties to share experiences and ideas with other women, is gathering support. Women's groups are becoming more of a reality (Atkinson and Williams, 1990; Sutcliffe, 1991) and a Women First Conference was held in Nottingham in 1992. This was the first national conference for women with learning difficulties (Walmsley, 1993a) and was attended by 240 women from England and Wales. It provided a forum where women could meet others and begin to develop a sense that their issues were important. Many women said it was the first conference they had ever attended, and some left determined to continue the work by setting up groups in their own areas.

A third development is the appearance of women with learning difficulties as 'stars' or role models for others. These include women who have gained a public platform through self-advocacy, and can demonstrate that women can be influential. At the time of writing Young People First has two paid staff, a woman with Downs Syndrome and a woman adviser. People First also has a paid worker whose job it is to encourage women's groups to develop. Alice Etherington and Jackie Downer won the Norah Fry Research Centre *Community Care* Award in 1993 for outstanding work in advancing the cause of people with learning difficulties. These developments suggest that self-advocacy in the UK has moved from its earlier reliance on male role models to encompass women and women's issues.

In terms of a future research agenda, more work needs to be done on the oppression of women, both in the past and in the present, and on women's strengths both then and now. We have quoted examples of women's work in caring for others; their resistance to oppressive regimes; and their support for one another. Research which illustrates the importance of personal identity, and which shows how women retain a sense of self in the face of conditions of life which appear from the outside to be overwhelmingly negative, has a place on any future agenda.

Williams (1992) makes the point that women with learning difficulties are women too. This reminder of shared concerns and commonalities between women is echoed more widely in the disability field. Morris (1991; 1993), Begum (1992) and Keith (1992), in the wider disability field, have shown that feminists have largely ignored the interests of disabled women. This may also be true of women with learning difficulties. In this chapter we have tried to show that while women with learning difficulties have some things in common with other women, they confront an additional set of oppressive barriers to full participation in society. Research on this aspect of 'a woman's place' would also be on a future agenda.

In recent years it has become possible to seek out, and portray, the views of people with learning difficulties. This chapter has drawn together women's accounts from a variety of sources where biographical research methods have been used. The next step is to use those methods to focus on the experiences of women and to involve women actively in the design, implementation and dissemination of the research. Only then do we begin to find out not just what a woman's place is but the means by which she may change it now and in the future.

Acknowledgements

We wish to thank Fiona Williams for her comments on an earlier draft of this chapter and to thank the participants from our respective research projects.

References

Atkinson, D. (1993). *Past Times*, Private publication, revised edition.
Atkinson, D. and Williams, F. (eds) (1990). *'Know Me As I Am' An Anthology

of Prose, Poetry and Art by People with Learning Difficulties. Hodder and Stoughton, Sevenoaks.

Begum, N. (1992). Disabled Women and the feminist agenda. *Feminist Review*, **40**, 70–84.

Board of Control (1943). *Annual Report on Bromham Hospital.* Filed in Mental Deficiency Papers (MDP) 27, Bedford County Record Office.

Booth, T. and Booth, W. (1992). Practice in sexuality. *Mental Handicap*, **20**(2), 64–69.

Booth, T. and Booth, W. (1993). A celebration of stories. *Community Living*, October, pp. 14–15.

Brown, H. and Smith, H. (1992). Assertion, not assimilation: a feminist perspective on the normalisation principle. In *Normalisation. A Reader For the Nineties* (eds H. Brown and H. Smith). Tavistock/Routledge, London.

Craft, A. (1993). *Parents with Learning Disabilities, BILD Seminar Paper No. 3.* British Institute of Learning Disabilities, Kidderminster.

Fernald, W.E. (1912). The burden of feeble mindedness. *Journal of Psycho-Asthenics*, **17**, 87–111.

Flynn, M.C. (1989). *Independent Living for Adults with Mental Handicap: A Place of My Own.* Cassell, London.

Graham, H. (1983). Caring: a labour of love. In *A Labour of Love: Women, Work and Caring* (eds J. Finch and D. Groves). Routledge and Kegan Paul, London.

Hutchinson, P., Nith Beeckey, L., Foerster, C. and Fowke, S. (1992). Double jeopardy: women with disabilities speak out about community and relationships. *Entourage*, **7**(2), 16–18.

Keith, L. (1992). Who cares wins? Women, caring and disability. *Disability, Handicap and Society*, **7**(2), 167–176.

Lister, R. (1990). Women, economic dependency and citizenship. *Journal of Social Policy*, **19**, 445–467.

Lonsdale, S. (1990). *Women and Disability.* Macmillan, Basingstoke.

Luton Society for Mentally Handicapped Children (1967). *Annual Report.* Luton Society for Mentally Handicapped Children, Luton.

Morris, J. (1991). *Pride against Prejudice.* The Women's Press, London.

Morris, J. (1993). Feminism and disability. *Feminist Review*, **43**, 57–70.

Noonan Walsh, P. (1988). Handicapped and female: two disabilities? In *Concepts and Controversies in Services for People with Mental Handicap* (eds R. McConkey and F. McGinley). Woodlands Centre and St Michael's House, Dublin.

Potts, M. and Fido, R. (1991). *A Fit Person To Be Removed.* Northcote House, Plymouth.

Richardson, A. and Ritchie, J. (1989). *Developing Friendships: Enabling People with Learning Difficulties to Make and Maintain Friends.* Policy Studies Institute, London.

Sutcliffe, J. (1991). *Adults with Learning Difficulties: Education for Choice and Empowerment.* NIACE and Open University Press, Buckingham.

Thompson, P. (1988). *The Voice of the Past. Oral History.* Second Edition. Oxford University Press, Oxford.

Thomson, M. (1992). *The Problem of Mental Deficiency in England and Wales c. 1913–1946*, unpubl. PhD thesis, Oxford.

Turk, V. and Brown, H. (1992). Sexual abuse and adults with learning disabilities. *Mental Handicap*, **20**(2), 56–63.

Walmsley, J. (1993a). Women First: Lessons in participation. *Critical Social Policy*, **38**, Autumn 1993, 89–99.

Walmsley, J. (1993b). Contradictions in caring: Reciprocity and interdependence. *Disability, Handicap and Society*, **8**(2), 129–141.

Walmsley, J. (1994). *Gender, Caring and Learning Disability*. PhD in progress, Open University, Milton Keynes.

Williams, F. (1992). Women with learning difficulties are women too. In *Women, Oppression and Social Work. Issues in Anti-Discriminating Practice*, Routledge, London.

Williams, P. and Schoulz, B. (1982). *We Can Speak for Ourselves* (eds M. Langan and L. Day). Souvenir Press, London.

Chapter 16

What kind of future? Opportunities for older people with a learning difficulty

Carol Walker, Alan Walker and Tony Ryan

One of the most important gains resulting from the social and economic development of the UK in the 20th century has been the increased longevity of its citizens. It has been virtually unnoticed by policy makers that this advantage of longer life is also shared by people with learning difficulties.

This chapter draws on the research we have recently completed on older people with learning difficulties in the north west of England. Our starting point is the general policy and service background against which good practice must be forged.

Although exact data on the number of older people in this group are hard to come by, the Department of Health has estimated that, in 1991, 47 per cent of people with learning difficulties were 45 or over and 17 per cent were 65 or over. Unfortunately, as far as the political debate is concerned the growing numbers of older people are frequently presented as a 'problem' – an economic 'burden' that the rest of the population has to carry, and a 'burden' which, it is claimed, the nation can ill-afford. This 'burden' is said to fall mainly on the health and social services, as well as on the social security system (Walker, 1990).

This extremely negative response to the triumph of population ageing is caused by, and gives rise to, organisational age discrimination or ageism. In the UK successive governments have consistently made assumptions about the inevitability of physical and mental decline in old age, arguing that it is a normal part of the ageing process. As a consequence the *additional* needs of older people with disabilities have not been recognised in the form of special social security benefits. Similar ageist or age discriminatory attitudes are common within social services, though they are usually covert. For example, it is commonplace for the needs of older people to be played down compared with those of children.

Within this context of overstretched resources and a long-standing bias against older people in service provision, a place must now be found for older people with learning difficulties – one of the least powerful and least vocal of user groups. With the emergence of growing numbers of older people with learning difficulties, there is a need for social service provision to bridge the gap between services aimed at older people and those for people with learning difficulties. Traditionally, these two sets of services have been segregated, and in some areas, there is a reluctance for services for older people to be opened up to those with learning difficulties. There have also been important differences in the way in which services for the two groups have developed.

In provision for older people the idea of a service continuum has prevailed – progressing from domiciliary care to day care to residential care. This in-built assumption of the inevitability of decline is ageist in conception; it is also contrary to many developments in service provision for people with learning difficulties. Despite a recent government emphasis on community care provision, considerable numbers of older people are still cared for in residential settings. During the 1980s moreover, there was a massive expansion in private residential provision for this group. Within the learning difficulties field, however, there has been an accelerating trend away from large, long-term institutional care towards small-scale living in the community. This has been underpinned by the principles of normalisation and the idea of enabling people with learning difficulties to lead 'an ordinary life', within and as part of local communities (see for example Towell, 1988).

There is an uncertainty however in both theory and practice, over precisely what an ordinary life means for older people, with the result that services and service providers tend to concentrate on the need to *care for* older people rather than to *support* them in independent living. Research by Hogg *et al.* (1988) has shown that older people with learning difficulties receive fewer opportunities in the community than younger ones, not as a result of lower functional capacity, but merely because of their age.

Fragmentation of service provision

Organisational fragmentation – the separation of service provision between different professional specialisms; for example the traditional distinction in health and social services between services for older people and those for people with disabilities, including learning difficulties has helped to create 'double jeopardy' for older people with learning difficulties (Sweeney *et al.*, 1979); they are inadequately served by both services for older people and those for people with learning difficulties. At present much mainstream provision for older people does not address the special needs of people with learning difficulties. For example, recent research we conducted in the North West Health Region (Walker *et al.*, 1993), found that some day centres for older people refused to accept people with learning difficulties. Six months after their move out of hospital into the community, none of the people with learning difficulties aged over 50 that we spoke to were using existing community facilities for older people, such as lunch clubs or day centres.

If older people with learning difficulties are not accepted into mainstream services for older people, then their segregation from other members of the community is exacerbated. However, caution must be exercised with regard to the proposal to offer older people with learning difficulties the same services that are provided for other older people (House of Commons Social Service Committee, 1985). On the one hand people with learning difficulties may be given entirely inappropriate services by, for example, grouping them together with those suffering from Alzheimer's Disease and, on the other hand, there is the risk that the specific needs of this group become submerged in those of the much larger group of older people and so become invisible. Any widening in the scope of services for older people to enable them to include older people with learning difficulties must be undertaken with special care to avoid alienating other service users and to prevent the ghettoisation of *all* older people. The success of this policy would depend on services for older people being adequately resourced to meet the different or extra needs of people with learning difficulties.

From the late 1980s onwards, and even before the government's push to accelerate the closure of long-stay hospitals, there was an established trend towards moving people with learning difficulties into the community. The North West Regional Health Authority produced a widely respected and pioneering strategy to shift from hospital-based to community-based services, which was published as *Services for People who are Mentally Handicapped: A Model District Service* (NWRHA, 1983). By the end of this decade over 2600 people with learning difficulties will have been moved out from the region's large long-stay hospitals into the community; a substantially better record than many other Regions (Collins, 1993). Research which we conducted to monitor this formidable undertaking (Walker *et al.*, 1993) showed that, despite imperfections and the need for further improvement and development, the transition enabled people to have a far higher quality of life than that offered previously by institutional care. Considerable effort was made by the researchers to obtain the views of the movers themselves and no one wanted to go back to hospital. Similarly positive outcomes have been found elsewhere (see, for example, Korman and Glennerster, 1990; Booth *et al.*, 1990).

This improvement in quality of life occurred: regardless of the level of dependency, regardless of the length of institutional living and regardless of age. However, the research did reveal discrimination against older people both at the point of resettlement and in the support and care they received after resettlement. Although the North West Regional Health Authority's strategy for community service provision for people with learning difficulties stressed that age should not be a barrier to resettlement from hospital, in practice older people were under-represented in the numbers who moved out. This disparity had been noted in an earlier study conducted in the same region by Hogg *et al.* (1988). Our research found that the average age of the people who moved out between March 1990 and March 1991 was 47.4 compared to an average age of the hospital population of 53. With the impending closure of all large long-stay hospitals, it is obvious that receiving health districts and local authorities cannot defer indefinitely their responsibility for older people with learning difficulties. Furthermore, any older people who might be reluctant to move will not be able to avoid this major life change.

Not surprisingly older people with learning difficulties tend to have lived in long-stay institutions for longer than younger people. Thirty-five out of 37 people aged over 50 in our sample had lived in an institution for 20 years or more, six out of ten had been there for 30 years or more. This is partly a reflection of age but also of the different admissions policies of earlier decades when admission to hospitals was made for the variety of social reasons, including homelessness and social stigma. As a consequence, although the older people in our sample were more likely to have a physical disability or long-term illness, they were *less* dependent than those under 50 in other aspects of everyday living. More were able to feed, wash and dress themselves independently or with only some supervision. The older group also tended to have better communication skills. There was little difference between the older and younger groups in their ability to shop and handle and understand money, but this was more a reflection of the impact of institutional living on everyone – with few opportunities to use and little necessity to acquire such skills – than an age difference. Despite this, the research on older people with learning difficulties we are currently undertaking for the Joseph Rowntree Foundation has revealed that care workers tend to *assume* that, while older people have the same level of need as younger people, the nature of those needs is different. For example, they reported that older people have higher physical and care needs but lower social needs than younger people. This seems to reflect ageist assumptions about what older people can and should do. In the words of one care worker: 'If you're younger you might need a lot of support to do things but older people need more care really. It's different.'

Thus, the greater personal competence of the older people in our sample contrasts with the opportunities given to them and the expectations made of them by support workers in the community. The first disparity in treatment between the younger and older age groups was found in assessments of the need for training. Care workers in the community reported that over four-fifths of older people (compared to three-quarters of younger people) would benefit from some training. However, only 49 per cent of older people had received or were receiving any training in the six months since resettlement, compared to 70 per cent of the younger age group. Thus, although more older people seemed to be in need of training, fewer were receiving it. Furthermore, the type of training provided also differed according to age; the need for speech therapy was the training need identified most frequently for the older group although, overall, their speech was better than that of the younger group whereas road safety topped the list for the younger people. Comments by hospital personnel working with people about to be resettled showed that they too seemed to identify different needs for older than young people and that these reflected a stereotypical dichotomy between the two groups. They suggested that, on resettlement, younger people would have benefited from improved educational and employment provision, while those over 50 needed better transport and outside recreational facilities. Not surprisingly then, two-fifths of the younger group were attending an adult education or other college compared to only a quarter of the older group. Twice as many in the younger group were receiving music or art therapy when compared to the older group. When two-thirds of this sample were interviewed more than two years later, there was little change. Only one-third of people over 60 were receiving any training at all, while all of those under the age of 50, and all but three of the 17 in the 50–59 age group were receiving some form of training.

Implicitly hospital and care workers seemed to operate an informal 'retirement policy' for both men and women which led to a concentration on support and skills development for the younger group but on care and recreation for older people. Care workers seemed to have lower expectations both of older people's ability to learn and of how much they needed to learn. One said of the 64 year old with whom he worked that he needed training but 'it was difficult because of his age'. The availability of adequate care and support was sometimes put forward as an alternative to training. Speaking of one mover aged 62, the care worker said: 'When she first arrived Joan had some basic skills, with some assistance. Those that she didn't have were not a problem because we were here to look after her'. Speaking of a man aged 69, another care worker said: 'I don't think Alistair's skills are at issue because he receives full support from staff'.

Such sentiments, while reassuring in terms of the level of care provided, do not help people to move towards greater independence. Indeed, they are counterproductive because they are based on the ageist assumption that old age is automatically associated with dependency. In the current Joseph Rowntree Foundation-funded research, we have again found that care workers have lower expectations of older people, regardless of their level of disability. All of the care staff working with younger people felt that they would be able to do more for themselves in the future, but almost half of the people working with older service users (some of whom were as young as 50) thought that there would be no improvement in the future and that some would be able to do less. Some care workers seemed to accept that older people had reached a plateau in their capabilities and level of functional capacity and could not be expected to make further progress. One said: 'I don't think we've got the staff and her age is something that holds her back. I mean the disabilities that come with age. For instance she's getting in and out of the bath OK at the moment, but we can foresee problems.' Another commented: 'I think Frank has reached the point where he won't really learn any more; it's his age.' In the first case, the assumption had already been made that this woman would experience increasing disability even though there was no evidence for reaching this conclusion at the present time.

Such discrimination against older people exists at an institutional as well as at an individual level, with the result is that older people with learning difficulties lose out all round. For example: 'Janet's keyworker would say that she should not be set goals because she is too old. I don't agree with this. I think everybody should have the chance. Also with the day centres, she's too old to go to a day centre for people with learning disability, but at the over 60s club they don't want her around because of her disability.' Another person said: 'Younger people look upon older people as being past it, with being disabled as well they get kicked into touch.' A care worker told us: 'People react to older people so when they have learning disability it must be twice as bad. They think both groups should be locked up.'

In our research in the North West, older people with learning difficulties also lost out in terms of structured day activities. While this was an issue of concern with regard to all age groups, older people fared particularly badly. Only two of the 15 people over 60 we interviewed had any organised day activity and that was for only one half day session per week. One of the reasons for the reduced participation of people over 60 lies in that fact that many day centres effectively operate 'retirement' policies, the cut-off point being 60. With a general lack of day centre places for older people there is a very obvious service gap. In one local further education college, places are geared towards the under 60s and age is an important criterion for entry. At least one man in our sample was refused a place on the course because he was over 60.

At a time of limited, and often inadequate resources, there is a danger that age will be used as a rationing criterion. It might be deemed more cost-effective to give younger people higher priority in the allocation of speech therapy services or educational opportunities which, even in adult education services, traditionally have been skewed towards the lower end of the age spectrum. However, because older people with learning difficulties will probably have been confined to an institution for longer periods than younger people, the reality may well be that they need, and would benefit most from, preferential treatment to compensate for their extra years of social disadvantage.

Re-institutionalisation

Such ageist attitudes and policies in the provision of services to older people threatens the extent to which older people with learning difficulties will benefit from the 'ordinary life' model. Not only is there sometimes greater reluctance to resettle older people from institutions; but there is a greater willingness in the medium or longer term to yet again exclude them from independent living. Preliminary findings from our current research in the North west, which gathered information approximately three years after resettlement, seem to indicate that older people's nursing or residential homes are considered as an acceptable option as people with learning difficulties get older. For example, one woman in the sample had already moved from her new home in the community to a residential home; and an older man was scheduled to make a similar move. The model district service (NWRHA, 1982) which sets down strict guidelines for the care of people with learning difficulties in the community, allows resettlement to residential or nursing homes only in exceptional circumstances, but in practice there is little to prevent re-institutionalisation after the initial resettlement.

In both of the above cases the move was justified by changes in the needs of the individual concerned: both were said to have become more dependent and to require 'care' rather than 'support'. Implicit in this approach is that the values of normalisation should be applied differently to older people. Residential care is considered an acceptable option for older people, when it would not be so for younger people, even where the level of dependency is similar. It is argued that such changes in people's living situations are appropriate: it is what happens to many older people as they become more frail, and the type of 'care' provided by residential or nursing homes will meet their needs more adequately. However, the philosophy of nursing homes is quite different to the principles of normalisation proselytised for people with learning difficulties. They are institutions whose role is only to care, and which therefore encourage and foster dependence rather than independence; where even the most basic decisions, such as when and what to eat, are taken away from people. This tendency to reinstitutionalise older people with learning difficulties seems to result from push rather than pull factors. The practice is, or could be, the response to inadequate staffing or levels of support in the community. Re-institutionalisation may be seen as a valid (not to mention an easy) response at a time of austerity in local services. In the light of a learning difficulties philosophy based on ordinary living, it is a strategy that is blatantly age discriminatory.

The development of a more coherent policy and one that reflects the needs of older people with learning difficulties, is unlikely to occur in the present context of provider domination. Currently, in the health and social services, definitions of need and the forms of service provision that are designated as suitable responses to identified need are determined primarily by the service purchasers and providers rather than the service users. Increasingly doctors and social services staff serve as the gate-keepers to services which, despite the rhetoric of the NHS and Community Care Act, inevitably puts the allocation of scarce resources before the needs of the individual. In the past such services have done little to give real power to the user. In such a system, people with learning difficulties are particularly disadvantaged. Of the 102 people we interviewed in the North west, a region which has given a very high profile to provision for people with learning difficulties, not one was in touch with a citizen's advocacy project or anything of a similar nature. Older people with learning difficulties are even more disadvantaged than younger people because they have often been isolated from the community longer and because they are less likely to have relatives who can speak on their behalf.

Even where there is an available relative, feelings of guilt in response to their own inability to care for their loved one, or of gratitude to service providers – almost regardless of the type of care provided – may make them unable or reluctant to challenge the views of welfare professionals. The role and response of families to new plans and services for their relatives is often seen in a negative light, as a conservative rather than a progressive force (Ward, 1990). The North west research found that this stemmed largely from fear and uncertainty about the outcome of change. If they were kept fully informed, and most importantly, if the package of care offered was adequate, then even those with reservations at the outset were very positive after the move into the community.

Positive futures

If older people with learning difficulties are to have positive futures, then, as an essential starting point, the implicit age discrimination that regards older people with learning difficulties as having lesser needs than younger ones should be tackled, root and branch, within all service provision agencies. A key aim of training and service guidelines would be to ensure that age is not a basis for discriminatory decisions that limit the potential of people with learning difficulties. Each person should be treated as an individual with special needs; some of which may be age-related. Service providers must break down their own prejudices and age-based stereotypes (as they have been encouraged to do with regard to race and gender) and see what progress can be made towards each individual achieving the central tenets of the 'ordinary life' philosophy: participating in the community, increasing competence, exercising individual choice, gaining self-esteem and sustaining and widening friendships (Towell, 1988).

Those involved in the planning and provision of services for older people and those responsible for services for people with learning difficulties need to join together on a regular basis to see what they can learn from each other. They need to seek out creative ways of enabling older people with learning difficulties to get the best, not the minimum and certainly not the worst, of both service sectors. Principles which might form the starting point for such a dialogue are:

- Older people and people with learning difficulties are individuals. Services must reflect that individuality and respond to individual needs. Stereotyping on the basis of age or disability is as unacceptable as doing so on the basis of race or gender.
- All older people with learning difficulties should be involved in a regular review of their care and support package, such as an individual programme plan. Service users should be enabled to express their own needs, and service providers should respond flexibly and creatively to those needs. The main goal of the review process should be to promote the independence of the individual, even if there is a growing need for care; the need for the latter should not mean the abandonment of the former.
- Older people have a right to training and skills development just as much as younger people with learning difficulties. The idea that older people need not or cannot learn new skills is false. Age should not be a factor in determining whether or not somebody is offered the chance to become more independent.
- Older people should be offered recreational and occupational activities. Assumptions about their ability to participate in or their interest in such

activities should not be restricted by ageist stereotypes. Individuals can only exercise choice if real alternatives are made available.

• Older people should remain in and be part of the community. Admission to residential care should not be considered only on grounds of age. Neither age nor disability should lead to segregation from the rest of the community.

Unfortunately the long-standing assumptions underlying services for older people have tended to work in the opposite direction to the strategy proposed above. Policies have separated and isolated older people from the community and taken away choice by fostering dependence rather than independence. There is a real danger that the service response to older people with learning difficulties will reinforce the double jeopardy they face (if racial disadvantage is added to this, it becomes triple jeopardy). The imposition of an arbitrary 'retirement age' on people with learning difficulties, few of whom have had any meaningful contact with the labour market, merely provides an excuse to reduce services. Thus, the positive and developing philosophy of an 'ordinary life' for a younger person with a learning difficulty gives way to the isolation and withdrawal from community which is the lot of many older people.

If the age discrimination implicit in many aspects of service provision is overlaid with the cost-efficiency imperative underlying the implementation of the NHS and Community Care Act, the result will be that older people with learning difficulties will not be given the opportunity to experience an 'ordinary life'.

The alternative is for the positive developments that have been made with regard to community living for people with learning difficulties to be continued into older life. If services are organised in ways that enable users to articulate their own needs and if service providers respond flexibly to these, rather than fitting people into pre-existing categories, then services for all older people will be enhanced.

References

Booth, T., Simons, K. and Booth, W. (1990). *Outward Bound: Relocation and Community Care for People with Learning Difficulties*, Open University Press, Milton Keynes.

Collins, J. (1993). *The Resettlement Game: Policy and Procrastination in the Closure of Mental Handicap Hospitals*, Values into Action, London.

Hogg, J., Moss, S. and Cooke, D. (1988). *Ageing and Mental Handicap*, Croom Helm, London.

House of Commons Social Services Committee (1985). *Community Care*, HC-1. HMSO, London.

Korman, N. and Glennerster, H. (1990). *Hospital Closure*, Open University Press, Milton Keynes.

North West Regional Health Authority (1982). *Services for People who are Mentally Handicapped: A Model District Service*. North West Regional Health Authority.

Sweeney, D. P. and Wilson, T. Y. (eds) (1979). *Double Jeopardy: The Plight of Aging and Aged Developmentally Disabled Persons in Mid-America*. University of Michigan, Ann Arbor.

Towell, D. (ed.) (1988). *An Ordinary Life In Practice Developing Comprehensive Community-Based Services for People with Learning Disabilities*, King's Fund, London.

Walker, A. (1990). The economic 'burden' of ageing and the prospect of intergenerational conflict. *Ageing and Society*, **10**, 377–396.

Walker, C., Ryan, T. and Walker, A. (1993). *Quality of Life After Resettlement*, North Western Regional Health Authority.

Ward, L. (1990). A programme for change: Current issues in services for people with learning difficulties. In *Better Lives: Changing Services for People with Learning Difficulties* (ed. T. Booth). University of Sheffield/ Community Care.

Chapter 17

Self-advocacy and inclusion: Supporting people with profound and multiple disabilities

Helen Sanderson

There is a definite need to better view the world from the perspective of an individual with profound handicaps and 'walk in their shoes' so to speak. By doing this, service providers may find that the goals and objectives, no matter how noble, might not be all that important to individuals with profound handicaps, if they could only more expressively communicate. In fact, quality of life for persons with profound handicaps might consist of greater opportunities to express their own preferences, likes and dislikes (Guess, 1989).

The essence of self-advocacy is being able to exert some control and influence over your life, and at a basic level this will involve indicating needs and desires, rejecting and refusing things, and making choices that matter. Self-advocacy and developing close, mutual relationships are key issues in the quality of people's lives. People who live in the same neighbourhood, share the same leisure activities, attend the same colleges, and work together are more likely to make acquaintances that lead to friendships (Hartup, 1975; Howes, 1983; Richardson and Ritchie, 1989). Just living in the community is not enough (Le Touze and Pahl, 1992; Ward and Kinsella, 1993). This chapter focusses on encouraging self-advocacy, supporting choice and discovering a positive future for people through circles of support and person-centred planning. These futures will involve including people who are labelled as having profound and multiple disabilities in communities, as work colleagues, neighbours, students and friends. This involves substantial changes to service provision and staff training, and begins with learning to listen to the slightest indications of preference and choice.

Self-advocacy: learning to listen

Everyone communicates. The challenge is to develop skills in recognising people's individual styles of communication, responding to them, and offering opportunities to make meaningful choices. Fitton (1994) describes how her daughter Kathy:

> communicated with us all by eye contact and a facial language of frowns, bad looks, smiles and raised eyebrows . . . She threw objects towards one that was out of reach, to show us she wanted us to fetch it; it took us years to realise that this was communication, not being awkward . . . People with severe learning disabilities go on trying to communicate in the face of constant frustration, misunderstanding and ignorance.

When a staff team support an individual it is easy to assume that everyone has the same understanding of how the person communicates. This is often not the case: in one study staff missed or misunderstood two-thirds of non-verbal communication (Campbell and Wilcox, 1986). There are several ways of identifying the individual's unique communication style so that people can be consistent in their understanding and response to it. *The Affective Communication Assessment* (Coupe *et al.*, 1985; 1988; Goldbart *et al.*, 1994) can be helpful, and video can be used to record people's responses to different experiences. *Assessing Communication Together* (Bradley, 1991) is also a very useful assessment.

Augmentative communication

When staff know how someone responds to positive and negative experiences, the individual can be enabled to communicate more clearly and effectively by using augmentative communication. This is the use of gestures, objects, signs or symbols (Baumgart, 1990; Kearns, 1993). An example of this is using objects of reference to help people develop an association between an activity and an object that naturally relates to it. This may involve giving the person car keys whenever they are going out, or a favourite essential oil to smell before a massage session. Depending on the person's abilities, the use of sounds of activities or pictures could also be useful references to help the individual to understand what is about to happen, and at a basic level indicate if they do not want it to continue (Kearns, 1993; MENCAP, 1994).

All behaviours can become communicative and people can learn to associate a particular movement with a particular response (response contingent learning). For example, staff can consistently offer a drink when the person makes a specific movement with their mouth, and by association, the person may eventually use this movement as a way of requesting a drink. The routine then 'belongs' to the individual, the initiator, rather than being led by staff (Evans and Scotti, 1989). Facilitated communication is another technique of augmentative communication that helps people to express themselves, through another person acting as a facilitator (see Chapter 18).

Mutual relationships

In helping people make choices the quality of their relationships are essential to success. Communicating and developing relationships are about more than just being able to satisfy needs, reject and refuse things; they also involve learning to interact, share activities and laugh together. People with profound and multiple disabilities often have a developed sense of humour (Latchford, 1989). Interactive approaches focus on learning to read and respond to subtle nuances of communicative behaviour and developing trusted, mutual relationships with people (Burford, 1990). Two approaches, intensive interaction (Nind and Hewett, 1994) and gentle teaching (McGee *et al.*, 1987) focus on developing positive, mutual relationships with people. These approaches move away from the power imbalance where professionals control and dominate people and stress the importance of working interactively with people rather than doing things 'to them'.

Essential lifestyle planning

Essential lifestyle planning is a type of person-centred planning that brings together the significant people and important choices in a person's life. Smull and Burke-Harrison (1992) describe this as 'seeking to understand the interactive set of circumstances necessary for the individual's happiness'. People who 'really know and care' about the person give information about their preferences and choices which are ranked as 'non-negotiables, strong preferences and highly desirables'. The group develops an action plan from this information and designs services to support the individual's choices.

In helping people to advocate for themselves, it is challenging to find a balance between informed choice and what is in the person's best interests. This involves achieving a balance between safety, health and freedom of choice; personal liberties and how society expects people to behave and encouragement without bullying (Bannerman *et al.*, 1990; Smull and Burke Harrison, 1992).

Self-advocacy is essential, yet there are times when everyone needs help to be heard, from a friend or someone who experiences similar difficulties.

> The best spokesperson for someone who cannot speak may be another person with a disability who can speak, may be a friend of that person. Another disabled person knows where the person is coming from: they've had similar experiences. Professionals may say they understand, but in reality they haven't lived as we have and haven't had the same experiences. (Kennedy and Killis, 1986).

Attridge (1995) describes this as 'paired advocacy' where another person with learning difficulties gets to know the individual and helps to communicate their choices. Another way of supporting self-advocacy is to form a group of committed people who listen and help the individual achieve a positive future. This is a circle of support.

Circles of support and person-centred planning

To achieve high quality lifestyles for people with profound and multiple disabilities requires enthusiasm and committed support from people over a long time. A circle of support (Mount *et al.*, 1988) is a group of people, outside of services, who meet regularly to help someone who needs extra support. A circle can use various tools of person-centred planning such as making action plans (MAPS; Forest and Lusthaus, 1989; 1990; Forest and Pearpoint, 1992), planning alternative tomorrows with hope, (PATH; O'Brien and Lovett, 1992), personal futures planning (Mount and Zwernik, 1988) or essential lifestyle planning (Smull and Burke-Harrison, 1992). Person-centred planning styles begin by establishing a 'dream' of how the person would like to see their future, extending expectations beyond what services are available. The circle develops action plans from this and meets regularly to monitor the plans, celebrate achievements, and attempt to solve any other difficulties. The members of a circle of support will usually include family, friends, neighbours, other local people, and sometimes service providers. The family or other people who care about the individual form a circle of support simply by inviting people to join them to focus on the person's future and collaborate to reach her or his goals and dreams. Meetings are held whenever the family or individual needs them, for example, monthly or quarterly. A circle of support is a practical expression of an inclusive community.

Nicola Elwell has had a circle of support for three years. It began after her mother, Lynne, heard of 'circles' during an inclusion conference. She was invited to join someone else's circle, which was a positive experience, giving her the courage to start one for Nicola. Lynne invited people whom she thought would be useful contacts and cared about Nicola. They were people who had been close to them as a family and included a tutor at a college, and a community nurse who had been helpful in the past. For the first few meetings they asked 'Who is Nicola?' and got to know Nicola and her parents better. Then the group worked with Nicola on a dream for her using the PATH technique. One of these was for Nicola to leave the day centre and find alternative ways of spending her days. This is now being achieved by a proposal to the local social services department for a pilot project where a worker will support Nicola individually to access a wide range of community-based activities. The circle of support will become a trust to manage and monitor the pilot. Another way in which the circle offered practical support was when the day centre was closed for two weeks. The circle members organised a rota of support for Nicola arranging for her to do something different each day.

Ideally, everyone with profound and multiple disabilities would have their own circle of support. Many people with profound and multiple disabilities still lead a impoverished existence in wards, hostels or even group homes without having opportunities to meet other people who could become part of a circle of support. One approach for helping people to make contacts and develop relationships is being developed by the Circles Network in Bristol. This is a voluntary organisation established to help people in the community develop and maintain circles of support. The Circles Network also provides a service to people with profound and multiple disabilities who are still living in a long-stay hospital, by getting to know each individual and making a portfolio for the person using photographs, pictures, or objects. The community inclusion facilitators support the person to regularly use community facilities, meeting people there and building bridges into community life. Eventually relationships and networks can develop which form the foundation of a circle of support for the person.

Services cannot be circles of support for people, but can focus on extending the individual's network of relationships and include 'community people' in planning with the person. Services can use different styles of person-centred planning, for example personal futures planning, PATH, and MAPS, to discover a positive future for and with the person. O'Brien and Lovett (1992) state that to be effective, organisations will take the lead from people with learning difficulties through person-centred planning. People would then agree goals based on achieving a full life with new experiences and opportunities to meet people, rather than listing deficits and identifying skills to be learned. Two important issues that contribute to these dreams of full, satisfying lives are people having real homes and real jobs.

Supported living and supported employment

> Though people with profound and multiple disabilities live every minute with the decisions others make, they can live in their own homes. (O'Brien, 1991).

Supported living programmes, (where people with learning difficulties are helped to live as they choose, see Chapter 1) have a policy of rejecting no one (Kinsella, 1993) and people with profound and multiple disabilities are being successfully supported by such initiatives. This can work either through agencies, for example Community Integration Care in Liverpool, or through small groups, for example those supported by the Federation of Local Supported Living Groups in the North west. The federation employs two development officers who work with groups to achieve supported living for their sons or daughters. Lillian and Albert Doyle are part of a group of parents in Manchester who are being supported by the federation. They intend to move from their council property to allow their daughter Alison, who has profound and multiple disabilities, to take over the tenancy. Her parents will then employ and manage support staff on her behalf.

Community Integration Care supports people in rented accommodation, and will also look for 'room-mates' or 'flatmates', non-disabled people who live with the person and benefit from free accommodation in return for support. This is complementary to paid staff supporting the person at other times (Kinsella, 1993). This happens in the USA (Racino and Walker, 1988) and is beginning to happen for people with profound and multiple disabilities in Liverpool through Community Integration Care. This is a significant development from congregating two or three people with profound and multiple disabilities in group homes.

Assumptions about people with profound and multiple disabilities being incapable of doing paid work are also being challenged by the experiences of supported employment (Nisbet and Callahan, 1987). In the 1980s real opportunities began to be developed for people by innovations such as Blakes Wharf Employment Service in London which was one of the first to use training in systematic instruction to help people with severe learning difficulties to work. Training in systematic instruction is a value-based teaching framework involving a structured approach to job analysis. It is used by employment agencies such Bridgeworks in Liverpool and the Barnardo's A Chance to Work project. This project offers a service to school leavers with severe and profound disabilities, who each have an individually designed pro-gramme that is usually full-time and lasts for two years. Nearly all service users complete their programme with a job and a vocational qualification. Other work initiatives include involving people in co-operatives and small companies. Essentially Celtic is a small company in Clwyd that employs 11 people, seven of whom have learning difficulties and one of whom, Julie, has profound disabilities. The company sells a range of aromatherapy oils and products as well as running workshops and courses in aromatherapy. Julie works there full-time, and is involved in the office, displays and deliveries. She also takes advantage of the on-site aromatherapy massage offered by the company.

Supported living and supported employment have significantly changed Shirley Davies' life from when she existed in a long-stay hospital in Liverpool. Shirley is an attractive, smartly dressed woman in her thirties who lives in a luxury rented flat in the Sefton area of Liverpool. Those who know Shirley understand her by reading her facial expressions, her noises and body language. Sandra, the manager of Community Integration Care, is considering a flatmate for Shirley. She says: 'Our focus in the beginning was for Shirley to live where she wanted and when that had been established to concentrate on what she wanted to do during the day. Once we had accomplished this the next priority has to be to find a flatmate, someone who lives with Shirley out of choice. This will give Shirley the chance to meet new friends and also having someone permanent to support her.'

In 1992 Shirley started work at the Body Shop for two mornings a week. Shirley is visually impaired and consequently relies on her other senses for information. The Body Shop seemed an ideal place to experience wonderful smells! Shirley's work involved pricing products and making up baskets. Kerry, her job support worker from Bridge-work Employment Agency, worked 'hand-over-hand' to help Shirley as she has limited movement in her hands. Shirley seemed to enjoy sampling new products and having facials with the rest of the staff. She received goods in return for her work. Shirley and Kerry both wore the Body Shop uniform, and became familiar faces in the area, particularly to people who used the same cafe for lunch.

After a while Shirley's support workers thought that she would benefit from a job that was more predictable and where she would not have to work around customers in a busy shop. Shirley now works at the Girobank headquarters doing general clerical work, including photocopying and franking with Kerry's support.

Finding real homes for people, choosing flatmates and supporting work opportunities are achievable alternatives to the current, typical service provision of group homes and adult training centres for people with profound and multiple disabilities.

Day services

Day services for people with profound and multiple disabilities have traditionally been provided, inadequately, in segregated, 'special needs' groups within adult training centres. The focus is usually on sensory-developmental approaches featuring 'sensory rooms' in all their guises as dark rooms, light rooms, white rooms and soft play rooms. Considerable amounts of money and time have produced secluded areas filled with a range of sophisticated equipment (usually including a projector, bubble tube and fibre optics) within which people have 'individual sensory stimulation programmes' and relaxation. Critics suggest that it is staff interaction which is responsible for any perceived benefits of relaxation or improved skills from using such rooms (Orr, 1993). Other activities that are age appropriate and involve interaction with others, could produce equally beneficial responses.

The benefit of such a predominance of sensory stimulation is being questioned (Jones, 1993) for its crucial lack of emphasis on enabling people to lead full lives in the community. An alternative is the ecological approach which, whilst not denying the needs of people to experience and take pleasure from the world through their senses, focusses on how these experiences can help people to become part of their communities. The ecological approach features functional skills in ordinary, typical settings and these would include developments in the areas of leisure, work, community and domestic skills. Procedures are identified for helping set objectives that directly relate to the person's life at home and in the community (Brown *et al.*, 1980; Sailor *et al.*, 1986; Nietupski and Hamre-Nietupski, 1987). To fully facilitate this requires a radical departure from the traditional day centre type of provision.

One approach, demonstrated by The White Top Centre in Dundee (Seed, 1991), has been to design a service for a small number of people and significantly improve the staffing, physical resources and use of community facilities. Other services have developed which almost exclusively use community facilities with people on an individual basis (Hill-Tout, 1988; Allen *et al.*, 1989; Allen, 1990; Jones, 1994). One of these initiatives is the small scale day service in Cardiff (Allen *et al.*, 1989). This service consists of two staff teams operating in different areas in South Glamorgan, who support people on an individual basis to use community facilities. Allen (1990) evaluated the service by comparing it to a local, traditional day service using a matched control group design. He found that the number and variety of activities, the levels of engagement in activities, the amount of community presence and the age-appropriateness of the activities were all significantly greater in the new service.

Kidderminster service

A similar service has been provided in Kidderminster where people who have profound and multiple disabilities (and use wheelchairs) spend part of the week in the new project and the remainder using traditional day services (Jones, 1994). The new service is totally integrated in the local area, designed around individual needs and interests, and offers a variety of activities representing a balance of work, leisure and domestic activities. The work opportunities include working in a shop checking prices and stacking shelves; in a pub putting bottles on shelves and putting out beer mats; at a local park, potting, watering and pruning plants; and at riding stables cleaning saddles and reins. People also attend fully integrated classes at a local college and use a variety of leisure activities ranging from golf to using a jacuzzi. Service users also spend time shopping, cooking, and cleaning their homes.

The evaluation compared how people spent each part of the week. When people used the traditional day service, on average only 6.5 per cent of their activities took place in the community and these were largely restricted to shopping and never included work opportunities, as they did in the new service. Typical activities in the day centre included gluing and sticking, using a peg board, lying in a bean bag, pressing an adapted switch for music, sitting in a ball pool, having physiotherapy, and feeling a board covered with textured material. In the new service levels of engagement and the appropriateness of activities were also significantly improved. As Jones (1994) points out, 'Whenever people with multiple disabilities are grouped together, the basic physical and daily care needs tend to predominate.'

The Kidderminster service is particularly impressive as it provides a balance of work, domestic activities and leisure for people. In the future, more people may consider hiring their own support worker as Nicola Elwell is doing. The World Institute on Disability (1994) has shown that providing individual services in this way, rather than through an agency, can reduce the cost of the service by half because of reduced bureaucracy and administrative costs. These alternatives to day centres could include leisure activities in the community and further education.

Further education

People with profound and multiple disabilities have two main routes to further education; to join segregated special needs classes, which often focus on increasing daily living skills or be supported on an individual basis within a mainstream class. Supporting individual students to attend mainstream classes can be achieved by linking them with another person who is interested in the same activity, with further assistance from residential staff or family, from additional tutors or through support from staff based at the college. This is similar to the services provided by Studylink.

Studylink comprises 11 full-time and three part-time staff who are based at the Riversdale Centre, part of Liverpool's community college. Studylink staff, who are known as inclusive education workers support people on an individual basis to attend mainstream vocational courses. Over the last five years people have participated in hairdressing, vehicle maintenance and spraying, woodwork, beauty therapy, furniture restoration, horticulture, fashion, screen printing and photography.

The project is firmly rooted in helping the individual make choices about course activities, which is challenging considering the limited experiences and communication ability of many of the students. This is achieved by working closely with other carers and a lengthy 'getting to know you' process where the individual and worker spend time together. An appropriate course is then located. The worker then joins the course as a participant and assesses its suitability for the person concerned. If the course is suitable, the student joins the course supported by the worker. Wherever possible, support workers fade their presence in the class, according to the support that the person receives from other members of the group. Studylink has been working with the supported employment service of the health authority to find people jobs when their courses have come to an end.

The success of Studylink is best illustrated by Arthur Brotherton. He is in his early forties, and for two years he enjoyed attending a local carpentry and joinery class. Arthur was already interested in wood-work and seemed to enjoy working with the tools although he has only limited use of his left arm. Heidi, his worker found a carpentry and joinery class at his local college in Kirkby. Each week Heidi supported him in the class where Arthur learnt basic woodworking skills using a mitre saw, planes and chisels. Individual students were very supportive and would assist Arthur with tasks such as preparing and marking up the wood. Although Arthur only communicates using signs, gestures and a few words, he quickly struck up friendships with members of the class. He found that another student was also interested in drumming. His relationships with the other students extended out of the class room, and Heidi went with Arthur to hear the other drummer's band several times. After the course had finished, Arthur found a job working in a bank sealing envelopes and franking the post. He has now returned to college to complete a computer course to widen his chances of employment.

Further education courses extend people's opportunities to meet other people, find work and experience new leisure activities. The experience of Studylink questions the need for segregated provision to achieve this.

Leisure

Leisure for people with profound and multiple disabilities tends to be confined to passively watching television and listening to music. Hogg and Lambe (1988) found this to be the case for 75 per cent of people. While this might also be true for many other people without disabilities, people with profound and multiple disabilities are not making informed choices from a range of other options. Watching the television or listening to music without being able to indicate preferences for types of music or particular programmes or to switch off when the person has had enough is even more limiting.

People with profound and multiple disabilities have impoverished leisure experiences. McConkey *et al.* (1981) found that 50 per cent of people living with their families did not have any leisure activities outside of the home. Cavet (1989), in her European study on leisure for people with profound and multiple disabilities, also found inadequate and limited leisure provisions for many people. Mount (1994) identified one possible reason for this, that service providers were unaware of the importance of leisure activities for developing relationships and self-esteem and consequently tended to give leisure a low priority. Some staff were also not aware of the vast range of ordinary leisure activities in which people with profound and multiple disabilities can participate. *Leisure for People with Profound and Multiple Disabilities: A Resource Pack* (Lambe, 1991) illustrates a range of different activities, many of which are community-based.

Although developments in day services have been described, what people require for fulfilling leisure experiences is support to use ordinary facilities without necessarily providing a separate day service. When Shirley, who was described earlier, is not at work she spends her time shopping, eating out, using a jacuzzi, having a massage, drinking at the local pub, and swimming, as well as doing more mundane things like housework. She does not attend any form of day service and is supported in her leisure activities by Community Integration Care. There are other ways for people with profound and multiple disabilities to actively and creatively enjoy leisure with other people. These include new technologies, for example Soundbeam, and initiatives to help people share leisure, like Leisure Link and One-to-one.

Soundbeam

Soundbeam is an ultrasound beam attached to a keyboard and midi system that converts movement into an electronic signal and translates this into music. It was originally designed for professional dancers to make music from their movements and now allows people with only the slightest movement to produce sophisticated music. Recent research using Soundbeam (Ellis, 1994; personal communication) demonstrated an increase in interactive communication, longer attention spans and increased motivation to move. The potential for this to enable people with profound and multiple disabilities to create music and participate in public performances is starting to become recognised. A recital of Haydn's music recently featured a Soundbeam accompaniment played by an individual with severe disabilities. The musician involved commented: 'It is great fun for me as a musician to play with non-musicians who are as good as me'. Through Soundbeam there are opportunities for communication and creative expression that can enable people with profound and multiple disabilities to be creators rather than just consumers of music.

Leisure Link

It is people's relationships with others that give the most meaning to their leisure experiences (Gold and Crawford, 1988) and friendships are often built or strengthened through leisure (McGill, 1987). Leisure Link and One-to-one are examples of schemes that includes people with profound and multiple disabilities that link people with others who enjoy similar social and leisure interests. In some cases, this has lead to people forming a lasting relationship that has helped people to advocate for changes in their lives. Both schemes have paid co-ordinators operating from local bases.

One of the co-ordinators of Leisure Link, Sharon Barlow, describes how Simon Johnson (not his real name), goes swimming with a leisure sharer at his local swimming baths. Simon lives at home and did not have any friends. He uses a wheelchair and does not use spoken communication. Before joining Leisure Link, Simon had only ever used segregated services. He enjoys water and a local pool had a 'swim bus' to provide a transport service. Over a six month period Sharon worked with Simon and linked him to a leisure sharer called John. She also helped him to use the bus independently to meet John at the pool. John and the pool staff help Simon to change as he is very strong and needs two people to help him. The link worker spent much time working with Simon's mother to convince her that the sessions would be safe and that people would not discriminate against Simon because of his disabilities. Sharon involved his Mum in going with Simon on the swim bus, and introducing her to John and the pool staff.

One way to extend people's network of relationships is to review the role of support staff and move towards a role of community facilitators. Instead of the existing preoccupation with personal care, daily living skills and housework evident in many group homes, support staff or community facilitators would focus on making links into the local community (Knoll and Ford, 1987). This obviously does not deny meeting people's personal care needs, but acknowledges that another very real need is to be connected by relationships in the community. This would include staff developing close relationships with the person they are supporting and involving them in their network of family and friends. By contrast, staff and managers traditionally talk about the importance of 'maintaining a distance' which is also seen as 'being professional'. In group homes staff are often moved if it is perceived that they are getting too close to the person with profound disabilities, who may become 'dependent' on them. It is this interdependence and sharing of networks that services should be developing rather than discouraging. The staff of both Studylink and Community Integration Care actively and successfully involve people who use their service in their own social lives. Such a change in approach will have implications for staff recruitment and training.

Training and recruitment

Kinsella (1993) believes it is essential to employ local people and make knowledge and membership of the local community valid and necessary criteria for recruitment. Staff training also needs to change. People with profound and multiple disabilities have specific needs that vary dramatically from person to person. New workers should receive some basic instruction but receive most of their training from the family and existing support staff, learning directly how to support specific individuals (Racino, 1990). Training would then include mentoring. Ratzka (1990) suggests that the assumption that any support worker can work with any individual with disabilities amounts to a denial of an individual's uniqueness as a human being.

Professionals have been training people towards 'independence' for many years. O'Brien and O'Brien (1990) offers two definitions of independence. The first is the familiar rehabilitation model where people are trained to be able to meet their own basic needs with minimum assistance. The second is an independent living perspective which sees independence as choosing and living one's own lifestyle, regardless of the amount and type of assistance necessary. Independence would therefore not be measured by the number of tasks which people can do without assistance but the quality of life a person can have with whatever support they need. For people with profound and multiple disabilities to 'choose and live their own lifestyle' requires services to prioritise developing self-advocacy and communication skills for each individual. Essential lifestyle planning can help to identify strategies for ensuring that these choices are respected. Instead of assessments which measure people's deficits, and individual planning that looks at strengths and needs, effective organisations will use person-centred planning to produce longer term strategies for achieving positive futures. This will involve developing flexible, intensive and individual support and rethinking group homes, 'special care' day services, segregated further education classes and the role of support staff. Community Integration Care, Bridgework and Studylink have demonstrated how it is possible for people to participate in integrated leisure, work and further education and to live in their own homes. The challenge is to build on these experiences and extend these opportunities to everyone with profound and multiple disabilities.

References

Allen, D., Gillard, N., Watkins, P. and Norman, G. (1989). New directions in day activities for people with multiple handicaps and challenging behaviour. *Mental Handicap*, **17**(3), 101–103.

Allen, D. (1990). Evaluation of a community-based day service for people with profound mental handicaps and additional special needs. *Mental Handicap Research*, **3**(3), 179–195.

Attridge, C. (1995). *Self Advocacy for People with Severe and Profound Learning Difficulties*. Orca Computers Limited, Luxembourg.

Bannerman, D., Sheldon, J., Sherman, J. and Harchik, A. (1990). Balancing the right to habilitiation with the rights to personal liberties: the rights of people with developmental disabilities to eat too many doughnuts and take a nap. *Journal of Applied Behaviour Analysis*, **23**, 79–89.

Baumgart, D. (1990). *Augmentative and Alternative Communication Systems for Persons with Moderate and Severe Disabilities*. Paul H. Brookes, Baltimore.

Bradley, H. (1991). *Assessing Communication Together. A Systematic Approach to Assessing and Developing Early Communication Skills in Children and Adults with Multi-Sensory Impairments*. Mental Handicap Nurses Association, Penarth, South Glamorgan.

Brown, L., Bradston, M., Baumgart, D., Vincent, L., Falvey, M. and Schroeder, J. (1980). Utilizing characteristics of a variety of current and subsequent least restrictive environments as factors in development of curricula context for severely handicapped students. In *Strategies for Teaching Chronological Age Appropriate Functional Skills to Adolescent and Young Severely Handicapped Students* (Vol. IX Part 1) (eds L. Brown, M. Falvey, D. Baumgart, I. Pumpian, I. Schroeder, and L. Greunewald). University of Wisconsin and Madison Metropolitan School District, Madison.

Burford, B. (1990). *Children with Profound Handicaps: How Carers Can Communicate*. The Health Promotion Research Trust, Cambridge.

Campbell, C. and Wilcox, M. (1986). Communication effectiveness of movement patterns use by non-vocal children with severe handicaps. Paper presented at the 4th International Conference of the International Society for Augmentative and Alternative Communication, Cardiff.

Cavet, J. (1989). *Occupation and Leisure Activities for People with Profound Retardation and Multiple Impairments: A Study of the Use of Creative Activities to Facilitate Social Integration*. Hester Adrian Research Centre, University of Manchester.

Coupe, J., Barton, L., Barber, M., Collins, L., Levy, D. and Murphy, D. (1985). *Affective Communication Assessment*. Manchester Education Committee.

Coupe, J., Barber, M. and Murphy, D. (1988). Affective communication. In *Communication Before Speech*, (eds J. Coupe and J. Goldbart). Croom Helm, London.

Evans, I. and Scotti, J. (1989). Defining meaningful outcomes for persons with profound disabilities. In *Persons with Profound Disabilities – Issues and Practices* (eds F. Brown and D. Lehr). Paul H. Brookes, Baltimore.

Fitton, P. (1994). *Listen To Me*. Jessica Kingsley Publishers, London.

Forest, M. and Lusthaus, E. (1989). Promoting educational equality for all students: Circles and MAPS. In *Educating all Students in the Mainstream of Regular Education* (eds S. Stainback, W. Stainback and M. Forest). Paul H. Brookes, Baltimore.

Forest, M. and Lusthaus, E. (1990). Everyone belongs with the MAPs action planning system. *Teaching Exceptional Children*, 22(2), 32–35.

Forest, M. and Pearpoint, J. (1992). Everyone belongs: building the vision with MAPs – the McGill Action Planning System. In *The Whole Community Catalogue: Welcoming People with Disabilities into the Heart of Community Life*. Communitas, Manchester, Connecticutt.

Gold, D. and Crawford, C. (1988). *Leisure Connections: Enabling People with a Disability to Lead Richer Lives in the Community*. Roeher Institute, York University, Ontario.

Goldbart, J., Warner, J. and Mount, H. (1994). *The Development of Early Communication and Feeding for People who have Profound and Multiple Disabilities. A Workshop Training Package for Parents and Carers*. MENCAP, London.

Guess, D. (1989). *Forward in Persons with Profound Disabilities – Issues and Practices* (ed. F. Brown and D. Lehr). Paul H. Brookes, Baltimore.

Hartup, W. (1975). The origins of friendship. In *Friendships and Peer Relations* (eds M. Lewis and L. Rosenblum). John Wiley & Sons, New York.

Hill-Tout, J. (1988). Personal services. *Community Care*, 4 February, 22–24.

Hogg, J. and Lambe, L. (1988). *Sons and Daughters with Profound Retardation and Multiple Handicaps Attending Schools and Social Education Centres.* Final Report, MENCAP, London.

Howes, C. (1983). Patterns of friendship. *Child Development,* 54, 1041–1053.

Jones, L. (1993). Working with students who have profound and multiple learning difficulties. In *Innovations in Educating Children with Severe Learning Difficulties* (ed. J. Harris). Lisieux Hall, The Brothers of Charity, Chorley.

Jones, L. (1994). *Evaluation of the Kidderminster Day Services Project.* (Unpubl.). Wolverly NHS Trust, Kidderminster.

Kearns, T. (1993). Communicating with signs and symbols. In *Innovations in Educating Children with Severe Learning Difficulties* (ed. J. Harris). Lisieux Hall, The Brothers of Charity, Chorley.

Kennedy, M. and Killius, P. (1986). *Self-advocacy: Speaking for Yourself Materials on Self Determination.* Centre on Human Policy, Syracuse University, New York.

Kinsella, P. (1993). *Supported Living: A New Paradigm.* National Development Team, Manchester.

Knoll, J. and Ford, A. (1987). Beyond caregiving: A Reconceptualization of the role of the residential service provider. In *Community Integration for People with Severe Disabilities* (eds S. Taylor, D. Biklen and J. Knoll). Teachers College Press, New York.

Lambe, L. (ed.) (1991). *Leisure for People with Profound and Multiple Disabilities: A Resource Training Pack.* MENCAP, London.

Latchford, G. (1989). Towards an Understanding of Profound Mental Handicap. (Unpubl. PhD thesis), University of Edinburgh.

Le Touze, S. and Pahl, J. (1992). Facilitating friendships for people with learning disabilities. *Mental Handicap,* 20, 144–146.

McConkey, R. Walsh, M. and Mulcahy, M. (1981). The recreational pursuits of mentally handicapped adults. *International Journal of Rehabilitations Research,* 4, 493–499.

McGee, J., Menolascino, F., Hobbs, D. and Menousek, P. (1987). *Gentle Teaching: A Non-Aversive Approach for helping Persons with Mental Retardation.* Human Sciences Press, New York.

McGill, J. (1987). Our leisure identity. *Entourage,* 2(3), 23–25.

MENCAP (1994). *Learning for Life.* MENCAP, London.

Mount, B., Beehman, P. and Ducharme, G. (1988). *What are we Learning about Circles of Support? A Collection of Tools, Ideas and Reflections on Building and Facilitating Circles of Support:* Communitas, Manchester, Connecticut.

Mount, B. and Zwernik, K. (1988). *It's Never Too Early, It's Never Too Late:* Governor's Planning Council, St Paul, Minnesota.

Mount, H. (1994). *Report on the Survey of the First 500 Purchasers of the MENCAP/Gateway Leisure Resource Training Pack for People with Profound and Multiple Disabilities.* MANCAP, PIMD Section, Manchester.

Nietupski, J. and Hamre-Nietupski, S. (1987). An ecological approach to curriculum development. In *Innovative Program Design for Individuals with Dual Sensory Impairments* (eds L. Goetz, D. Guess and K. Stremmel-Campbell). Paul H. Brookes, Baltimore.

Nind, M. and Hewett, D. (1994). Access to Communication. David Fulton, London.

Nisbet, J. and Callahan, M. (1987). Achieving success in integrated workplaces: critical elements in assisting persons with severe disabilities. In *Community Integration for People with Severe Disabilities* (eds S. Taylor, D. Biklen, and J. Knoll). Teachers College Press, New York.

O'Brien, J. and O'Brien, C. (1990). *Design for Accomplishment: Responsive Systems Associates.* Atlanta, Georgia.

O'Brien, J. (1991). *Down Stairs that are Never Your Own: Supporting People with Developmental Disabilities in their Own Homes.* Centre on Human Policy, Syracuse University, New York.

O'Brien, J. and Lovett, H. (1992). *Finding a Way Toward Everyday Lives. The Contribution of Person Centred Planning*: Centre on Human Policy, Syracuse University, New York.

Orr, R. (1993). Life beyond the room?, *Eye Contact*. Royal National Institute for the Blind, London.

Racino, J.A. and Walker, P. (1988). *Supporting Adults with Severe Disabilities in the Community: Selected Issues in Residential Services.* Centre on Human Policy, Syracuse University, New York.

Racino, J.A. (1990). Preparing personnel to work in community support services. In *Preparing Personnel to work with Persons with Severe Disabilities* (eds A. Kaiser and C. McWhorter). Paul H. Brookes, Baltimore.

Ratzka, A. (1990). Design criteria for personal assistance programs. In *Design for Accomplishment* (eds J. O'Brien and C. O'Brien, 1989). Responsive Systems Associates, Atlanta, Georgia.

Richardson, A. and Ritchie, J. (1989). *Developing Friendships: Enabling People with Learning Difficulties to Make and Maintain Friends.* Policy Studies Institute, London.

Sailor, W., Halvorson, A., Anderson, J., Goetz, L., Gee, K., Doering, D. and Hunt, P. (1986). Community intensive construction. In *Education of Learners with Severe Handicaps. Exemplary Service Strategies* (eds R. Horner, L. Meyer and H. Fredricks). Paul H. Brookes, Baltimore.

Seed, P. (1991). The establishment of a day centre for young adults with profound learning difficulties. In *Innovatory Practice and Severe Learning Difficulties* (ed. J. Watson). Moray House Publications, Edinburgh.

Smull, W. and Burke-Harrison, S. (1992). *Supporting People with Severe Reputations in the Community. A Handbook for Trainers.* University of Maryland, Baltimore.

Ward, L. and Kinsella, P. (1993). Whose home is it anyway? *Health Services Journal*, August 12.

World Institute on Disability (1994). *Cost-effective Plan Recommended for Personal Assistance Services. Futurity.* Minnesota Governor's Planning Council, September.

Chapter 18

A challenge to change: Better services for people with challenging behaviour

Mary Myers

In the field of learning difficulties, there can be no area which so profoundly challenges our assumptions, beliefs and value systems, as the planning and providing for those individuals who confront us with desperate, destructive and self-injurious behaviours. For their committed supporters, to ensure the eventual inclusion in ordinary community life of such individuals presents a huge challenge: they are having to think and work much harder, with more empathy, with more imagination. For commissioners and planners of services, the closure of long-stay hospitals has brought forward the residents of the 'back' wards; those people living deprived, violent, useless lives, who are identified as 'difficult to place' and so expensive to contain that planning must expect to include those very economies of scale which have so failed the individuals in the past. Day services, neither staffed nor skilled for the tasks, are trying to deal with young adults leaving special schools, who in the past would have been admitted to hospital.

This challenge to think and operate in fresh ways is being faced and met with much success in many places. Far more is known about the possible causes of challenging behaviours, about their relief and replacements and many other related issues, than was known 10 years ago.

But the application of this expanding knowledge and understanding presents fundamental questions about the perceived value of people who do such 'challenging' things, and about the ultimate goals of any interventions. The basic question is: do we believe that the individual who performs bizarre and frightening acts is nevertheless a full human person, one of us, with reasons for the behaviours, and in need of help to live among us? Or do we, in our hearts – however kind – really believe that '*they*' must be fundamentally different from '*us*', as past adjectives 'defective' and 'subnormal' emphasised? It is the answer to this question which will dictate the foundations and directions of service developments.

In the debates about community care in the 1980s in the UK, it was often argued that there was not scientific proof that being in the community worked better for people with severe disabilities. But as Biklen (1985) pointed out, did Abraham Lincoln ask for *scientific proof* that ending slavery was the right thing to do? Human rights, social inclusion, are not *scientific* issues; they are *moral* ones. Thus the recognition of mutual humanity with those of us with severe disabilities, including behavioural ones, is at its core, a philosophical and emotional one.

However the perception of people with severe disabilities as being somehow not real people is very pervasive. Such individuals suffer from 'diagnostic overshadowing', which means that the diagnosis of learning difficulties prevails over the recognition of common conditions or issues which may affect anybody. This is illustrated by the way many behaviours identified as 'challenging' in people with learning difficulties are interpreted differently when performed by people of 'ordinary' intelligence. Young adults without learning difficulties, for example, who are lonely, lack close relationships, have no job, no vision for the future, can be violent to themselves with wrist-cutting, overdosing, alcohol abuse, or be violent to others. They can sometimes describe their difficulty in expressing feelings because of inadequate language, the lack of a receptive listener and their sense of worthlessness and hopelessness; and sometimes there is a real response to their 'cry for help'. Often people with clinical depression are irritable, agitated, miserable, aggressive, violent to themselves or others. What is recognisable in people of 'ordinary' intelligence and communication abilities, is not, however, automatically considered in people who are perceived as different from us.

Although humans are social and communicating beings, the central role of communication problems in the lives of people with learning difficulties gets little everyday attention. It is another example of diagnostic overshadowing. Being identified as 'mentally handicapped' means you are not expected to say much, if anything.

When people with learning difficulties cannot describe or explain why they do desperate or bizarre things, they are labelled as unpredictable, non-complaint or mad.

This book is about visions and values, and this chapter is based on the belief that all human beings matter: that we are all capable of growth and change; that we all share basic needs in common and a role in helping to meet them in each other.

Universal human needs

Maslow (1987) described a hierarchy of human needs, with which most of us can identify, and it provides a helpful structure with which to consider the lives some individuals experience.

The basic level of need is *physiological*. Human beings need nutrition, fluids, sleep, movement, visual and hearing stimuli, touch, sex, relief from pain and discomfort, stimulation. Individuals who experience continued deprivation of food or sleep become totally preoccupied with obtaining it.

The second level of need is for *environmental safety*: freedom from dangers, fear, anxiety and chaos. Individuals can be dominated by the need for structure, predictability, familiarity.

Third, we need *relationships, reciprocity, love and affection, a sense of belonging*.

Fourth, we need a *sense of competence and self-esteem*, to experience a sense of worth, responsibility.

And finally, there is the need for *self-actualisation*, 'to become everything one is capable of becoming', which can emerge as the earlier four levels of needs are met. These levels of need are readily recognisable in ourselves in raising our children, who are dependent on us for care, protection, love and our interest and pride in their growing achievements. The various levels, of course, are interwoven, and meeting some needs will meet other needs at the same time. The ability to create a meal provides nutrition, opportunity for social interaction, and a sense of competence. Needs can be met in excess of course, producing for example obesity, overprotection, emotional smothering, and smugness or arrogance.

However, major deficits in meeting levels of need are clearly damaging. Chronic malnutrition, or chronically restricted movement can certainly impair health and functioning, for example. We try to create safe environments for our children and ourselves with vaccinations, car seat belts, smoke alarms. We easily recognise that failure to meet either of the first two levels can lead to damage and even death.

Individuals whose early needs to feel loved and wanted 'for themselves' have not been adequately met grow into adults with an insatiable hunger for meaningful relationships, who experience chronic depression and often injure or kill themselves. We all know the occasional experience of making an embarrassing mistake, of feeling stupid, mortified. How does it feel to be reminded by all the events in your life that you are incompetent, incapable, inferior? We know that 'learned helplessness', from the sense of permanent entrapment in one's situation (be it poverty, ignorance, brutality or other) underlies chronic depression in many deprived people who feel powerless to alter their world.

It is clear then, that failure to meet any of the four levels of need can lead to physical and emotional damage, and this certainly applies to those whose behaviours took them into hospitals in the past.

Much emphasis in this chapter is on the needs of adults who live or have lived in institutions, because their lives have been complicated by the abnormal influences of institutional life, and a long time in which to practise their behaviours. It is very painful to acknowledge that verbal, physical and sexual abuse has been more common than people have wanted to believe: Post-Traumatic Stress Disorder is now considered as possibly underlying the behaviours of some individuals with learning difficulties who have experienced or witnessed bad things. The lessons which can be learnt from addressing such complicated and chronic needs are all available to help those adults and children who have remained in the community.

It might be said that the hospitals met the first two levels of need with residents being fed, kept clean, inoculated against diseases and protected from the hazards of the outside world. The need for close reciprocal relationships was certainly not acknowledged, and commonly they were prevented and broken up, accidentally or intentionally. As for needing to feel competent and have a sense of self-worth, that was not a consideration for people at the bottom of the power pyramid. The language of some older people on leaving hospitals is revealing. A woman of 78 had settled well into a new flat, after a half-century in an upgraded workhouse. When a previous staff member visited to celebrate the event, Ellen Atkins wept. 'Don't take me back, don't take me back, I'll be a good girl', she said. A 50 year old woman had done some excellent baking. She offered a sample, and asked pleadingly: 'Are you pleased with me?'

Institutional life often failed the first two levels of need as well. Consider nutrition: 'Pica' is the label for the behaviour of collecting and eating inedible things, cigarette ends being a common favourite. Pica was very common in institutions in the past. It is a very complex subject, but for some people at least the problem has been reduced by offering nutritious items of food at frequent intervals. Many residents in hospitals were restlessly on the move, and whether that was due to neurological impairment, or the expression of their feelings, it consumed a lot of calories. At the same time the nutritional value of food offered in long-stay hospitals has been challenged at intervals over the years. People of 'ordinary' intelligence when chronically malnourished are preoccupied with thoughts of food; could this not present as pica? And may not the nicotine of cigarette ends suppress hunger? Reference has already been made to the fact that life within institutions was anything but safe for some.

To younger care staff, who never worked in the big institutional environments, these descriptions may feel morbid, out-of-date or irrelevant. But for any adult who did live thus, however good their new home is now, their past experiences are part of them, and we have to take account of that when offering support. Efforts to do the 'right thing' by people with challenging behaviours are still evolving, and it is important to identify and understand the changes made over time in these interventions, but especially the changes in *posture* and *expectations*. The term 'posture' here means the set of attitudes, values and beliefs that define and direct the judgement and actions which one applies to a situation, and its use has come from the liberation theology of South America with its efforts 'to be alongside' the poor and oppressed in their efforts to become empowered. Thus the institutional posture of hierarchical control, descending from the superintendent down to the 'inmates', (sometimes congregated on wards of 100, less than 20 years ago) expected people with enormous unmet needs to be co-operative, patient, obedient, unselfish, and thoughtful of the needs of all the other residents and the overstretched staff. When individuals failed at this, they were labelled non-compliant, disruptive and in need of extra control.

During the 1980s, a visitor to an old hostel for men noticed a middle-aged man wandering around at midday in dressing gown and pyjamas. On enquiring if the gentleman had been ill recently, the confident response from the person in charge was no, it was to stop him absconding: 'He's a nuisance he is, he thinks this place is run for his benefit!' This is a good example of a very maladaptive posture. The more 'difficult and disruptive' people were, for whatever reason, the more they were segregated, congregated and left to destroy their environment. The organizational posture was authoritarian, paternalistic, and usually punitive. The maximum expectation was that the individual might stop assaulting himself or others; nothing more. The interventions used to control and restrict individuals became increasingly sophisticated over time, and took three main forms.

First, there was physical restraint. This included the hospital boundaries, padded cells and seclusion rooms. Tying people to chairs and beds is no longer tolerable practice in the UK, and strait-jackets are museum pieces; but there are individuals with learning difficulties who remember them. Second, there were drugs. Bromides and barbiturates were in use long ago, but the major tranquillizers were much stronger. They could not always suppress behaviours, but were widely used as a chemical cosh. They were often applied because the behaviour was automatically interpreted as psychotic. Third, psychological techniques were employed. The use of rewards – and even more so of punishments – was nothing new of course, but new techniques to target them were seized upon to change behaviour, mostly just to stop it. Where there were more positive behavioural goals, they were chosen and prioritised by staff. Antecedents and consequences of behaviour were talked about, but really only consequences were considered. Individuals could not only 'earn rewards' (like more cigarettes paid for out of their own money, and a chance to talk to the ward doctor!) but could also lose 'privileges' like meals, or visits from relatives. The need for, the morality, and the effectiveness of punishment has always been taken for granted, and although the deliberate infliction of physical pain is illegal in the UK (unlike parts of the USA where electric cattle prods are on sale for challenging behaviour management), verbal abuse and sarcasm is still widespread. (The sad fact is that humiliation is a common tool in ordinary childrearing and social control.)

It is hardly surprising that when the concepts of values, dignity and human rights came to be applied to people with learning difficulties, there was a revulsion against technologies used in their abuse. Psychotropic drugs and behavioural expertise were widely rejected and are only now being rehabilitated as the very real help they can be.

Technology by itself of course is neither good nor bad; it is the application which is to be judged, which is why examination of posture is fundamental. Do we believe that this person needs control and supervision from someone in charge, who knows best? Or do we believe she needs someone alongside, to help her gain control over her self and her environment? The technology is there to achieve either. One chair may be a trap, to restrict movement; another can provide mobility and access to living. Medication can be a chemical cosh, or provide relief from emotional torment. Psychological techniques can manipulate and control by fear and pain, or they can empower people to learn and grow, to be included and respected.

Not all work done with people with challenging behaviours has been punitive of course, although a benign paternal posture has been the norm. Individuals have been put on careful programmes planned for outcomes the *staff* believed were desirable. The expectations were limited by the scale of vision, but nevertheless individuals grew in competences and staff improved in teaching. For some people with challenging behaviours this has been a major step forward; they have become able to live quieter lives in their special environments while their damage to themselves and others diminished. But just as the developments of systematic industrial skills training and group homes in the community have been an improvement on the past, such provisions do not lead to inclusion in ordinary local social networks and activities. So Emerson *et al.*'s (1987) description of challenging behaviour 'as likely to seriously limit or delay access to and use of ordinary community facilities' points towards the outcomes hoped for in our interventions.

Dealing with challenging behaviours

The first need is to confirm our posture towards the individual, to acknowledge him or her to be fully human, with immense needs both ordinary and special; to confirm that we want to help that person take charge of his or her life, to enjoy relationships and feel good about themselves; to offer the skills experience and insights we have in learning alongside the person.

Although it is likely that the individual as yet has no vision of a satisfying future, the direction of developments will be guided by his or her choices indicated over the course of time.

The second stage is to ask, *Who is this person?* What is his or her life story? (Sometimes nobody seems to know, which already says a lot). Have there been significant episodes and losses in his or her life? Have they been explained to them and understood by them? Might there have been any physical or sexual abuse? How well can this person communicate? How well do others understand and respond? How much do you believe he or she understands? What is the content and rhythm of their days and weeks? Do they have activities they enjoy, and how often, who with? Does he or she have sensory, movement or spatial problems? What strengths and resources does he have, what are the attractive things about and who really loves them? Are there situations where he or she seems happy, and the challenging behaviour does not occur?

Third, there need to be positive interventions which aim to understand the behaviour; replace damaging behaviours with others which fulfil the same function; and build new skills and experiences.

The next step is the careful observation and recording of the behaviours, without any instant interpretations ('she's attention-seeking', 'he can't get his own way'). Video recording of complex situations can help analyse events, but a much wider understanding of the person's whole self and situation than just the 'antecedent–behaviour–consequences' records of the past, is needed.

The *functional analysis* of behaviour is the process of asking what function it fulfils for the person, and that function must be incorporated in the positive planning. The analysis asks such questions as: 'What would cause a person to do this? What was life like up to this point? What does he or she think is happening? Why should this person need to bite him/herself to get attention? It is now recognised that challenging behaviours very commonly serve a communicative function, and by rushing in to stop bizarre or even dangerous behaviours before analysing them, we may actually be blocking an important message.

Herb Lovett (1985) describes Martha and her obsession with the staff's mugs of coffee and the endless power struggle which went on. He suggested that the need for the struggles would become unnecessary if Martha was able to acquire her own coffee supplies and the skills to make it when she wished. It would then cease to be a conflict. We, too, had a Martha, called Doris, and we loved Lovett's approach. Doris was capable of making coffee already, so she was provided with the ingredients and encouraged to make her own coffee rather than trying to grab the staff's. She did so successfully . . . then she started faecal smearing. We had not first analysed the function that coffee-grabing had performed for Doris before we intervened. When we weakened her communication, she found a stronger one and became even more unpopular. Doris had been subjected to institutional abuse about 20 years ago.

Some common messages identified about the here-and-now fall into groups, and have been listed in the mnemonic SEAT (ranked for memorising, not priority!):

- Stimulation (for example: 'I'm bored out of my mind, I need something meaningful to do.').
- Escape. ('I want to get out of this task/place/noise/company. I want to stop. I don't understand what you want, the anxiety is unbearable.').
- Attention ('I need some undivided attention, some personal interest, someone to belong to. I feel insecure.').
- Tangible ('I'm hungry/thirsty/tired/cold/in pain/I want the music off/TV on. My mother has not come, I'm disappointed and angry.').

It is not difficult to identify these messages with Maslow's hierarchy of need, nor recognise that past experiences may leave individuals with inadequate, idiosyncratic or painful perceptions of the world, which need long-term management.

Hearing such communications presents the biggest challenge of all, because it raises the issue of power and authority. Is the demand to get away from appointed tasks or individuals – or for free access to food – legitimate or tolerable? Do people with learning difficulties have a right to get angry? What are the 'permitted' ways to express it?

Food and drink are quite a common focus for challenging behaviours. In an old institutional ward, Brian Davies, a middle-aged man with little speech, was referred because of his behaviour, which consisted of aggressive and destructive behaviours which were at their worst in the busiest part of the morning. Their cause was not difficult to guess. He was a fairly active individual, who always woke about five in the morning. Breakfast was not until 8 am, and those individuals going out to day centres in transport had to eat first. Put simply, Brian had to wait four hours, meanwhile smelling the food, before he could eat. His behaviour was hardly surprising. But the staff's was: 'No, there was no way that his breakfast could be brought forward.' It was then proposed that Brian could be taken to the shops to buy his own tin of biscuits and help himself if he was hungry but 'That wouldn't work, the other residents would steal them from his locker.' The tin could have Brian's name on it and live in a cupboard in the kitchen? The response: 'Oh no, residents are not allowed in the ward kitchen, it is too dangerous.'

Leslie Plant provides another example of this type of behaviour. He was 22, strong and had a history of explosive violence. He had little speech, but was developing good skills in electronic assembly work which he clearly enjoyed. He lived in a hospital ward the rest of the time. He was referred to the psychiatrist (again) because of his rising aggression. The story was fairly simple. On returning to the ward at 3.20 pm, he wanted a cup of tea. However, tea was not for another half hour, and he was known to get one at work at 3 pm. But don't most of us have a cuppa on getting in from work? The response: 'Well, if he had one, they'd all want one.' Leslie lives in a self-contained part of the ward with three others; he's probably already able to, so could he not make and serve tea for the four of them? There were reasons, of course, why this couldn't happen either.

These stories illustrate the underlying priorities for the staff employed to 'serve' the two men. It was more important to keep control, 'not let them get away with it', than to find ways to agree to quite simple requests. Meanwhile the two men continued to earn their negative reputations, of course.

The reasons we continue to hold onto power have to be examined and understood, if carers and others are to change posture and grow as well. A change to a person-centred approach, a different posture, some human insights and creativity, can sometimes be enough. James Humphres was 30, a little bit 'slow', very shy, and lived in a hostel for people with mental health problems. He had become increasingly irritable and uncooperative, and eventually kicked a staff member, breaking a bone. One choice was to have him charged with assault, but it was agreed that he should be admitted to a psychiatric unit for assessment instead. After two months there, doing nothing much, not being aggressive but with no cause identified for his assault, the hostel was afraid to have him back. An outside adviser started a 'getting-to-know-you' exercise and took a look at James' daily life and environment at the hostel.

James had always had limited language and been a bit slow at school. His father had tried to urge him on, and after one of their frequent rows, had a heart attack and died. This was seen as James' fault, and he was sent into residential care. He lost his father, his home, and his beloved brother all together. His life then contained many more losses as favourite staff moved on and he changed hostels. He had no job, no role, no relationships, no purpose in living. The day he kicked the staff member he was being told to get out of bed and go down for breakfast. He was not going on anywhere else. James' bedroom was dreary, but the communal day room was much worse. It was aesthetically horrible, and occupied with numerous people, restless and agitated or staring into space.

The staff were caring people, uncertain how to act, and welcomed discussion about James. The adviser summarised James' life story to date, and suggested how depressed and defeated he must be feeling. As James had no day programme, and given the limited choice of where to spend each day – the awful dayroom or bed – was not the choice of bed very reasonable?

Discussion of the possible ways in which to provide interesting activities for James revealed his huge enthusiasm for cricket and staff quickly drew up some creative suggestions involving library books, videos and outings (even though it was winter). The staff talked in uncomplicated language to James, explaining that they understood he was unhappy and that they would help him to do interesting things. A few months later he did not need to be called in the mornings, and had developed a satisfying round of activities in town. Supported employment, had it been available, would have made life even better.

Viewed through the framework of 'SEAT' (which he wasn't), James wanted escape from demands to get up, stimulation with enjoyable activities and the attention of someone really interested in him. All needs were eventually met.

Every effort must be made to build up the person's life story, which sometimes continues while new behaviours and experiences are growing. Ancient case files stored in hospitals hold sad and awful histories; quiet revelations of bizarre family behaviours give sudden insights. Dennis Harris, who took a long time to stop throwing televisions and other objects through the windows of his house, later commented that his grandfather had thrown things through the window when he was cross; this was confirmed by his family. Sam Jones, whose obsession with his bowels took us some time to relieve and replace with creative activities he enjoyed, unexpectedly murmured at a party that his late father used to stick Coca Cola bottles up his bottom.

While not all challenging behaviours are a message, they can give important information about the person's internal environment, that is part of the antecedent analysis. Flushing, sweating, overbreathing; this may indicate anxiety. *Stereotyped behaviours (twiddling, pacing, flicking) often serve a self-regulatory and tension reduction function.*

Autism is a disorder in which language and speech are always affected in varying degrees. Recent developments within the field of autism are providing new insights into the nature and causes of much challenging behaviour. Unfortunately, for years many British services and professionals denied the existence of the syndrome, and needful individuals have been failed by organisational disability and blindness. The lessons being learnt extend beyond autism alone. Some adults with autism have given vivid descriptions of their painful childhood experiences; for example, an excruciating sensitivity to high volume and pitch of sounds. Grandin (1986), now a successful professional consultant in animal management, describes the 'sandpaper' torment from wearing new clothes, the agony of small engine noises, and at the age of three having no speech with which to explain it, so throwing herself on the floor and screaming. She describes how stereotyped rituals (rocking, spinning), blocked out her tidal wave of sensory stimulation. Physical pain resulted from touch and embraces, and as a youngster she found how to desensitise herself by organising deep pressure for her skin, to produce relaxation: she recommends massage and deep pressure to help children with autism.

Grandin's descriptions, combined with her professional knowledge, contribute to the growing recognition of autism as a neurological disorder with movement disturbances. (Possible fresh insights come from Oliver Sachs' writings, in particular *Awakenings* (Sachs, 1990).) We now know that individuals may have quite different perceptions of environments; 'global pictures', rather than sequences, written ones better understood than spoken ones. One very active man registered his environment as 'not like a photograph' but a 'constant running film'. The knowledge that more able individuals with autism find *written* words more useful than *spoken* ones could be more widely applied. Derek Slater for example, who lived in a special unit for years and frequently destroyed his clothing, had virtually no speech. He was perceived as exasperatingly non-compliant when he 'pretended' not to understand what was asked of him, because he was able enough to read the newspaper. Written requests might have been more effective. Elaine Parker, 18, had mild autism and was extremely shy and found it difficult to talk in other than a monosyllabic way. However, when she wanted to convey information which was emotion-laden to her sympathetic employer, she wrote it down fluently.

Confusion and anxiety are commonly present where there are challenging behaviours, and positive interventions are concerned to reduce them, and provide individuals with 'durable' and 'portable' methods they can apply themselves in stressful situations. It is essential to develop *alternative coping mechanisms* to handle anger and stress, for example, before trying to reduce stereotyped behaviours which currently fill that role. (Some stereotyped behaviours create an emergency – such as eye poking – and require skilled urgent interventions.) Anxiety management can include relaxation training (it may take two years in children, but is both durable and portable) and the judicious use of medication. 'Snoezlan' rooms, with relaxing images, lights and sounds are gaining in popularity as calming environments, but unless the relaxation becomes more 'portable' and some positive behaviours are developed from the relaxation, they are perhaps of limited long-term value.

Other coping skills will need development, tolerance, strengthening patience and sharing, but this will take time, when individuals have never had their personal needs and wishes attended to consistently.

Some challenging behaviours should not be eradicated but indeed modified. Excessive talking or touching, for example, need to be reduced and redirected, but not totally eradicated: there are effective and positive ways to do that and often to build such modified behaviour into employment or social routines.

The communication issue remains a focal one. Our ability to convey feelings and information, to control our environment, to talk, write and draw symbols, marks us out as human beings. Many people with learning difficulties have major language impairments, but as the saying goes: 'Because I can't speak doesn't mean I have nothing to say'. Alternative methods of communication have been developed and refined for a long time. Signing by deaf people has been adapted in the UK as Makaton, a simple manual system quite widely used in special schools, but without application in the wider world. People with movement disorders, especially cerebral palsy, are of course better served with symbol systems (which also includes writing and pictures). An *awareness* of the need for communication in order to make sense of the world and have some control over daily life, has encouraged the development of pictorial systems. A portable card which says: 'I've had enough now, please stop' can be offered, instead of a physical assault. Wall diaries give understanding of the week's activities.

Alan Richards had limited speech and occasional seizures which frightened him, and he had a past history of explosive actions. One evening he was in the local pub and was noticed to be increasingly agitated. He was invited by his support worker to return home: on getting there, Alan rushed to his wall diary and tore off the picture of a swimsuit for the following morning. 'You don't want to go swimming tomorrow?' 'No,' he said emphatically. 'OK, we won't go, put the picture away.' Alan immediately looked relieved, and staff were convinced of the importance of pictures for information.

The use of keyboards with unicorn helmets or blow devices for people with cerebral palsy is no novelty as a form of augmentative communication, and electronic voice synthesisers have improved further.

Facilitated communication is another strategy for improving motor skills to enable someone to point to or touch objects, pictures or letters for communication purposes, and was originally developed for people with cerebral palsy. The technique is basically hand-over-hand or hand-on-forearm support while the person points. The contact is often faded back to upper arm or shoulder. The facilitator provides support and a resistant back pressure to the pointing action, and encourages a rhythmic movement. The intervention of the facilitator is providing 'accommodation', a phenomenon long familiar to people with Parkinson's Disease, who use light or heavy touch, rhythm, singing or visual cues to assist their difficulties in moving, thinking, perceiving or speaking.

The introduction of facilitated communication a few years ago identified many mute untutored adults and children with autism across the world, who were able to express themselves on keyboards with physical support. The communications typed have challenged our understanding of autism to its foundations. Not surprisingly, there is professional resistance, with sceptics suggesting the typing is that of the facilitator, and others alarmed that unsubstantiated claims of abuse are being typed out.

The 'criterion of the least dangerous assumption' states that 'in the absence of conclusive data, educational and clinical decisions should be based on assumptions which if incorrect will have the least dangerous effect on the learner' (LaVigna and Donnellan, 1986). On this basis, offering an individual communication possibilities is likely to do less harm than denying them the opportunity.

Organisational issues

As challenging behaviour becomes better understood, so more issues emerge. In the USA, punitive methods are permissible, because systematic electric shocks or ammonia squirts stop eye-gouging and other serious behaviours. But that is *all* punishment does: *it stops behaviour while applied*; it does nothing to build alternative strategies for coping. Punishments do not provide good role models, and their effects can be very reinforcing to the user.

A Department of Health Project Group chaired by Professor Jim Mansell, addressed the needs of people with learning difficulties and challenging behaviour or mental health problems. The report (DoH, 1993) laid out issues facing commissioners and senior managers of services, recognising that their past lack of understanding of necessary supports had resulted in the failure of numerous good projects.

Despite the initial expense of most challenging behaviour interventions, economies of scale are likely to be self-defeating because to make progress, each person needs an environment of sustained, consistent and individually focussed staff behaviours. The presence of other needful people with their own staff supports, means that sheer numbers alone renders environmental consistency impossible. Successful organisations seem to keep themselves small, with short and flexible lines of communication and supports, and containment of anxiety.

For a time in the 1980s it was believed that kindly, non-institutionalised, untrained people were enough to meet these very special needs. It became obvious that staff needed many skills, from good housekeeping to teaching skills. The highly detailed analysis of long-standing behaviours needs very special professional skills, which can of course be shared. Individuals may then be recognised as in need of treatments (psychotherapy, psychiatry or medication), and staff in need of further training and support. The work is extremely draining, and makes a variety of emotional challenges. We do not know whether it is possible or desirable for staff to remain in such work for prolonged periods.

This chapter has not discussed the needs of children and their families. In the UK service organisation badly fails to offer them the expertise and insights already available. For all individuals whose behaviour challenges us and them, there are numerous therapeutic approaches to be borrowed from other fields of work. At the same time, fresh understanding in this area of learning difficulties is capable of informing and encouraging development in many other services.

References

Biklen, D. (1985). *Achieving the Complete School: Strategies for Effective Mainstreaming*. Teachers College Press, New York.

Department of Health (1993). *Services for People With Learning Disabilities and Challenging Behaviour or Mental Health Needs: Report of a Project Group*. HMSO, London.

Emerson, E., Toogood, A., Mansell, J., Barrett, S., Bell, C., Cummings, R. and McCool, C. (1987). Challenging behaviour and community services: 1. Introduction and overview. *Mental Handicap*, 15, 166–169.

Grandin, T. (1986). *Emergence Labelled Autistic*. D.J. Costello, Tunbridge Wells.

LaVigna, G.W. and Donnellan, A.M. (1986). *Alternatives to Punishment: Solving Behavioural Problems with Non-Aversive Strategies*. Irvington Publishers, New York.

Lovett, H. (1985). *Cognitive Counselling and Persons with Special Needs*. Praeger, New York.

Maslow, A.H. (1987). *Motivation and Personality* (3rd edn). Harper and Row, New York.

Sachs, O. (1990). *Awakenings* (2nd edn). Pan Books, London.

Pseudonyms have been adopted in this chapter.

Chapter 19

No more double standards: Sexuality and people with learning difficulties

Michelle McCarthy and David Thompson

Few people would disagree that service providers have some responsibilities in the sexual lives of people with learning difficulties. In many
settings these responsibilities have been formalised through the development of guidelines and the provision of sex education, with sexual
abuse and HIV prevention curently major focusses. But very often
work concerning the sexuality of people with learning difficulties is
lacking on two counts. First, by failing to acknowledge the reality of
people with learning difficulties' sexual lives. Second, by being ill-
informed or even ignorant of wider debates on sexual behaviour and
gender. Staff concerned with these issues must learn from people with
learning difficulties about their experiences and locate their work
within a framework of sexual politics.

There is a common assumption that opportunities for both consented sexual expression and sexual abuse are greatest for those people
with learning difficulties living in community settings rather than
within institutions (Marchant, 1993). In fact, there is no evidence to
support this and the opposite may be true (Crossmaker, 1991;
McCarthy and Thompson, 1993).

It should be obvious that living in a large hospital which has spacious
grounds, with scores of other people with learning difficulties accords
more opportunities for sex than living in a small house with a few other
people, and higher levels of supervision. So, despite living in a far more
'normal' and normalised setting, opportunities for sex in the community are usually reduced and service providers need to acknowledge the
effects of this. While it has the obvious negative effect of taking away

desired opportunities for some people, the effects are by no means all bad. Much sex between people with learning difficulties is abusive (Elfrida Rathbone Women's Group, 1988) with men with learning difficulties making up the biggest single group of abusers of other people with learning difficulties (Brown and Turk, 1992). It follows that a reduction in opportunities to have sex will produce a reduction in the opportunities for sexual abuse.

People with learning difficulties (most commonly men) do have sexual relationships with people of the same sex, yet services are typically reluctant to face this reality. Resources are still produced which do not mention the possibility of same sex relationships (BIMH *et al.*, 1989). Those resources which do give the subject some attention either marginalise it (Kempton, 1988; Craft, 1991) or are only comfortable presenting intimate contact between people of the same sex as abusive (Kempton, 1988; Lifefacts, 1990). Clearly these are inadequate tools when required to support, for example, women with learning difficulties who seek relationships with women (Elfrida Rathbone Women's Group, 1988) or the significant numbers of men with learning difficulties who visit public toilets for sex (McLeod, 1993 (unpubl.); McCarthy and Thompson, 1994).

The authors' own sex education package is an attempt to address equal opportunities with respect to sexuality (McCarthy and Thompson, 1993). However, even with this resource and the commitment to equal opportunities of those using it, equality is immensely difficult to achieve. In group settings participants' own prejudices about same sex relationships are likely to surface. This can become apparent from an agenda set by people with learning difficulties which excludes same sex relationships, or individuals taking the opportunity to make homophobic statements. The authors' experience of men's groups is that, even when the majority of participants are privately known to have sex with men, they never feel able to talk about their own experiences in this context.

Recent challenges to traditional models of service provision

Finding a model of sex education which faces the reality of a multicultural society has been a very real challenge for many service providers. A good model needs to go beyond including images (but not stereotypes) of people of differing ethnic origins in resources, and should extend to including an awareness of cultural conventions and beliefs concerning sexual behaviour and the employment of service providers who reflect the racial diversity of the client group (Baxter, 1994). While these are laudable aims, it is however essential to recognise that some cultural beliefs about sex conflict with other equal opportunities perspectives. For example, most religions do not respect women's fight for control over their own sexuality or lesbian and gay equality (this includes the dominant white Christian culture within the UK).

Baxter does recognise this dilemma and urges people with learning difficulties to make a choice about how far they wish to go along with their families' religious beliefs. However, this does not solve the problem for three reasons. First, some religions have been adamant that matters related to sex should not be the subject of individual choice (for example, the Roman Catholic Church's refusal to sanction the use of artificial methods of contraception). Second, not all people with learning difficulties are in a position to make such complex moral decisions; the disabilities of some may prevent them from doing so. Finally, if a person with learning difficulties decides to go against the religious beliefs of their culture, then in providing support to that individual a service will itself be set in opposition to those beliefs. For example, the Sex Education Team at Harperbury Hospital was in touch with a Jewish man with learning difficulties who continued to have sex with men in public toilets knowing that sex between men was not sanctioned by orthodox Jewish doctrine. To offer him effective safer sex work it was necessary to provide him with a space where he was given the message that sex between men was acceptable. If a service does choose to disregard the cultural background of a person with learning difficulties with the justification of acting in that individual's best interests, it should openly acknowledge that its own values about sexuality have taken precedence, rather than claim the decision is value free, or 'professional'.

Examining the role self-advocacy can play in responding to sexual needs is difficult and controversial. The sex education, and particularly the staff training, that we have provided has been criticised by one or two people who believe that all such work should only be carried out by, or at the very least, with people with learning difficulties themselves, as nobody else can speak from their perspective. This is a reasonable stance that other disadvantaged people have taken, for example, many women and black people have rejected being defined and discussed by those who do not share their experiences. While it is true that the Sex Education Team has not worked alongside formal self-advocacy groups, its work has nevertheless been informed by intimate discussions with hundreds of people with learning difficulties. There is more than one way of consulting and involving people with learning difficulties in service provision. Moreover, we have been concerned that almost all the self-advocacy groups we have come into contact with have been dominated by men. Working with people with learning difficulties as individuals has been one way of preventing men with learning difficulties having a disproportionate influence on the service.

Although having a learning difficulty means being disempowered in many ways, it does not automatically give people with that label an awareness of the inequalities experienced by other disempowered groups; for example, women or gay men and lesbians in their sexual lives. People with learning difficulties should have the right to sex education from people, with or without learning difficulties, who will challenge these social and sexual inequalities. An ideology which suggests that people with learning difficulties are always best placed to undertake this work, simply because they have a learning difficulty, without regard to the political perspective of the work, is not likely to produce the best service.

Changing ideas about sexuality

Recent decades have seen changes in ideas about sexuality, many of which have been forced by social and political changes such as feminism, the campaign for lesbian and gay rights and the disability rights movement.

It is a sad irony that while some services have fought hard for the right of people with learning difficulties to sexual expression, very few have simultaneously accepted political perspectives which might lead them to be concerned for equality between people with learning difficulties with regards to sexual matters. For example, most residential and day services that we have come into contact with have reflected the widespread prejudice of society towards same-sex relationships. Regardless of whether they are run by private individuals, voluntary agencies, social services departments, health authorities or trusts, very few appear, as a service, to have been influenced by the political campaigns and the social movements which encourage a positive view of sexual relations between men or between women. Instead, outdated ideas which pathologise same-sex behaviour or apologise for it as being inevitable in single-sex environments are still very strongly held. There are, however, individual women and men working within these services who do have positive attitudes. The only *organisations* known to us which take a positive view of same-sex relationships are typically small and autonomous. Here the personal beliefs of key people can influence the service.

Another example of the way in which changing ideas about sexuality have failed to influence service provision to people with learning difficulties is in the area of gender power relations. There is generally little recognition of how they both reflect and shape women's and men's sexuality. Very few of the women and men with learning difficulties with whom we have worked have been made aware of the changes which have taken place regarding both attitudes to, and the reality of, women's sexual opportunities. Many staff are in the same unenlightened position. Women with learning difficulties' experience of sex continues to be largely a passive experience devoid of sexual pleasure (McCarthy, 1993). Sex for many many women with learning difficulties means little more than providing a sexual service to men.

Service providers, including those like psychiatrists and psychologists who might be more expected to have kept up with current thinking and to have developed insights into sexuality, often have a very poor understanding of some crucial issues. It is well accepted that sexual behaviour does not fit neatly into dated medical categories – that is homosexual, heterosexual – neither does it necessarily determine a person's sexual identity, for example, lesbian, gay, bisexual (Weeks, 1985). Yet professionals working with people with learning difficulties seem largely to be ignorant of this; a simplistic link is often made between sexual behaviour and sexual identity. Service providers continue to attempt to label their clients – 'is he homosexual?' – or pressurise people with learning difficulties to label themselves.

Our experience of work with men with learning difficulties who have sex with men is that issues of sexual identity are incredibly complex. Overwhelmingly, these men have picked up society's prejudices towards same-sex relationships. This is demonstrated by their reluctance to talk about these relationships compared to their willingness to talk about sexual contacts with women. In addition, their predominant understanding of the words 'gay' and 'homosexual' are negative. Many of these men have had, or continue to have, sexual relationships with women and almost all state that they would like a girlfriend. Some staff will naively ask men with learning difficulties who have sex with men whether they prefer men or women. When a man answers 'women' staff satisfy themselves that he is not really 'homosexual', instead of recognising that this answer is more likely to reflect the men's desire not to be stigmatised than give any indication of their actual sexual interests. After all, having a female partner offers all men a socially valued status in addition to the opportunity for sex.

Only one or two of the most able men with whom we have worked have been able to openly acknowledge a distinct sexual attraction to men; for them a gay identity might have been a possibility. But they were isolated both from other gay men (gay staff members largely feel inhibited from revealing their sexuality to clients) and from the gay culture (based round clubs and bars which are largely inaccessible for those with a physical disability or for financial or geographic reasons). Hardly surprising then, that these men did not see themselves as gay. What chance is there for a man with learning difficulties to take on a gay identity if he knows no gay men with whom to identify?

Cross-dressing or transvestism also highlights how thinking on sexuality issues for people with learning difficulties often lags behind the times. For men with learning difficulties it is suggested that not having wives or girlfriends may be a significant contributory factor in the development of this behaviour and the 'promotion of heterosexual relationships is important if the behaviour is to abate' (Bowler and Collacott, 1993). Men without learning difficulties who cross-dress do not cite an absence of a heterosexual partner as a significant factor in their transvestism (Beaumont Society, undated). Indeed, the availability of advice and support groups for the wives and girlfriends of transvestite men testifies to the fact that it is very common for men who cross-dress to already have heterosexual relationships and that this does nothing to diminish their desire to wear women's clothes.

Sexual abuse

It is in the area of sexual abuse, perhaps more than any other, that there have been both very significant changes in attitudes in society and also very long delays while services for people with learning difficulties catch up with these changes.

For 20 years or more feminists in particular have devoted much time and energy into exposing the reality of sexual violence. (Brownmiller,

1975; London Rape Crisis Centre, 1984; Hall, 1984; Kelly, 1988). The result is a wealth of material both from the perspective of the people (largely women and children) who have experienced sexual abuse and that of the perpetrators.

In the UK sexual abuse only really started to be addressed on any scale as an issue for people with learning difficulties in the late 1980s; there had, therefore, been ample time for informed ideas about sexual abuse generally to have been absorbed by service providers. Yet even as we head towards the mid-1990s it is still common to find influential professionals within services for people with learning difficulties who still promote very outdated and (to many) offensive ideas about the sexual abuse of, and by, people with learning difficulties. These outdated opinions (sadly often presented as facts) match almost exactly the traditional myths about rape and sexual abuse which have now been generally discredited. Only recently, for example, we have heard service providers say that women with learning difficulties commonly make false allegations about sexual abuse; that women with learning difficulties enjoy sexual and physical violence from men; that sexual abuse which takes place within an established relationship is not real abuse; and that the experience of being sexually abused has no significant or lasting effects.

Compared with the attitudes informing services run by women from a feminist perspective (like rape crisis centres and incest survivors groups) these attitudes are far behind the times. But they also compare unsatisfactorily with other statutory care provision. In child care and child protection services, mental health services, parts of the probation service and (in large part due to *Community Care*'s 1993 campaign to raise awareness of elder abuse (*Community Care*, 1993)) parts of service provision to elderly people, clients are receiving a better informed, more respectful and responsive service in relation to sexual abuse than many of their counterparts with learning difficulties. People with learning difficulties are already among the most disadvantaged in society and are being further disadvantaged in this way.

Many assumptions made about the behaviour of men with learning difficulties who sexually abuse are equally disturbing and ill-informed; for example, service providers saying that men with learning difficulties who sexually abuse others do so because they have no 'normal' heterosexual 'outlet' for their sexual feelings, that physical injuries (severe bruising and bitemarks) caused by a man with learning difficulties during sexual activity were not due to his aggression but to his sexual excitement. Perhaps the two most common justifications made for the men's abusive behaviour are that they don't know it is wrong, and that it is a consequence of their own sexual abuse. But the vast majority of sexual abusers are men, whether they have learning difficulties or not (Brown and Turk, 1992) and women with learning difficulties (who as women are more likely to be sexually abused) do not themselves abuse in any significant number.

Not facing up to the reality of men with learning difficulties as perpetrators of sexual abuse allows services to avoid dealing with such behaviour. There is perhaps an emotional resistance on the part of service providers to seeing these men outside the disempowered status of 'having a learning difficulty'. There is no organisation which focusses on men with learning difficulties who are abusers, though there are a number which specifically address the needs of people with learning difficulties who have been abused. However, in recent years there have been some significant developments focussing on men who abuse and it is in the interests of men with learning difficulties who sexually abuse that there is research and service development in this area. One area of great concern, for example, is the extent to which anti-libidinal medication is prescribed to men with learning difficulties whose sexual behaviour is problematic; medication which is often rejected by other men, not least because of its side effects.

The way forward

Although criticism has been made of the attitudes and practices of many learning difficulty services on sexuality, it is nevertheless important to acknowledge that standards are rising. Over the past four to five years in particular, much commendable work has been developed in the areas of staff training, research, policy development and, most importantly, direct service provision. Staff training is now available on sexuality, sexual abuse and sexual health issues from an informed equal opportunities perspective. This training seeks to enable service providers actively to challenge the inequalities faced by many service users.

Developments in the research field are also encouraging: an example of innovative research which fits into the above framework is the assessment of needs of men with learning difficulties who have sex with men in public toilets (Cambridge et al., 1993). Further detailed research is also currently being carried out by the authors into the sexual experiences and sexual abuse of both women and men with learning difficulties. Meanwhile, an analysis of gender inequalities is becoming more common (see, for example, Williams, 1992; Burns, 1993).

In recent years, too, there has been a huge increase in the number of voluntary and statutory organisations which have developed guidelines and policies regarding the sexuality of service users. Even more recently a number of agencies have started to produce policies specifically on providing a good response to instances of sexual abuse. This is clearly a move in the right direction. However, an evaluation of a selection of these sexual abuse guidelines (conducted by the Tizard Centre at the University of Kent) shows that there is a long way to go. Of the 13 sets of abuse guidelines evaluated, seven failed to acknowledge that there was a good chance that the perpetrators would be male service users themselves and consequently no suggestions were made as how staff should respond in such cases, two of the remaining six sets of guidelines which did acknowledge the potential of abuse by service users offered responses which were less than satisfactory (Brown and Stein, 1995; in preparation).

Clearly there is little point in improving staff training, research and policy developments if the benefits of these do not filter through to direct service provision to clients. In many ways, this is the most difficult area of work to evaluate. By its very nature it is personal and often confidential and so it is hard to know just when effective work is taking place. Despite these difficulties, evaluation tools need to be developed which measure the outcomes of sexuality work with people with learning difficulties. Without these tools there is a risk that scarce resources will be misused and people with learning difficulties will, at best, receive support which is believed to be in their best interests, rather than that which has been demonstrated as being the best possible intervention to meet their needs. For example, all practitioners providing safer sex education to people with learning difficulties need to assess sensitively that individual's ability to negotiate safer sex once that education has ended. Without this some people will inadvertently be left very vulnerable to HIV infection, as assumptions may be made that they are in a position to act in a certain way, when they are not able to do so.

Evaluating the support offered to people with learning difficulties in relation to sex means recognising that the work will not necessarily have achieved its initial aims. If this is the case, workers must then face the dilemma of how far services have a responsibility to protect people with learning difficulties from the risks of sex. These include the risk of

HIV infection as well as the risks of sexual exploitation and abuse. If after extensive work with him, a man with learning difficulties lacks the assertiveness, rather than the motivation, to insist on safer sex with men who expose him to a very real risk of HIV, should the service take measures to prevent the sex which puts him at risk? Similarly, if a woman with learning difficulties experiences sex with her boyfriend as physically painful and emotionally distressing and the work with both her and the boyfriend fails to change the situation, should the service actively stop the relationship? Practitioners have said that to answer 'yes' in either of these situations is to apply a different standard to the sexual lives of people with learning difficulties than those without as intervention would not be made to protect other people in these positions. It is our view that for some people with learning difficulties, protection from unreasonable risks which may have devastating consequences is the only responsible course of action and that this is an instance where a double standard is desirable.

Because of the complexity of the issues that are raised in working with people with learning difficulties on sexual issues, it is important that service providers get a chance to inform each other honestly about the work they are doing. When individual practitioners write up their work this can inspire others. The latest book edited by Craft (1994) contains some excellent descriptions of good quality services provided to individuals and groups of people with learning difficulties (see for example, Baum's very moving account of the service provided to a pregnant woman with severe learning difficulties in that volume).

The series of seminars which we co-ordinate provide another model for good practice. These are informal seminars where practitioners have a chance to present their ideas and practice to colleagues. Feedback from the participants has been very positive with comments that it provides an excellent opportunity to hear about others' work in a supportive and encouraging environment.

Good practice dictates that when people with learning difficulties have a specific need or problem relating to their sexuality, sexual abuse or sexual health, then service providers should look at what their clients have in common with other people who have similar needs or problems. This means a shift in focus from the learning difficulties themselves as the issue or problem, to the life experience. For example, we should think of a person who has been sexually abused who also has a learning difficulty, rather than a person with a learning difficulty who has been sexually abused. The change of emphasis is subtle but crucial.

It will force service providers to put the experience of people with learning difficulties into a wider social and political context. This in turn will force a recognition that much of what happens to people with learning difficulties regarding sexual matters is very similar to what happens to other people. Where there are significant differences, then, it is to be hoped, service providers will seek out the reasons for these differences and no longer accept without question that they are due to the learning difficulty itself. Only in this way will it be possible to dispense with double standards.

References

Baum, S. (1994). 'Interventions with a pregnant woman with severe learning difficulties: A case example', in *Practice Issues in Sexuality and Learning Disabilities* (ed. A. Craft). Routledge, London.

Baxter, C. (1994). Sex education in the multi-cultural society. In *Practise Issues in Sexuality and Learning Disabilities*. (ed. A. Craft). Routledge, London.

Beaumont Society Leaflet No. 3 *Transvestites, Partners and Families: Some Questions and Answers*. Beaumont Society, London.

BIMH (now British Institute of Learning Disability), Brook Advisory, MENCAP and the Family Planning Association (1989). *AIDS: What It Is and How to Protect Yourself*, BIMH, Kidderminster.

Bowler, C. and Collacott, R. (1993). Cross-dressing in men with learning disabilities. *British Journal of Psychiatry*, 162, 556–558.

Browmiller, S. (1975). *Against Our Will*. Secker and Warburg, London.

Brown, H. and Stein, J. (1995). *A Matter of Policy: Policies on Sexual Abuse of Adults With Learning Difficulties* (in preparation).

Brown, H. and Turk, V. (1992). Defining sexual abuse as it affects adults with learning disabilities. *Mental Handicap*, 20, 44–55.

Burns, J. (1993). Invisible women – Women who have learning disabilities. *The Psychologist*, 6, 102–105.

Cambridge, P. *et al*. (1993). Men with learning difficulties who have sex with men in public places. Tizard centre, Canterbury.

Community Care, 6 May–23 July 1993 inclusive.

Craft, A. (1991). Living Your Life, Learning Development Aids, Cambridge.

Craft, A. (1994). (ed.) *Practice Issues in Sexuality and Learning Disabilities*. Routledge, London.

Crossmaker, M. (1991). Behind locked doors: Institutional Sexual Abuse. *Sexuality and Disability*, 913, 201–219.

Hall, R. (1984). *Ask Any Woman*. Falling Wall Press, Bristol.

Kelly, L. (1988). *Surviving Sexual Violence*. Polity Press, Cambridge.

Kempton, W. (1988). *Life Horizons I & II*. James Stanfield and Co., Santa Monica, California.

Lifefacts I and II (1990). James Stanfield and Co., Santa Monica, California.

London Rape Crisis Centre (1984). *Sexual Violence: The Reality for Women*. Women's Press, London.

Marchant, C. (1993). A need to know issue. *Community Care*, 28 October.

McCarthy, M. and Thompson, D. (1993). *Sex and the 3Rs: Responsibilities and Risks*. Pavilion, Brighton.

McCarthy, M. and Thompson, D. (1994). HIV/AIDS and safer sex work with people with learning disabilities. In *Practice Issues in Sexuality and Learning Disabilities* (ed. A. Craft). Routledge, London.

McCarthy, M. (1993). Sexual experiences of women with learning difficulties in long-stay hospitals. *Sexuality and Disability*, **11**(4) 277–85.

McLeod, J. *More than One Barrier. HIV & AIDS and Men with Intellectual Disabilities Who have Sex with Men: An Education Needs Assessment*. Victoria AIDS Council, Melbourne. (Unpubl.).

Weeks, J. (1985). *Sexuality and its Discontents: Meanings, Myths and Modern Sexualities*. Routledge, London.

Williams, F. (1992). Women with learning difficulties are women too. In *Women, Oppression and Social Work* (eds M. Langan and L. Day). Routledge, London.

Chapter 20

For better, for worse: Professionals, practice and parents with learning difficulties

Tim Booth and Wendy Booth

What can be done to bring about a closer alignment between professional practice and parents' perceptions of their own needs, and what is the likelihood of this happening?

The study on which this chapter draws (Booth and Booth, 1994a) was designed to explore the experience of child-rearing and parenthood as recounted by mothers and fathers with learning difficulties. The aim was to provide a parent's view of parenting using a life story approach. Thirty-three parents (20 mothers and 13 fathers) from 20 families took part in the study of whom 25 (18 mothers and 7 fathers) had learning difficulties. Between them these parents had 50 children of whom 26 belonged to partnerships in the study. Contact with the families was extensive: 126 interviews were conducted over a period of 18 months.

Standing back from the detail of people's lives, five themes emerge from their common experience of the health and welfare services.

- Service workers and practitioners occupied an ambivalent status in the eyes of parents. They were a valued source of support for some. For others they brought little but heartache and trouble. All the families were receiving support of some kind from the statutory services. While recognising they needed help in order to cope, they often complained bitterly about the terms on which it was delivered.
- A signal feature of much professional intervention was its inconsistency. A change of service worker frequently entailed a change in practice. A few families received intensive support where others were left to fend for

themselves until a crisis erupted. Blatant disparities were found in the contact that parents were allowed with children who had been removed from home. Some parents were required to maintain standards of child care or cleanliness in the home that were not applied to others.

- Support varied from competence-promoting to competence-inhibiting in character (Tucker and Johnson, 1989). Competence-promoting support allows parents to feel in control, encourages them to handle their problems on their own, and reinforces and develops their skills and sense of self-worth. Competence-inhibiting support assumes the parents are incapable of managing on their own and tends to be demotivating, crisis-oriented and unresponsive to the parents' view of their needs.

- A good deal of work with parents who have learning difficulties is infused with moralistic overtones. Good parenting is a vague concept (Brantlinger, 1988). There are no agreed minimal requirements of adequate child care. Consequently, practitioners often base their judgements and assessments of parental adequacy on value-laden comparisons with middle-class standards (Tymchuk, 1990) and parents are often left 'striving to meet standards of care which are not made explicit'. (Painz, 1993)

- Too often the problems of families are made worse by the services intended to provide them with support. Such an effect is sometimes referred to as 'system abuse' in the literature (Prosser, 1992). System abuse describes institutional attitudes, policies and practices that 'hurt children, harm family integrity, and infringe basic rights' (Gil, 1982). Parents with learning difficulties are especially vulnerable to its manifestations because of prejudicial assumptions about their fitness for parenthood.

These points come out of the parents' experience of the services but not out of their mouths. They represent the viewpoint of the observer, summing up people's stories, rather than the authentic voice of the parents themselves. It is in the small change of people's lived encounters with social workers, community nurses, doctors, support workers and the like that the makings of good and bad practice are found. Working from the personal accounts of the parents we interviewed, we have pieced together a users' guide to how current practice must change before a new partnership between parents and practitioners can develop.

Features of bad practice

Bad practice is not confined to work with parents with learning difficulties. Many of the examples cited by parents in our study could also be found among other service users. Its significance and impact, however, are mediated by the lives people lead. Parents with learning difficulties live with the ever-present fear their children may be taken away (Andron and Tymchuk, 1987). Such worry is well-founded. Of the 20 families in our study, 14 had had one or more of their children placed in short-term or permanent care, including six who had none of their children living at home with them. Moreover, the evidence points to the fact that children are too often taken away because professionals fear harm may befall them rather than because of parenting breakdown (Booth and Booth, 1994b). Against this background, bad professional practice further increases the stress on parents' coping resources.

With these points in mind, let us look more closely at the key features of bad practice as seen by our parents.

Practitioners with book knowledge only, who lack personal experience of parenting

Many families in our study had been allocated social workers or support workers who were young, inexperienced and had no children of their own. These parents felt they needed 'somebody that's got a bit of age on their back, you know, a bit more experience of life, a bit of understanding.' Mr Stewart spoke for many when he said: 'the welfare . . . send kids of about 25, if that, not qualified. They were giving me all this advice about children and I says to them, "Have you any children, love? Are you married?" I thought, they're trying to give me all this advice with no children. They might know all the theory of the job but they haven't the practical experience. When you're bringing up children and that, and you're tired, you've to really experience it.' Parents are victims of their label: practitioners were reluctant to allow that people with learning difficulties had anything to teach them. Consequently, the parents felt their workers often failed to understand their needs and the pressures in their lives and were unresponsive to them.

Lack of continuity in service delivery

High levels of staff turnover caused a lot of problems for families. Mrs Armstrong could name eight social workers she had seen over the past seven years. Cathy Pollock commented: 'We've had that many social workers I can't remember them all.' Parents found themselves continually having to explain the same things over again. More seriously, such frequent comings-and-goings inhibited the formation of trusting relationships, made parents reluctant to confide or talk openly, and increased the stress which the services themselves imposed on families. Even in child protection reviews, parents reported finding 'quite a few away, not actually involved in [the] case but just standing in'. Indeed, most families were aware that any support they received might easily be withdrawn. When Mr and Mrs Derby moved to another part of the city, the new social services team in whose area they now lived did not allocate them a replacement family aide and, in fact, a year after the move, they still had not been assigned a new social worker. Such lack of continuity lessened the effectiveness of the services, heightened the vulnerability of parents and their families, and threatened their ability to cope.

Undermining the parents' authority in their own home

Many parents complained about practitioners bossing them about, telling them what to do, and generally not showing enough respect for them as people. There was a widespread feeling among parents that workers too often overstepped the mark in the way they treated them. Julie Burnley voiced these complaints forcefully: 'I just want them to leave me alone, let me get on with my life. I don't like social workers on my back. They interfere with us. I don't want anybody telling me what to do. Only your mam should tell you off, not social workers. They treat me like I was one year old and I'm nearly 26.' Mr Stewart expressed similar frustrations: 'We had a health visitor that was very domineering. She came that often I thought she were my wife. She really did wear me down.' Mr and Mrs Derby's support worker was 'quite jolly' but: 'She'll not let you get away with owt, not let you slack. She's got a list of different things to do for days of week and what should be done on a certain day, and she'll tick you off if they're not done. She'll say, "Oh, I'm not pleased." ' Families generally had no say in when support workers came and went, and felt it as an intrusion on their privacy. The frequency with which workers arrived late or failed to show at all was also a cause of annoyance ('When I clean the place up for them, they don't turn up'). Incidents such as these reinforced parents' own perception of their devalued status.

Attributing deficits in the services to the inadequacies of the parents

Negative assumptions about parents' coping abilities combined with deficiencies in support frequently tip the balance of judgement in child welfare proceedings against the parents. Stella Richards is a case in point. Looking back on the reasons for her difficulties in trying to look after a young baby, Stella said: '. . . not being learnt in the early stages how to look after a child and that, I think that's what it was. We was shown this film about sex and that but I wasn't taught how to cope. If they'd have give me summat, like learn me, taught me how to look after a baby, I'd been all right.' Joan Pointer told a similar story. For the first three months after her son was born she lived with a couple who helped her look after him. 'It were when I went back to my own flat I couldn't cope. It were getting on top of me. She didn't even bother to come and see me, my social worker. I would have liked to have looked after him, if I had somebody near me what could help me like. But with living up other end of city it were too far for my family to come and see me.'

Judging parents by inappropriate standards and values

Parents were widely expected to maintain standards of child care and housekeeping that were foreign to their neighbourhoods, family and friends. As Julie Burnley complained: 'They want me to get my house perfect but I cannot get it perfect. I'm not like other people, them posh people. It's just like other houses round here.' Discipline too was another area where parents' and professionals' views did not match up. Many study families reported having been warned against smacking their children. However, generally lacking powers of verbal reasoning (or a warm bedroom where a child could be sent), they were left with no effective method of discipline and began to encounter problems of control. Similar differences in expectations were also evident in such things as diet ('They've got us eating meat, and I don't even like meat.'); playing with the children ('They said they were there to try and help like, how to play with Sue. They were more or less doing it for me. What I usually do . . . is get the toys in the middle of the floor and let her play with them. They probably expected me to play with her . . .'); smoking (one family had been told not to smoke when the child was in the room); children's bedtimes ('Jeremy's to get to bed at right time'); and routines (one couple were instructed to move their toddler out of their bedroom into a room of his own). One mother and father were even forbidden to give their children sweets at contact meetings on the grounds that they'd come to expect them. As Grant (1980) has pointed out, parents with learning difficulties are often placed in a kind of double jeopardy. Subjected to a closer level of scrutiny than most other poor parents, they are also required to meet higher expectations.

Diminishing the importance of family relationships

Practitioners tended to undervalue the strength of family bonds. Partly this comes about because their principal focus of concern is usually the welfare of the children rather than the well-being of the family, and partly too because of ingrained attitudes that prevent us from seeing people with learning difficulties as capable of loving and being loved. Such attitudes showed in the practice of treating people as individuals rather than as a family unit. Mrs Spencer, temporarily resident in a local authority hostel following her recent estrangement from her husband, complained bitterly that her family had not been present when a case review had been held to consider her future living arrangements: 'I would have liked my husband and daughter to come to my review but they didn't ask me. And nobody phoned them afterwards. They wouldn't let me.' The same attitudes were also revealed in casual responses to the feelings of parents whose children had been taken away. Mrs Armstrong recalls meeting her children's headmistress shortly after they had all been put in foster care. 'She said, "It turned out for the best, didn't it?" I said, "Maybe you think it did." She said, "Because Mark was hard work for you." I said, "Yes, but I wouldn't say it turned out for the best." ' Failing to see that families are more than the sum of their parts can lead to skewed judgements about parental competence and what is best for the child.

Interfering in matters that have no bearing on the reasons for intervention

A regular complaint was that practitioners meddled in things that were not their concern ('They're watching you all the time'). Often these complaints concerned money – which many parents saw as a touchstone of their independence. Mrs Pollock contrasted her social worker unfavourably with her community nurse: 'When you have a social worker they ask you how much money you get, stuff like that, and what you're spending it on, how much clothes, how much food you're getting. But community nurse never does that. It's up to us what we do you see.' Parents objected to what they saw as interference dressed up as help. For instance, some practitioners used their legitimate concerns about child welfare and protection as a pretext for intervening in people's sexuality. Mrs Hardy recalls, 'When I was having Alice, the social worker said I had to have an abortion with her. I told her straight. I says I'm having her, and that's it.' Ms Trevelyan had been receiving contraceptive injections since the birth of her child five years before even though she was no longer in a relationship and had no social life. Social services decided that one father should have a vasectomy. As his wife said, 'They told him he'd to have it done and they arranged it.' He was escorted to the clinic and they waited while he had the operation. Parents' lack of power and their need for support make it very hard for them to resist the encroachments of practitioners who wish to run their lives for them.

Taking advantage of people's learning difficulties: treating the parents as less than fully adult

Parents with learning difficulties straddle two worlds. As parents they occupy a socially valued role in the wider society. As people with learning difficulties they are stigmatised and excluded. All too often the services reinforced their subordination rather than their citizenship. Generally speaking, this showed most clearly in the way parents were treated by frontline staff on a day-to-day basis. Mrs Spencer was not allowed to make her own appointments to see her GP but had to go through the community nurse who restricted her to a maximum of one visit every six weeks. Julie Burnley and Neville Fletcher had five different workers visit during the course of a week to check on their baby. All visits and attendant observations were recorded in a book kept in their living room ('Julie was in a bad mood today and I had to tell her off for not hoovering the carpet'). Julie and Neville could not read the handwriting and the book annoyed them intensely: 'If they keep writing in that book I'm going to put it back of the fire. I'm sick of seeing it.' Mr and Mrs Hardy's son was placed for adoption after their social worker told the court that Mr Hardy (who does not have learning difficulties) would not be able to care for him adequately given that his existing parental duties extended not only to his baby daughter but also to his wife. In the minutiae of parents' encounters with practitioners it is possible to see how their learning difficulties are used to reinforce their dependency as a way of managing their lives.

Using parents' fears of losing their child to secure their acquiescence

Parents with learning difficulties 'live in constant fear that someone will come to take their children away' (Andron and Tymchuk, 1987). Practitioners were not averse to using these fears to ensure parents went along with their decisions. Julie Burnley confessed to being frightened of losing her young son, 'if I argue with social workers'. Her sister backed up her point: 'Sometimes they say to her, "Your baby's not clean enough. If you don't clean him up, we'll have to take him off you." ' Several fathers (without learning difficulties) were told that their children would be taken into care unless they gave up work to look after them. When Mr Baker asked to see the ID card of a social worker whom he hadn't met before, the social worker (who couldn't produce any identification) accused him of being awkward and threatened to go to the local police station to get a search warrant and a child care order. All the parents knew their hold on their children was fragile and this put them under enormous stress. It also fostered a suspicion of the motives of professionals that made them reluctant to seek or use help when it was needed.

Gender bias

Gendered assumptions about the role of mothers and fathers infused a lot of work with parents and sometimes locked them into ways of living that failed to make the best use of their personal resources and skills. It was invariably the mother who received what little training in parenting skills was given. One father recalled his wife coming home from hospital with her first baby: 'They must have tried to show her how to care for him, how to put nappies on or something like that. The point is they didn't show me. No one were there to help me you see. When she came home with him he were put into my hands and no one ever came and told me how to make a bottle or anything. So what I had to do, I had to take notice of how I took the nappy off, I had to ask how to make a baby's bottle.' Equally, mothers were often expected to cope where fathers were given support. Molly Austin was angered by the fact that she'd had to look after two young children all day in a broken-down caravan while the community nurses had provided her partner, Kevin, with day care for two days a week (even though he was out of work) when she left him briefly. The other side of the coin is that practitioners often failed to encourage parents to think beyond the stereotypes they had grown up with and took for granted. This was most evident where they went along with the parents' assumption that contraception was the woman's responsibilty even when she had problems.

Failing to respond to problems until a crisis erupts; failing to respond to parents' concerns; failing to involve parents in decisions affecting their lives.

Several families in the study accumulated large debts despite having support workers who were supposed to help them with their finances. Parents were often left to cope on their own until things went wrong. Mr and Mrs Pollock are a case in point. They both have learning difficulties and their two sons, Stewart aged eight and Justin aged six, go to a special school. They have had almost no support from social services. 'They always said that when your kids are growing up you can cope on your own.' Stewart had recently been giving them problems. 'I went up to school [and] told them we couldn't cope with our Stewart because he was swearing and biting and saying these "f" words like that. Might be his ways, they says, because he's getting older now.' The Pollocks are now being told their children might have to go into care. They don't want that, but neither the school, their community nurse nor the social services have helped them deal with Stewart's behaviour. The Pollocks, it seems, are being left to struggle on until a decision about what to do is taken out of their hands.

Failing to recognise parents' emotional needs

Parents frequently talked about incidents where their feelings had been disregarded. Nobody in the study who had had a child taken away received any guidance or counselling to help them cope with their loss. Despite repeated requests, Mrs Gore's social work assistant kept forgetting to bring her some recent photographs of her two youngest children who were in care. Mrs Gore's sister commented, 'They're supposed to send them every year but they don't. We've just got a few about two years since.' When Mr and Mrs Hardy said their final goodbyes to their son prior to his adoption, their social worker made them a video of the parting. Although critical of the idea ('It's not the same as your child being here or seeing him'), they wanted the video. Two months later it had still not arrived. Mrs Armstrong told how she broke down at a birthday party given by her children's foster parents: 'I cried and all [the social worker] said was, if you come and upset the kids you'll not see them again. It's all right for them to say hold it back, don't cry in front of kids. I couldn't help it.' Countless similar examples in the study suggest that many practitioners find it hard to respect the authenticity of parents' feelings for their children or to accept their capacity for love. At times of emotional stress for parents, a good practitioner was someone who could respond to them in ordinary human terms.

Features of good practice

Our parents voiced more criticisms than compliments. Inevitably, perhaps, for they had all had a tough time. Listening to their stories, however, we have been able to pick out some features of good practice that resonate with their experience. In one sense, of course, good practice means avoiding the mistakes discussed above. But this merely fixes a baseline. The real challenge is to go on and build a more positive partnership with parents.

Assigning a worker with a genuine liking for the family

The attitude of those delivering support is a crucial factor determining its effectiveness. As Andron and Tymchuk (1987) comment, a 'professional must be really committed to working with these families'. One father conveyed the same point when he praised the family support worker by saying, 'It's not just a job she does for a wage at end of day.' Kingsley Stewart's wife, Lois, attended a special care unit and what impressed him most was the quality of the staff: 'I says there's one thing that all these other places haven't got. They've got good staff and there's a load of love there, and there is you know, heck of a load of love and they share it out equal.' The most effective kind of support was consistent, non-intrusive and non-threatening. Molly Austin said as much when talking about her community nurse: 'Oh no, [she] doesn't interfere. . . . If I have any problems I just say "Can I have a talk to you?" when she come, and she'll say, "Yes, if you like," and I'd have ten minutes or something like that with her. And sometimes she'll say, "You're better off doing it that way instead of this way." ' Another mother simply summed up the qualities of the family's support worker by saying, 'She's like a mam to us'.

Practical support that is sustained over the longer term and directed towards reinforcing and developing parents' own skills

Having children and running a household puts a premium on skills like coping with money, budgeting, time management, and basic literacy.

Poverty adds to the pressures and problems. Parents, like Mrs Jennings, valued support with everyday tasks which they found hard to manage: 'She just comes to sort my money out, help me with my shopping, and help me with my housework. Then she sorts out, like, money in the bank, and telephone bills, and television licence, and electric bills.' To be effective, however, such help must not smack of interference. Julie Burnley and Neville Fletcher were aggrieved at having no say over how much they saved or spent since social services stepped in to sort out their debts: 'They said, we're not going to take money off you. And what've they done? They've took money off us. They give us pocket money.' The more positive comments about the services came from parents, like Mrs Stephenson, who had never seen them as intrusive: 'They've helped me a lot. They're there when I want them.' It is also important for support, once provided, to be sustained as long as it is needed. Training in the acquisition of new skills was often either not carried over from the classroom into the home, or withdrawn before parents had learned to manage on their own. For example, although Mrs Derby was attending skills classes at a local adult education college her family support worker failed to reinforce her learning at home. Instead, she helped Mr Derby – who does not have learning difficulties – to look after the house, even rearranging one of her twice weekly visits to a day when Mrs Derby was at college. As Mr Derby said, 'We can only get owt done in house when I'm here.'

The mobilisation of community supports, including the extended family

The presence of a benefactor has been found to be crucial in enabling parents to continue looking after their children (Kaminer, et al., 1981; Tymchuk, 1992). Indeed, a key feature of successful parenting is the presence of other adults able to give support as required with tasks beyond the parents' own coping resources (Espe-Sherwindt and Kerlin, 1990). According to Zetlin et al. (1985), informal networks exhibit a number of advantages over formal services in the delivery of support to parents. They are local, familiar, reliable and the help given is based on standards rooted in the common cultural and class experience of members. Significantly, the only person in our study who reported having no difficulties bringing up her child was a single mother living with her own parents. Many people's troubles began when their supports broke down. One father (without learning difficulties) was able to 'go out to work more at ease knowing my mother was looking after things.' When his mother died, his wife was unable to maintain a domestic routine alone and the family was pitched into a succession of crises.

Close integration of formal services and informal support networks

The failure to co-ordinate formal and informal supports can impair parents' ability to cope and add to their troubles. Mrs Pollock explains how in her case: 'Len lost his mother last year. He was close to her. She used to live close by us. She give us a lot of help and she gived Len a lot of help, and she used to look after kids for us . . . And then it started. Len was in hospital for two months with his depression . . . I couldn't cope . . . We asked for a social worker but they wouldn't give us one.' Leaving Mrs Pollock to cope alone without the support of Len's mother and with the additional burden of a depressed husband is now threatening to break up the family (Booth and Booth, 1993).

The other side of the story is illustrated by Jill Trevelyan. She lived alone with her father until her baby was four years old when Mr Trevelyan requested day care for his granddaughter to allow him to return to work. The visiting social worker found that Jill was unhappy at home. She was completely under her father's thumb and expressed a desire for more independence. A comprehensive programme of support was initiated culminating in Jill moving into a council flat near to her father's house. She has been much happier since her move and has gained confidence in her abilities. Her relationship with her father has improved and they visit one another regularly. It is expected that home care support will gradually be withdrawn.

Provision of independent advice or advocacy

As Harris (1990) observes, families in difficulty 'typically turn to the very professionals who have the main statutory responsibility for child protection.' In their 'policing' role, social workers are responsible for defining good-enough parenting and for determining if parents meet these standards. In their 'enabling' role, they command the resources with which to influence the outcome. Without independent advocacy support for parents, the negative views held by many practitioners about the parenting abilities of people with learning difficulties make actions and decisions that are detrimental to their interests more likely. Ms Pointer was unable to speak up for herself in court when the hearing to determine the future residence of her child was held 'because they had social worker, health visitor and doctors from hospital . . . I couldn't do it.' Mrs Armstrong felt the same: 'It really is a bit much in court'. Independent advocacy is also an important check against system abuse. When Mrs Hardy's baby was born, the social services put in home helps who almost took over. According to her advocate, she 'saw it as interference' and 'felt threatened by people coming into her home and telling her what to do.' He was able to set up a support group of volunteers from the local church. Good professional practice should include facilitating the involvement of an independent advocate with the parents' consent.

Changing practice

Creating a new partnership between parents and professionals entails shifting the balance between the good and bad features of current practice as revealed by the experience of parents themselves. The three following major obstacles lie in the way of progress in this direction.

- Prevalence of discriminatory attitudes and, in particular, the widespread presumption of incompetence (based on the mistaken belief that good-enough parenting is a function of intelligence) which so often marks the response of practitioners to parents with learning difficulties.
- The organisational division that exists between child protection work and services for people with learning difficulties. The Children Act 1989 has reinforced this split by bringing neglect as well as abuse under the purview of child protection teams. As a result, parents with learning difficulties are at risk of investigation because the presumption of incompetence provides sufficient cause for concern about the welfare of their child. At the same time, the danger of them being assessed as inadequate is increased because the practitioners involved generally have little or no experience in the learning difficulties field.
- The current slant given to the 'welfare balance' in child protection work (DoH, 1989). Child care practice is about balancing the right of parents to bring up their children against the need to protect children from harm (Hayes, 1993). Ever since the Maria Colwell case in 1974, the emphasis within social work has shifted more and more from supporting families to protecting children. The effect, as Prosser (1992) has observed, is that professional practice too often 'seems to see the good of the child requiring the sacrifice of the family.' Until the balance is corrected, parents with learning difficulties and their children will continue to be disadvantaged.

Tackling these obstacles is a stiff challenge. The first step must be to ensure that fewer and fewer parents have occasion to say what Joan Pointer said of her social worker: 'She wouldn't listen to me.'

References

Andron, L. and Tymchuk, A. (1987). Parents who are mentally retarded. In *Mental Handicap and Sexuality: Issues and Perspectives* (ed. A. Craft). D.J. Costello, Tunbridge Wells.

Booth, T. and Booth, W. (1994a). *Parenting Under Pressure: Mothers and Fathers with Learning Difficulties*. Open University Press, Buckingham.

Booth, T. and Booth, W. (1994b). Parental adequacy, parenting failure and parents with learning difficulties. *Health and Social Care in the Community*, **2**, 161–72.

Booth, W. and Booth, T. (1993). How Cathy copes. *Community Living*, **6**(4), Apri, 18–19.

Brantlinger, E. (1988). Teachers' perceptions of the parenting abilities of their secondary students with mild mental retardation. *Remedial and Special Education*, **9**(4), July/August, 31–43.

Department of Health (1989). *An Introduction to the Children Act 1989.* HMSO, London.

Espe-Sherwindt, M. and Kerlin, S. (1990). Early intervention with parents with mental retardation: do we empower or impair? *Infants and Young Children*, **2**, 21–28.

Gil, E. (1982). Institutional abuse of children in out-of-home care. *Child and Youth Services*, **4**(1–2), 7–13.

Grant, C. (1980). Parents with defined intellectual limitations. In *Sterilization and Mental Handicap: Proceedings of a Symposium*. National Institute on Mental Retardation, Toronto.

Harris, R. (1990). A matter of balance: power and resistance in child protection policy. *Journal of Social Welfare Law*, **5**, 332–339.

Hayes, M. (1993). Child care law: an overview. In *Parents with Learning Disabilities* (ed. A. Craft). British Institute of Learning Disabilities, Kidderminster.

Kaminer, R., Jedrysek, E. and Soles, B. (1981). Intellectually limited parents. *Journal of Developmental and Behavioral Pediatrics*, **2**(2), June, 39–43.

Painz, F. (1993). *Parents with a Learning Disability*. Social Work Monographs No. 116, University of East Anglia, Norwich.

Prosser, J. (1992). *Child Abuse Investigations: The Families' Perspective*. Parents Against Injustice (PAIN), Stanstead.

Tucker, M. and Johnson, O. (1989). Competence promoting *vs.* competence inhibiting social support for mentally retarded mothers. *Human Organisation*, **48**(2), 95–107.

Tymchuk, A. (1990). *Parents with Mental Retardation: A National Strategy*. Paper prepared for the President's Committee on Mental Retardation, SHARE/UCLA Parenting Project, University of California, Los Angeles.

Tymchuk, A. (1992). Predicting adequacy of parenting by people with mental retardation. *Child Abuse and Neglect*, **16**(2), 165–178.

Zetlin, A., Weisner, T. and Gallimore, R. (1985). Diversity, shared functioning, and the role of benefactors: a study of parenting by retarded persons. In *Children of Handicapped Parents: Research and Clinical Perspectives* (ed. S. Thurman). Academic Press, New York.

Chapter 21

Healthy lives: The health needs of people with learning difficulties

Jackie Rodgers and Oliver Russell

Health is a positive concept: 'a state of complete physical, mental and social well-being and not merely the absence of disease or infirmity' (World Health Organisation, 1946). There is much more to health than the diagnosis and management of illness. During the past two decades we have come to realise that it is social processes that are of critical importance in determining the health status of individuals and communities. (Davies and Kelly, 1993). Social influences, such as deprivation, poor environmental conditions, and discrimination through class, race and gender are among the key issues which define peoples' health experience.

Meeting the health needs of people with learning difficulties

Many people with learning difficulties are interested in health and keenly follow any training which is offered. One of the most common requests to the Women in Learning Difficulties network[1] is for accessible information about health. People First, the London based self-advocacy organisation, has a group which is learning about how health services operate and talking about how to make them better (see Chapter 12).

There is worrying evidence that the health needs of people with learning difficulties are not being met, even in countries where there is

[1]WILD (Women in Learning Difficulties), c/o National Development Team, St Peter's Court, 8 Trumpet St, Manchester M1 5LW.

an otherwise sophisticated health service. Evidence comes from a series of studies which have been undertaken in the UK, USA and Australia. Nine years ago, Howells (1986) reported the results of health screening for 151 people with learning difficulties who were attending an adult training centre in Wales. A large number of common medical problems were identified which were not known to the individuals' GPs and/or were not being adequately managed.

In the same year Cole (1986) undertook medical examinations of 53 'trainees', almost all male, in a social education centre in England. Thirty five people were found to need medical attention, four urgently. Thirty eight people had not visited their GPs since they had left school, either because they had not complained of feeling ill (it was not known whether they had actually *been* ill) or because their parents were reluctant to take them. Similarly, Barker and Howells (1990) emphasised how, when a person with learning difficulties leaves the umbrella of the school medical services, their contact with medical and dental services appears to decrease.

Four years later, Wilson and Haire (1990) reported the results of a study in another English city in which 65 people attending a day centre for people with learning difficulties were given a physical examination, including tests of their vision and hearing. Most of the people concerned were under 45 years of age. In this study, 57 people had an appreciable problem brought to light, and there was no evidence that people had been screened for common medical problems.

Beange and Bauman (1990) reported a study from Australia which aimed to determine the frequency of medical problems in people with learning difficulties and to examine their need for health care. The study concerned 251 people who attended a health promotion clinic for people with learning difficulties. They were mainly young adults, mostly living in the community and obtaining their health care from GPs. High levels of unrecognised and untreated medical conditions, and medical risk factors, were identified. New diagnoses of previously undetected medical conditions were made in 66 per cent of the cases. For many people, these physical difficulties were more limiting than the learning difficulty, and the study emphasised the need for regular, accessible comprehensive health care.

Langan, Russell and Whitfield (unpubl.) studied the primary health care offered to 90 British adults with learning difficulties living in an English city, compared with that offered to matched controls. They found that preventive health procedures, such as routine screening of blood pressure, recording smoking status and observation of obesity were not performed as frequently for people with learning difficulties as they were for other patients.

Hayden and DePaepe (1991) reviewing the American literature on the health needs of people with learning difficulties found that, of the 47 studies and reports reviewed, about half recommended improvements in community health care. Some people were found to have unmet medical needs and for others the availability and accessibility of community based services were a problem. They noted that a lack of adequate health care contributed to resistance to moving people with learning difficulties into the community, or placed them at risk of re-institutionalisation. They said: 'It behoves advocates of community integration to acknowledge current barriers in the provision of medical services, to determine what services are needed, and to develop strategies and assurances that quality medical care is available in the community.'

Dental health

Another area of concern is the dental health needs of people with learning difficulties. Clevenger et al. (1993), in common with other studies reviewed in their paper, found a higher incidence of poor dental health and poor oral hygiene in people with learning difficulties living in hospitals and in the community. Some reasons for this are suggested, such as a greater consumption of sweet foods and drinks (sometimes as a reward in behaviour modification programmes), difficulty in maintaining oral hygiene, teeth grinding, and more frequent accidents to the teeth due to epilepsy or poor motor control. Certain anti-epileptic medications also have an adverse effect on gums. A further reason suggested was the lack of preventative care, including the lack of regular visits to the dentist. Manley and Pahl (1989), found that although children with learning difficulties do not appear to have more dental disease than other children, they do have more untreated decay and have had more teeth extracted. Similarly, Hinchcliffe et al. (1988) concluded from their research that: 'The predominant form of treatment given to mentally handicapped people with decayed teeth has been extractions . . . for the more severely handicapped there was an even greater likelihood that extractions would have been the form of treatment undertaken.' The undesirability of extractions as a first option is stressed particularly in view of the finding that nearly half of those examined had problems with the use of dentures. Participants in the Langan *et al.* study (unpubl.) reflected this: 'I did go [to the dentist] but they gave me dentures but I don't wear them. They made my gums sore.'

Problems may be made worse if paying for dental work is difficult. The high costs of treatment and the difficulty of obtaining suitable insurance for people with learning difficulties contribute to the problem in the USA. In the UK, many dentists, in dispute with the government over fees for treatment, are refusing to take NHS patients. In some areas no NHS dentists are now available (Dobson, 1992), and travelling further afield for dental care is not always an easy option for people with learning difficulties.

Health care for people from ethnic minorities

There has been little discussion of the health care needs of people with learning difficulties from ethnic minority groups, but the evidence which is available does not encourage optimism that their needs are being met. We know that there are health needs specific to particular ethnic groups, such as tests for monitoring for sickle cell disease and thallassaemia. Other diseases which are experienced by people of some ethnic minority groups more frequently than the population as a whole include ischaemic heart disease, cirrhosis of the liver, strokes, diabetes and accidents (Whitehead, 1988). Reports such as those by the National Association of Health Authorities (NAHAT, 1988) and Baxter *et al.* (1990) indicate that health and social services authorities often fail to meet the particular needs of this client group.

Women's health needs

As Atkinson and Walmsley reflect in Chapter 15, women with learning difficulties have particular needs as *women*. This means they have women's particular health needs, and like other health needs these may be inadequately met. Langan *et al.*'s (unpubl.) research found that women with learning difficulties were much less likely to have had cervical cytology (the smear test) performed than their counterparts without learning difficulties. This was in part due to the problems GPs had in performing the procedure: 'An attempt was made in 1990 but she became very distressed. We had to desist'; or because of an assumption that a woman with learning difficulties is not sexually active and therefore at low risk of developing cancer of the cervix. One carer interviewed for the same study was unhappy with this blanket assumption: 'I do feel that because a person has some sort of learning difficulty their sexual life is dismissed. They should be given the same screening as any person has.'

A service user, interviewed in Langan *et al* (unpubl.), explained her distress at the way a vaginal examination was carried out: 'I like the doctor better because they don't hurt you. I did cry once though – I don't like it when they mess you about down below. My boyfriend got very angry because I was upset. The doctor used one of those silver things [gestured with hands shaped like a speculum] and didn't tell me what he was doing. It's not right to do that. He shouldn't have done that. I hope I haven't offended you. Are you a doctor? I don't mean to be rude but I don't want anyone messing me about down there.'

Some service providers (Rosen, 1991) have suggested the use of pre-examination sedation, but this is not routinely offered to women generally, and is no substitute for careful preparation. Such situations require the teaching of relaxation skills, the use of user-friendly, easy-to-understand resources (with pictures and illustrations) and familiarisation with the personnel, equipment and surroundings that will be experienced. Similarly, it is important that a sympathetic breast screening service should be provided. In the UK, breast screening is offered nationally for women in the 50–65 age group. The Langan *et al.* (unpubl.) study found that this service, too, was less likely to be offered to women with learning difficulties.

Breast screening personnel and carers have discussed the difficulties of providing a service for more profoundly disabled women, in a local women's health group. Carers may not have experienced breast screening themselves, and, without accessible information to guide them, can find it difficult to prepare women for the procedure. Screening may be carried out in cramped, inaccessible premises. The radiographer has to work quickly and may use few words of explanation as she manipulates the woman's breast between metal plates for the mammogram to take place. It is not surprising that some of the women the carers accompanied were unable to benefit from the service. One can only imagine how such a situation is experienced by a woman who does not understand what is happening, and is unable to communicate what she is feeling.

In one English county (Avon), service providers have responded by producing an accessible pack for staff and service users in conjunction with the breast screening service. They are also providing information to GPs which will support the screening of women with learning difficulties who live at home with their families.

Maintenance of reproductive health may be particularly problematic for women with learning difficulties. Their womanhood is at risk of denial. Menstruation may be presented as 'unmanageable' for hygienic reasons. The elimination of menstruation, through drugs or surgery, is the approach favoured in the medical literature (Carlson and Wilson, 1994). The assumption is made, unsupported by research evidence, that women who cannot care for their own personal hygiene needs will find menstruation distressing. In their study of 30 mothers of women with learning difficulties, Carlson and Wilson (1994) found that, in the absence of practical support or good information about menstrual management, most mothers supported this approach. More than half of these mothers were given initial advice about menstrual elimination without it being sought. There are training materials available which are specifically designed, or suitable for, helping women with learning difficulties and their supporters cope with menstruation. For example, Learning Development Aids have produced 'Coping with my period', a set of colour photographs illustrating aspects of menstrual care (O'Boyle, 1986), and the Simplicity Advisory Service offers 'Growing up young', with information about menstruation for parents and teachers of girls with learning difficulties.

Little consideration is given to other reproductive health needs, such as those related to premenstrual tension and the menopause. There is no accessible information covering such topics.

> Do you know much about the menopause? I've had terrible hot flushes
> . . . I can't sleep at night . . . I've been really flooding.
> Have you seen your doctor?
> Yes, he gave me a leaflet about the menopause.
> Was it helpful?
> I don't know – I can't read.
> (Woman with learning difficulties in conversation with Jackie Rodgers.)

If the womanhood of women with learning difficulties is not denied, they may be subject to another extreme, which seeks to control their fertility, suggesting the influence, whether conscious or not, of eugenic ideas. Women may be denied the right to have children and be steered toward long-term contraception and sterilisation. Whichever half of the double bind women with learning difficulties find themselves in, they are the women least likely to have 'a woman's right to choose'.

Health promotion

Health promotion has been defined as 'the process of enabling people to increase control over, and to improve, their health' (World Health Organisation, 1986). Community participation has become a central feature of health promotion in recent years with particular attention being paid to work with disadvantaged and marginalised groups. Such work aims to increase self-confidence, self-esteem and self-knowledge with a view to empowering individuals and groups to enable them to define their own health needs. (Smithies and Adams, 1993).

Stewart and Beange (1994), undertook a survey of nutritional status and dietary problems in adults with learning difficulties living in the community in Australia. They found that the frequency of overweight and obese women (and for people with Downs Syndrome both men and women) was more than twice that of their counterparts without a learning difficulty. Higher blood pressure and cholesterol levels were found in the overweight and obese women with learning difficulties than in the control subjects.

Little attention has been paid to health promotion activities aimed at meeting the needs of people with learning difficulties. Healthy eating, regular exercise, stopping smoking and avoiding excess alcohol constitute the healthy lifestyle message disseminated to the public at large. But how far are these messages accessible to people with learning difficulties? An innovative project in England (Richardson, 1993) focussed on encouraging healthy eating, looking at weight control and how eating affects health. The project leader reflected upon a number of possible reasons why people with learning difficulties tended to be overweight or unhealthy. She suggested that people with learning difficulties often live in situations where they have little or no choice over what they eat, decisions being made by those who care for them, who in turn may have little awareness of nutritional matters. If people are offered choice they may not know what constitutes a healthy diet and its importance. This may never have been an important part of their education. Income levels are influential, as are cooking skills and facilities. This project attempted to increase the participants' awareness of the importance of exercise, healthy living and maintaining a healthy diet. The results varied but for some participants there were great benefits.

A novel attempt to provide an alcohol education service for people with learning difficulties who had moved from an institution to live independently has been described (Lindsay *et al.*, 1991). Workers providing support noticed that some individuals had increased their alcohol intake since moving into the community. The authors suggested that drinking in pubs is seen by many as a highly desirable and valued activity and, together with the greater freedom of life in the community, leads to greater self-esteem. The project workers, rather than aiming for abstinence, devised an alcohol education programme, discussing aspects of alcohol and role-playing alternative ways of behaving and drinking in pubs.

At the time of writing, there are no studies focussing specifically on smoking or exercise habits of people with learning difficulties, though the Langan *et al.* (unpubl.) study asked service users what advice they had been given by their doctor about keeping fit. Much of the discussion centred around food: 'The doctor has never told me what's good for me. I know fruit is healthy. Sometimes I have to ask what I can have for lunch, I don't know what's good or bad.' Some respondents smoked, but hadn't been advised not to by their doctor: 'I smoke like a trooper. No, he [the GP] hasn't told me to stop.' Others were against smoking, and were knowledgeable about its effects: 'It's bad for your health – I think it causes cancer.'

There is little advantage in carers and professionals dictating the health behaviour of people with learning difficulties. The result may be healthy or unhealthy, but the process will inevitably undermine the person's independence. If a person with learning difficulties makes her or his own decisions about health behaviour, in the light of knowledge gained through accessible information, the results may be similarly healthy or unhealthy, but will maintain the precious (and healthy) element of free choice. Unfortunately, this seems to be missing from many people's lives.

Barriers to good health care

Clearly, there is strong evidence that there are significant barriers to the health care needs of people with learning difficulties being met, and we need to explore what these barriers are. Some people with learning difficulties find it difficult to recognise and report illness, explain distress or express unhappiness with the care or treatment they are given. This means their parents and other carers have a greater influence on how well people's health needs are met. Langan *et al.*'s (unpubl.) report discusses what this means in practical terms. Carers become responsible for recognising illness and the effects of drugs, deciding when access to health services is required, and representing the person in dealings with health professionals. There is little information to support unqualified carers in this role. Much of the literature on health care needs has a medical emphasis, not taking into account the important role of carers. There are very few published examples of practical health care advice to carers, or of training in health needs for parents or paid carers. Carers' lack of knowledge is sometimes compounded by a feeling that a person with learning difficulties has such insurmountable problems that 'minor' health issues are insignificant (Barker and Howells, 1990). If carers are undertaking their role in understaffed facilities or under supported family homes, day-to-day pressures may not allow the care which is necessary to successfully address a person's health needs.

Role of health professionals

Health professionals may be similarly unprepared for their role in ensuring that the medical care needs of people with learning difficulties are met. Professionals may be unaware that particular medical conditions are more common for people with learning difficulties, such as sensory disabilities, hypertension, chronic bronchitis, epilepsy, cerebral palsy, gross obesity, spinal deformities, skin disorders and mental health problems (CRIMD, 1990). They may also be unaware of the possibility of nutritional disorders, dental problems and 'polypharmacy', or new health challenges such as HIV and AIDS. Downs Syndrome is associated with particular medical concerns, which may not be recognised. These include a higher incidence of thyroid disorders, Alzheimer's disease and atlanto-axial subluxation (a weakness in the neck which can put people at risk of serious injury if they participate in certain sports) (Rubin, 1987). As has been suggested, insufficient attention is given to the need which people with learning difficulties have for preventative care and advice. Primary health care professionals may not have the skills needed to overcome communication difficulties within a consultation, and may not be aware of the need to provide information about health promotion in an accessible form. Training about the particular needs of people with learning difficulties is unusual for general health professionals, and they do not necessarily see a need for more.

Psychotropic medication

The prescription of anti-psychotic drugs is another area of urgent concern. People with learning difficulties are often prescribed anti-psychotic drugs as a means of controlling their behaviour. Such medications may have been overprescribed on inadequate indications, and without any relationship to any other treatments such as behavioural therapy (Einfield, 1990). Hubert (1992) undertook an in-depth study of 20 families with a young adult living at home who had been classified as having severe learning difficulties and challenging behaviour. Many of the young people in this study were prescribed one or more anti-psychotic drugs over many years without a diagnosis of mental illness. One parent described his experience of this: '[The psychiatrist] never to my satisfaction actually explained why he was on drugs in the first place. She kept explaining what the drugs did and why there was a concoction of drugs but never got back to the basic question which I raised . . . I said: "I'm only a layman, I may be a bit thick even, but could you tell me why he's taking drugs in the first place?" '

It is not only the blanket prescription of drugs that is the problem, but the prescription of drugs in multiple combinations. In general psychiatry, the maxim is that giving more than one or two psychotropic drugs in combination is unlikely to be beneficial and may be harmful (Lynch, 1989), but this caution often seems to be ignored for people with learning difficulties.

One of the parents interviewed by Hubert (1992) said: 'They've got him high on drugs . . . he's very, very dosey . . . they're mixing drugs apparently because they're using one mainstream drug which has side effects so therefore they have to use another drug to minimise the side effects he then has to have another drug . . . he's started to have hand tremors, he's never had hand tremors before, and . . . he's asking to go to bed at six at night, I mean, he's 20 years old, and you don't find many 20 year olds going to bed at six at night.'

Side effects of heavy dosages of certain anti-psychotic drugs can be serious and produce permanent harm, such as retinal damage, softening of the bones, gum disease and weakening or loss of muscle control. There may be more temporary, but unpleasant side effects, such as nausea, double or blurred vision, dizziness and mental confusion (Hubert, 1992). People may be unable to explain what is troubling them. Deterioration or behavioural changes may not be noticed in those living in residential accommodation which is understaffed, or which has a high staff turnover. Staff will not be able to recognise such changes in people they hardly know. Side effects can be controlled by careful monitoring and review of the drugs prescribed but this, too, can be neglected. Wilson and Haire's study (1990) of 65 people in a British day centre found 26 people were taking antidepressant or anti-epileptic drugs, and most of these were given by repeat prescription with no review.

In some cases the side effects of drugs may not be life-threatening, but are equally unacceptable. One of the parents in Hubert's study (1992) took their son off drugs while he was at home, to see what happened: 'When he was small his eyes used to glow, it was an outstanding feature, these glowing eyes, and in the last couple of years they've dulled, but all of a sudden he had these glowing eyes again. It was like having him back with us – it sounds ridiculous I know . . . and he was happy – it's the little things, the stupid things – I hadn't heard him laugh, not for a long long time. That weekend he was home not only did his eyes start glowing, but he started laughing.'

Some of the barriers related to the role of health professionals could be overcome by better collaboration with other workers who *do* have the skills and knowledge which are lacking. In the UK community learning difficulty teams have existed since the early 1980s. They are organised separately from primary health care teams and involve professionals with special skills and experience in supporting people with learning difficulties. There is a core membership of a community nurse and social worker, often supplemented by other specialist workers such as speech therapists, occupational therapists, pysiotherapists, and psychologists. A psychiatrist with a special interest in learning difficulties is usually involved. The skills and experience of these team members could be utilised to offer people with learning difficulties the best possible health care in the community. Good interprofessional collaboration between community learning difficulty teams and primary health care professionals could play a part in improving the service offered, but this, as several studies point out,

(RCGP, 1990; CRIMD, 1991; Langan *et al.* unpubl.) does not appear to be happening.

There have been major changes in the organisation of British health care in recent years. The government White Papers *Promoting Better Health* (1987), *Working for Patients* (1989) and *Caring for People* (1989), embodied in the NHS and Community Care Act 1990, have transformed the delivery of health care. *The Health of the Nation* (1991) formulated, for the first time, a health strategy for England.

An important element of the changes is to introduce competition by creating a market in health care, with the aim of increasing efficiency. A split between purchasers and providers of health care has been created. Some providers have become self-governing trusts, responsible directly to the Department of Health and able to retain budget surpluses to invest in their provision of services. Some larger GP practices have become fund holders, able to purchase specified services for their patients. Since April 1993 they have been able to buy services for people with learning difficulties.

Under these new arrangements, providers of care are motivated to produce care in the most 'efficient' way, thereby winning contracts, staying within their budgets and retaining any surplus. Glennester (1990) found that in the USA this entailed a strong emphasis on getting rid of expensive or time-consuming patients. This has implications for all vulnerable groups, including people with learning difficulties. Efficiency may be judged in primarily financial terms, and quantity, not quality, emphasised in the drive for efficient use of resources. If GPs are not aware of the particular needs of their patients with learning difficulties they will not be able to refer effectively for specialist health care when it is needed.

The barriers which have been outlined are specific barriers to the meeting of health care needs. The most important barrier, however, is the position of people with learning difficulties in society. People with learning difficulties are an oppressed group, and, in common with other oppressed groups, are socially and materially disadvantaged. Socio-economic circumstances are related to health (Townsend *et al.*, 1992; Blaxter, 1990); people who are largely socially isolated and have little income to call their own, will feel the adverse effect of this. If there is a prevailing attitude that people with learning difficulties do not count for much – that they are not 'proper' women and men – their needs will never be adequately met. Such attitudes are a very real and difficult barrier to overcome.

Empowerment and advocacy

How can, and will, change be achieved? It is essential that people with learning difficulties gain more control over their health. This means real empowerment (not just consultation) achieved through advocacy and mutual support. People with learning difficulties can be supported to speak up for themselves on health issues, and allies can speak up for and with them. Women's groups can provide a safe place for women to discuss health and find out more about it.

Gaining more control over health must also entail the provision of accessible information, with people with learning difficulties having a central role in its production. The written word, symbols, pictures, photographs, audio and video cassettes and, not least, personal contact, can be used to inform people about their bodies, prepare them for routine procedures and increase their knowledge about health services.

Further research based on aspects of health identified by people with learning difficulties as important, can increase understanding, support moves for change, and identify ways of achieving it. To improve health and health care, we need a much better understanding of people and their health. If we do not know what people's health needs are, policy and provision may be misguided. We need to consider how health should be defined in research, and how any such definition can be operationalised and measured.

In the short-term, policies can be effected which will improve the experience of health care for people with learning difficulties. Local policies can be explicit about what is acceptable in services. For example, the learning disability service in south east Kent has introduced a policy which prohibits the use of major tranquillisers for the control of behaviour. In the absence of a major psychiatric disorder no such drugs would be prescribed (Walsh, 1993).

National policies can identify areas where health gain can be achieved. The Welsh Office has recently produced a protocol identifying a strategic approach to health gain for people with learning difficulties (Welsh Health Planning Forum, 1992). This document outlines opportunities where good health care is likely to produce significant health gains, including sight, hearing, communication, mobility, epilepsy and other specific conditions. The targets outlined could be translated to a clinical level as a basis for individual service provider's standards. In line with the original aims of the NHS, policy needs to be geared towards a health service which is equitable for all, so that people with learning difficulties, in common with other oppressed groups, can benefit fully from it.

In the long-term, what is needed to meet the health needs of people with learning difficulties, in common with the other unmet needs identified in this volume, is adequate support and social justice.

Acknowledgements

We wish to thank Joan Langan and Michael Whitfield for permission to quote from an unpublished report to the Department of Health. Parts of this chapter are drawn from a paper, J. Rodgers, Primary health care provision for people with learning difficulties, *Health and Social Care in the Community*, vol. 2, No. 1, January 1994.

References

Barker, M. and Howells, G. (1990). The medical needs of adults. In *Primary Care for People with a Mental Handicap*. Occasional Paper **47**, 6–11, Royal College of General Practitioners, London.

Baxter, C., Poonia, K., Ward, L. and Nadirshaw, Z. (1990). *Double Discrimination: Issues and Services for People with Learning Difficulties from Black and Ethnic Minority Communities*. King's Fund Centre/Commission for Racial Equality, London.

Beange, H. and Bauman, A. (1990). Health care for the developmentally disabled: is it necessary? In *Key Issues in Mental Retardation Research* (ed. W. Frazer). Routledge, London.

Blaxter, M. (1990). *Health and Lifestyles*. Routledge, London.

Carlson, G., and Wilson, J. (1994). Menstrual management: the mother's perspective. *Mental Handicap Research*, **7**, 51–63.

Clevenger, W.E., Wigal, T., Salvati, N., Burchill, R. and Crinella, F.M. (1993). Dental needs of persons with developmental disabilities in Orange County. *Journal of Developmental and Physical Disabilities*, **5**, 253–264.

Cole, O. (1986). Medical screening of adults at social education centres: whose responsibility? *Mental Handicap*, **14**, 54–56.

CRIMD (1990). *Primary Health Care for People with a Learning Disability*, Policy paper no 1. Centre for Research and Information into Mental Disability, University of Birmingham.

Davies, J.K. and Kelly, M.P. (eds) (1993). *Healty Cities: Research and Practice*. Routledge, London.

Dobson, J. (1992). A tooth for a tooth. *Health Service Journal*, **102** No. 5311, 16 July, 15.

Einfield, S. (1990). Guidelines for the use of psychotropic medication in individuals with developmental disabilities. *Australia and New Zealand Journal of Developmental Disabilities*, **16**, 71–73.

Glennester, H. (1990). *Community Care in a Mixed Economy*. Papers from the Social Services Research Group, London.

Hayden, M.F. and DePaepe, P.A. (1991). Medical conditions, level of care needs and health related outcomes of persons with mental retardation: a review. *Journal of the Association for Persons with Severe Handicaps*, **16**, 188–206.

Hinchcliffe, J.E., Fairpo, C.G. and Curzon, M.E. (1988). The dental condition of mentally handicapped adults attending adult training centres in Hull. *Community Dental Health*, **5**, 151–162.

Howells, G. (1986). Are the medical needs of mentally handicapped adults being met? *Journal of the Royal College of Practitioners*, **36**, 449–453.

Hubert, J. (1992). *Too Many Drugs, Too Little Care, Parents' Perceptions of Administration and Side Effects of Drugs Prescribed for Young People with Severe Learning Difficulties*. Values into Action, London.

Langan, J., Russell, O. and Whitfield, M. (1993). *Community Care and the General Practitioner: Primary Health Care for People with Learning Disabilities*, Report to the Department of Health, Norah Fry Research Centre, Bristol, (unpubl.).

Lindsay, W., Allen, R., Walker, P., Lawrenson, H., Smith, A.H.W. (1991). An alcohol education service for people with learning difficulties. *Mental Handicap*, **19**, 96–100.

Lynch, S.P. (1989). Prescribing practice in a mental handicap hospital: psychotropic medication from 1978–1987. *Mental Handicap*, **17**, 123–128.

Manley, M.C.G., Pahl, J.M. (1989). Dental services for children with mental handicaps: policy changes and parental choices, *British Dental Journal*, **167**, 163–167.

National Association of Health Authorities (1988). *Action not Words: A Strategy to Improve Health Services for Black and Ethnic Minority Groups*. National Association of Health Authorities, Birmingham.

O'Boyle, E. (1986). Learning Development Aids. Coping with my period. Duke Street, Wisbech.

Richardson, N. (1993). Fit for the future. *Nursing Times*, **89**(44), 36–38.

Rosen, D.A. *et al.*, (1991). Outpatient sedation: an essential addition to gynecologic care for persons with mental retardation. *American Journal of Obstetrics and Gynecology*, **164**, 825–828.

Royal College of General Practitioners (1990). *Primary Care for People with a Mental Handicap*, Occasional Paper 47. Royal College of General Practitioners, London.

Rubin, L.I. (1987). Health care needs of adults with mental retardation. *Mental Retardation*, **25**, 201–206.

Simplicity Advisory Service. Growing up young. Kimberley Clarke Ltd, Kent.

Smithies, J. and Adams, L. (1993). Walking the tightrope: issues in evaluation and community participation for health for all. In *Healthy Cities: Research and Practice* (eds J.K. Davies and M.P. Kelly). Routledge, London.

Stewart, L., Beange, H. and Mackerras, D. (1994). A survey of dietary problems of adults with learning disabilities in the community. *Mental Handicap Research*, 7, 41–50.

Townsend, P., Davidson, N. and Whitehead, M. (1992). *Inequalities in Health, The Black Report and the Health Divide*. Penguin, London.

Walsh, P. (1993). Drugs may meet service needs – but they fail the clients. *Community Living*, 7, 18–19.

Welsh Health Planning Forum (1992). *Protocol for Investment in Health Gain, Mental Handicap (Learning Disabilities)*. Welsh Office, Cardiff.

Wilson, D.N. and Haire, A. (1990). Health screening for people with mental handicap living in the community. *British Medical Journal*, **301**, 1379–1381.

World Health Organisation (1946). *Constitution*. World Health Organisation, New York.

World Health Organisation (1986). *The Ottawa Charter for Health Promotion*. WHO, Canadian Public Health Association, Health and Welfare Canada, Ottawa.

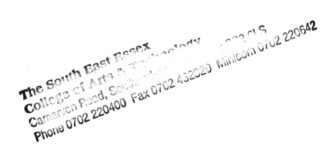

Chapter 22

Clearer visions and equal value: Achieving justice for victims with learning difficulties

Christopher Williams

'To no one deny or delay right of justice' – how true are the words of the Magna Carta for victims with learning difficulties? Does our vision of the victimisation of people with learning difficulties ensure that it is accorded the same value as for others?

Mary and Usha were, in separate incidents, shouted at and threatened by drunken men – offences under the Public Order Act 1986. Within a few weeks Mary had received £50 compensation through the courts and the offenders were fined.

When Usha told her parents, they said she would have to put up with verbal insults because she had learning difficulties. But Usha insisted that the police were called. They had to be persuaded to interview her, and were reluctant to report the incident to the Crown Prosecution Service (CPS) or even record it as a crime. Finally, when this was achieved, the CPS would not prosecute because they concluded that Usha would not be an adequate witness; a decision based on an IQ assessment made fifteen years' earlier.

Had Usha appeared in court, it is possible that she would have had to wait in the same area as the offenders, and might have suffered further abusive insults, relating to her disability, from the defence solicitor. The case may have been thrown out because she could not give an instant definition of 'truth'; something that is only expected of witnesses who bear the label, 'learning difficulties'.

The purpose of this chapter is to outline what currently happens to victims with learning difficulties, what needs to be changed to ensure equitable justice, and to provide the basic knowledge for bringing about that change. The material derives from a two-year research project supported by the Joseph Rowntree Foundation (Williams, 1995).

Victimisation

Sexual victimisation was the first area of crime against people with learning difficulties to receive significant attention from researchers and policy makers. The result is some excellent training material, numerous policy guidelines, and voluntary support organisations (Brown and Craft, 1992; NAPSAC/ARC, 1993; NAPSAC, 1993; 1994). Sexual offences against men deserve special attention because we less readily take notice of a report from a man. One young man who repeatedly said, 'This girl kissed me' did not attract immediate concern, yet he was reporting a serious sexual assault. The very conservative parents of a man assaulted by another man were very slow to seek help because they were embarrassed and ashamed that the act was homo-sexual.

Abduction became a particular concern following the disappearance and death of a young woman with learning difficulties, Jo Ramsden, in 1991. Many women with learning difficulties will relate stories that are probably abduction attempts, but it is not only women who are at risk. One man reported that he was taken by two (female) prostitutes, who then ransacked his flat looking for money. Fear of abduction should prompt the teaching of effective coping skills to people who may be at risk. Fear should not be a justification for restriction of liberty. People with learning difficulties often employ very effective strategies. One woman who was propositioned responded with great effect: 'Not bloody likely. I don't fancy *you*. I'm not that hard up.'

Life in the community can be dangerous for people with learning difficulties, but this is true for anyone else. The murder of a Bristol man on his way home from the pub, for the sake of stealing a few pounds, is distressing but does not provide an argument for re-institutionali-sation. After many years in hospital, the value of having a regular drink with his father probably far outweighed the risk of such an event happening. More pertinently, long-stay hospitals were, and remain, equally dangerous. Shortly after this murder, a woman died because nurses had left her tied to a toilet by her bib, whilst they went for lunch (Brindle, 1992).

Assault in public places is a significant problem. People with learning difficulties frequently end up in hospital needing stitches, and there are many reports of muggings with victims losing handbags, bumbags and personal stereos. The lesson for victims is not to display stealable items; the question for the community is why do most of these incidents happen in full view of passers-by and no one offers help? Even less excusable are the frequent assaults on people in service settings. Bites, bruises, and hair-pulling are commonly suffered, yet *staff rarely conceptualise these events as criminal acts*. Parents and carers are not informed; police involvement is not offered as an option; double standards abound. A man who was hospitalised because another service user threw boiling water thrown over him concludes appositely: 'Now if *I* had done something like that to someone *outide*, I would have been sent down.'

The most commonly reported forms of victimisation are public order offences, that is, threatening, abusive or insulting words or behaviour. Being called names such as 'spastic', 'cretin' and 'imbecile' are daily events in the lives of many people. This can be compounded by racial abuse. If the perpetrator intended to cause fear of violence, or the victim is likely to fear violence, an offence has been committed. Yet, there is not one single instance of a Public Order prosecution on behalf of a victim with learning difficulties. Again, the public and police perception is that this type of victimisation is something that people with learning difficulties must tolerate.

Crimes that feature significantly in the crime statistics, namely theft, damage, and car crime are, by comparison, minor in the lives of people with learning difficulties. They own relatively little property, particularly cars. By contrast, false imprisonment is a rarely considered aspect of crime amongst the general community, but is common in the lives of service users. The perpetrators are usually staff who are often unaware that locking people in rooms, or even telling them to stay there under threat, could be an offence.

The nature of victimisation against people with learning difficulties does not, therefore, always fit our vision of 'crime'. Even if it does, such victimisation does not feature in national crime surveys because data is not collected from group homes. An hour's discussion with any group of people with learning difficulties about 'the bad things you suffer', is usually enough to inspire the change in attitude that is needed to start the fight for equitable justice.

The perpetrators

Who are the perpetrators? Motivation in individual cases is hard to assess, but it is possible to identify perpetrator *groups*.

The most worrying of these groups is staff and volunteers. Of course most staff do not victimise, but the breach of trust involved in *any* victimisation by staff makes it serious. A police report of 500 alleged offences in a single residential unit shows that the scale is sometimes far from insignificant (*The Independent*, 1994). Abuse of power is a common weapon, wielded not only over the victim but over junior colleagues and other service users who may be tempted to report.

Service users constitute another significant victimiser group. The 'challenging behaviour' label can cloud the fact that many incidents between service users are, from the perspective of the victim, criminal offences. Similarly when the perpetrators are children, incidents are seen as naughty rather than unlawful. Incidents are not restricted to verbal abuse, and include the theft of walkmans, being burnt with cigarettes, and muggings involving knives. It is not just 'problem children' who offend. One day centre had to change its opening hours to avoid coinciding with abusive children from a local Catholic girls' school.

Family members are a particularly invisible perpetrator group. Incidents often concern step-parents and distant relatives who take advantage of the trust bestowed in them as occasional carers. Victims are often very fearful of reporting because they are told that they will 'get taken away by social services.' Financial offences are especially difficult to unravel. One man, who inherited a considerable sum of money, was immediately removed from his group home to live with the family. Was the new conservatory, new car, and redecoration of the house really what he wanted to spend his money on?

Few discussions about victimisation with people with learning difficulties do not contain a story of what they experience as victimisation by the people. Tim Hart (1992) of People First writes in *Disability Issues*: 'Policemen always pick me up. Why is that when I haven't done anything wrong? They often think I have run away from home.' At the serious end, a number of miscarriages of justice have emerged, such as the case of Stephan Kisko who was jailed for murder, later to be freed when officers were charged with perverting the course of justice.

Finally, the least tangible victimiser 'group' is the organisation. Deaths in care settings due to lack of care or breakdowns in communication, on-going petty problems with services leading to suicide, and infringements of human rights and liberties that would be unacceptable in any other walk of life are all part of an elusive pattern of organisational victimisation. Laws are often broken, vulnerable people suffer, yet because the standard victim–perpetrator relationship is not evident, justice is rarely achieved. Care in the community legislation does not embody a duty to care.

Staff, service users, families, police, service providers; these perpetrator groups do not fit our preconceived visions of criminals. Detection, effective prevention and the achievement of justice are often hindered because of this.

Prevention

Learning about prevention best derives from the personal experiences of people with learning difficulties. There is often a high awareness of crime from TV programmes such as *Crimewatch*. Newspaper cuttings provide another route for opening discussions. People with learning difficulties have produced videos such as the *Walsall Women's Group Safety Video – No Means No* (WWG, 1994). The learning pack *Cracking Crime* contains another video by people with learning difficulties and ideas for using role-play and drama to develop coping skills (Williams, 1994).

Specific incidents are also an excellent basis for developing personal preventive strategies. Following the murder of a Bristol man, a group of friends discussed the circumstances and concluded the following.

- Don't stand at bus stops late at night unless you know a bus is due.
- Remember, you can use a bus if you have no money, just tell the driver your name and address.
- Tell someone where you are going and when you expect to be back.
- Don't dress in expensive clothes for walking in the street. Don't show expensive watches, wallets, or anything people might want to steal.
- If people start bothering you, try not to look scared. Get help quickly by going into a shop or public building.

Service providers can contribute to prevention through *avoiding advertising vulnerability*. A basic check list might include the avoidance of things that suggest the physical weakness of residents such as disability logos; signs such as 'ambulances only'; hand rails; conspicuous ramps; ambulances or mini buses.

Avoid giving an 'institutional look' to buildings such as social/health service or local authority notices; unaesthetic placing of dustbins; gardens without any 'human touches'; obvious staff car parks (which can also advertise when there is no, or only one, staff member on duty); and regularity such as 'lights out' at the same time each night should also be avoided where possible. Finally, refrain from using interactions which suggest vulnerability. These include making people walk in 'crocodile' lines; unnecessary shouted warnings about traffic or behaviour; over-protective care concerning the use of money; and patronising or 'baby talk'.

Encouraging a police presence can be extremely effective. As one woman explained: 'I had a lot of trouble with school kids. We told the police and next day, when I was waiting at the bus stop, this police car pulled up and the officer said to me, "Hello. Are these the kids that are bothering you? Don't worry, I've had a good look at them." There's been no more trouble.'

The protective use of transport is a vital area of prevention: How to minimise the time waiting at bus stops and train stations; how to plan journeys for safety, and what to do when things go wrong; what to do if you have no money (it is possible to use most forms of transport by giving a name and address); and when and how to make an 'emergency' decision to use a taxi. These are all important points which need to be considered.

Prevention takes on a more specific aspect in care settings. A priority policy of preventing peer victimisation would make a radical difference to many people's lives. 'They are all as bad as one another' is a common response from day centre staff. In one centre, a man was observed walking round in circles and regularly clipping a woman behind the ear. When challenged the manager said, 'Oh, they always do that.' What did the manager mean by 'they', when there was such a clear victim–victimiser relationship?

The single most effective strategy to reduce the level of victimisation in people's lives is increasing the awareness of staff as to what might constitute a crime (see Ashton and Ward, 1992). This would equip staff to respond more readily when police involvement is appropriate, insist on an adequate police response, and prompt them to question some of their own actions more closely. This awareness should include the following.

- Any deprivation of liberty, without consent, could be 'false imprisonment', if not imposed under the Mental Health Act or for safety reasons in an emergency.
- Any form of touching, without consent, might be a common assault unless done for safety reasons in an emergency. Assault can result from an act that is intentional *or reckless*.
- Aggressive shouting or gestures, which may cause a person to fear violence, outside a 'dwelling' may be an offence against the Public Order Act 1986. Staff should assume that public areas such as staff rooms, offices, garages, gardens and sheds may fall under this Act.
- A manager or staff member, who knowingly permits, or encourages, a man to have sexual intercourse with a woman with severe learning difficulties in a residential home within their jurisdiction may commit an offence. (Sexual Offences Act, 1956 Part 1 s27 [1]).
- Any male member of staff who has sexual intercourse with any client, within a Mental Health Act setting, may commit an offence (Mental Health Act, 1959 sec. 128 [1]).
- Punishments, such as depriving people of meals, would probably constitute 'wilful neglect' under the Mental Health Act 1983 (sec.127) and contravene conditions set out under the Registered Homes Act 1984.
- A person with severe learning difficulties cannot give consent, whenever there is a consent element concerned in determining an offence (for example, opening mail, assault, abduction, 'false imprisonment', sexual acts).
- Authorisations that give power to third parties to manage the financial affairs of someone with learning difficulties are usually restricted. For example, authorisation to collect a person's social security benefits (as an appointee under the Social Security Act 1987, reg.33) does not give permission to deal with earnings or gifts of money (which would require authorisation under the Mental Health Act 1983, s.142). A Social Security appointee must use state benefits for the direct benefit of the claimant – maintenance to a residential unit, unwanted holidays, day-trips, or parties may not be considered as such.
- Opening people's mail or intercepting phone calls, without the consent of the recipient or a court, may be an offence against the Interception of Communications Act 1985. This can be so even if the intent is helpful, for example intercepting cheques and putting them in a bank account.
- 'Counselling' or 'inciting' people to do something that is unlawful may itself be unlawful. This may include setting up and encouraging sexual relationships that are not clearly consensual.
- Most service users cannot be compelled to undergo medical treatment, which would include minor things such as taking an aspirin. There is particular confusion concerning people who are transferred from long-

stay hospitals, and are under Section 8 Guardianship Orders. Guardianship does not sanction compulsory treatment.

- Managers and staff, not directly employed by the NHS, may still be working within the Mental Health Act which makes clear a duty to care. The terms 'in-patient' and 'mental disorder' used in the Act are defined very widely, and almost certainly embrace people with learning difficulties in community settings (Gunn, 1990). Service providers contracted by the NHS to provide residential care, are probably operating a 'mental nursing home' on behalf of the NHS and are therefore covered by the Act.

- Staff in residential homes are sometimes bound by the Registered Homes Act 1984. This includes a duty to notify the registration authority within 24 hours of 'any event in the home which affects the well-being of any resident; and any theft, burglary . . .'

- Service users may sue for damages if they have not been protected from bullying and other victimisation. This is a very new area of litigation, but is likely to increase, and cases may be based on events from many years before.

- An unproven allegation that someone (staff member *or service user*) has committed an offence may amount to a defamation. In the case of libel (written defamation) the plaintiff need not show that there was loss or damage; this must be shown in the case of slander (verbal defamation) except when the alleged offence is imprisonable. For example, if a staff member said, 'Yuk-chung hit David', and this assult was unproven, there could be a straightforward claim for damages without the need to demonstrate the Yuk-chung's character had been affected, because assault is imprisonable.

- Staff may be guilty of an offence if they impede a report to the police. Impeding a prosecution by omission (simply not reporting a crime) is not an offence. But any 'act' which impedes a prosecution may constitute an offence. A manager who, for example, instructs, verbally or in writing, that a probable crime should not be reported may commit an offence.

- Staff may be dismissed lawfully if there are 'reasonable grounds' for believing that an offence has been committed, which relates to their work. The circumstances do not have to be 'proven' and a single, probable offence is sufficient grounds for dismissal.

- Corroboration, by third party witnesses, of an offence is not necessary. Although it is desirable to corroborate a victim's story, a court may still convict if the victim's version of events is believed to be true. A conviction can be achieved solely on the word of a victim with learning difficulties.

Most importantly, people with learning difficulties should be seen as part of our community resistance to crime. An employee at a do-it-yourself store pointed out a man who looked suspicious to the manager, and sure enough the man did steal something. The employee says he took note of the man because, 'He looked just like a Gizmo gangster – just like those criminals on *Crimewatch*.' A woman who discovered burglars next door, because her dog was barking, alerted the police who made a quick arrest. When asked how she managed to achieve such a quick response from the police, she replied, 'I just told them to shift their arses and get here quick.'

Reporting

At present in the UK, there remains a feeling that reporting to the police should be discretionary. Staff often express the view that 'it will make things worse' or that it would be an abdication of responsibility by a professional carer. But such judgements can look very different in the light of subsequent events. The decision by a doctor, not to involve the police when a woman had tried to kill herself and her daughter with learning difficulties with an overdose, may have seemed reasonable at the time of the incident. But it appeared less valid when, later, the mother and father did kill themselves and their daughter.

In North America, reporting is becoming mandatory. In Connecticut, for example, mandated reporters must *ensure* that a report reaches the official agency, not just inform a line manager. Reporters are then protected from any actions against them, provided the report was not malicious.

In addition to ethical and moral questions, there are pragmatic reasons, as the following points convey, for reporting to the police and pursuing cases through the courts.

- Success in the courts often depends on the police gathering evidence *immediately*. Forensic evidence, for example relating to a sexual assault, usually must be obtained within 48 hours. Photographs taken by police photographers are now a very strong part of the evidence used to prove assault. Where victim and defendant are the only witnesses to assault, cases can hinge on a police photograph of injuries, taken soon after the event.
- Criminal Injuries Compensation does not cover claims under £1000. Compensation under £1000 can only be achieved through a court.
- Criminal Injuries Compensation can only be claimed when someone is the victim of a 'violent' crime and the crime is reported to the police 'without delay'.
- While the police cannot keep official records of unproven allegations, they do maintain an informal knowledge of suspected offenders. This can influence the seriousness with which they treat subsequent reports. At a period when economic constraints lead to strict prioritisation of police resources, the importance of this should not be underestimated.
- Police involvement can help reinforce crime prevention lessons for victims.

In an instance in which £2000 went missing from a man's Building Society account, the local police were very helpful, but it was decided not to pursue the case because evidence was weak. Despite this, the parent concluded: 'I think the police had an entirely beneficial effect on John. Nice as they were, they made him realise it was a serious matter and he had to take some responsibility for looking after his own affairs.'

- Staff protect themselves against allegations of negligence or of impeding a prosecution if they make a report.
- Perpetrators cannot usually be helped unless their actions are formally recognised.

Future debate should not concern whether or not to report, but how the police should then respond.

The starting point for ensuring that offences are reported is to teach people with learning difficulties to recognise and conceptualise crime *before* they are victims. Do they know the difference between crime and something that is simply disliked? Do they have the relevant vocabulary? Do they know what happens when a report is made so that their opinion about police involvement is an informed choice? Two booklets, *Jenny Speaks out* and *Bob Tells All* (Hollins, 1992) provide an excellent pictorial basis for helping people to report sexual offences or harasssment or to conceptualise the process of reporting. The video *Crime Against People with Learning Difficulties* (Williams, 1994) presents victims talking about their experiences, which provides a basis for discussion.

The main reason for reports not reaching the police is the linear, 'chain' nature of reporting routes within service settings (victim – worker – house manager – line manager – senior manager – frontline police – specialist police). One missing link in the chain and the report fails. It is more useful to develop reporting 'webs' in which all relevant parties have direct access to specialist police and senior service managers. In one region, all service users have a printed card with an identifying number. All they need do is post it and a senior manager will investigate. It is good policy to ensure that in every residential unit at least one service user is able to conceptualise crime and communicate clearly. Other strategies include helping everybody to know at least one police officer personally. The NAPSAC booklet *Who can I Tell? Blowing the Whistle on Sexual Abuse* (NAPSAC, 1993) is an example of the type of document that should be available to all carers, parents, and people with learning difficulties.

When a report has been made, there is no guarantee that the police or

CPS will treat the complaint equitably. Most cases that have reached the courts have experienced attempts to block their progress by police officers or the CPS or both. In one instance a man was, on separate occasions, gored by a bull and the victim of a hit-and-run driver. The police were informed but did not go to interview him, presuming that he was unable to tell them what happened. As his sister was a police officer in another force the situation was soon rectified. Often the CPS base their decision not to proceed with a case on the assumption that a victim–witness with learning difficulties will not be able to tell a court what happened; a decision usually taken without even meeting the victim.

The process of reporting is therefore frustrated in four main ways where: victims sometimes do not know what or how to report; there is often a service ethos of not involving the police quickly; 'chain' reporting routes often fail and perpetrators can often create the missing link in the chain; and those who control the formal paths to justice block reports either because of prejudice or a guess about what will happen somewhere else in the system.

Every decision in the reporting system can have a kick-back effect. The CPS block cases on a guess about what might happen in court. Police fail to report to the CPS because they presume the case will be blocked. Professionals fail to report to the police because of a belief that nothing will happen. Victims find that reports to staff are not worth making. And the message to perpetrators is that people with learning difficulties are easy victims because their reports will be ignored.

Using the courts

Very few cases concerning victims with learning difficulties end with successful court convictions. But this should be viewed in the light of what happens generally; only 3 per cent of all crimes result in convictions.

Appearing in court as a victim–witness can be very traumatic for anyone. The best way to help people with learning difficulties overcome natural fears is to visit courts *before* there is a need to go as a formal witness. Visits to observe from the public gallery should be part of the routine programme of day centres, schools and education projects.

Should an individual need to attend formally? Court 'witness support services' now undertake to show vulnerable witnesses around empty court rooms, to let them stand in the witness box and practise reading the oath. If possible this should be in the same court as the hearing will take place. Court rooms vary and differences can be very disturbing for people with learning difficulties, for example if the defendant appears where the victim thought the press would be sitting.

Courts may also assist in other ways. Given warning, the listing officer can usually avoid excessive waiting periods for vulnerable witnesses. In some cases, judges have agreed to lawyers removing wigs and gowns, and to screens between defendant and victim.

The most important aspect of preparing victim–witnesses is to make it clear that a case may not succeed for many reasons, and that a 'not guilty' verdict is not a reflection on their performance. Coaching concerning the facts of a case must be avoided, but witnesses can practice repeating or reading an oath or affirmation, saying and recognising their name, address and date of birth. Witnesses can be taught that they can ask for questions to be repeated, can ask to go to the toilet or to have a glass of water, and should always say if they do not know the answer to a question. The National Society for the Prevention of Cruelty to Children *Child Witness Pack* (NSPCC, 1993) provides an excellent preparation for *any* witness be they child or adult. *Going to Court* (Hollins, 1994) is specifically for people with learning difficulties.

Alternatives to the criminal system

For many victims, a criminal court may not be the best route to justice. Civil action is the main alternative. Cases are proven on a less strict standard of proof and the rules of evidence are different. Someone with learning difficulties can sue through another person (a 'next friend'), and legal aid may be available.

Staff disciplinary proceedings provide a route for remedying victimisation by staff. An employee may be dismissed if an employer has 'reasonable grounds' to suspect that an offence may have been committed. Establishing this in the case of a single incident would be sufficient. Even if an employee is later acquitted by a court, a dismissal may still be lawful. The drawback with dismissal proceedings is that hearings are not as efficient as in court, they can be very protracted, and union representatives can frustrate the process on the basis of technicalities which are unfamiliar to those hearing the case.

The Criminal Injuries Compensation Board may make payments, irrespective of a court case, but only if the injury results from a 'violent' criminal offence and the police have been informed 'without delay'. However, claims for less than £1000 will not be considered. In contrast a court may order payments for any amount and compensation will be paid for minor injuries such as bruises, scratches and even trauma.

Victimisation in domestic settings can be addressed by withdrawal of Registered Homes status where any person with reasonable grounds for concern can apply to the clerk at the local magistrates court for an emergency order. The National Assistance Act 1948 is another protective measure. On the advice of two doctors, a magistrate could order the removal of a victim from a residential home for offences of 'act' or 'omission' (for example neglect). Guardianship under the Mental Health Act 1983 can be used to similar effect to protect the welfare of someone who is technically a 'patient', but this can be very restrictive of the person's freedom. Invoking an inspection is another useful power within the Mental Health Act (Sec.115). It is an offence to prevent such an inspection. In some cases Health and Safety regulations have been used against negligent service providers, if, for example, someone has an accident due to a failure to assess the risk of a particular activity.

Voluntary mediation projects can provide an excellent means to resolve minor disputes, often providing a well-trained mediator. Usually mediation is only appropriate if the relative power of the two parties is about equal, and there is an agreement that the outcome will be accepted. Day centres might consider operating a similar system, but punishments (as distinct from reparation) should never be imposed.

Changing our vision of victimisation

The current perception of victimisation against people with learning difficulties is embodied in the language we use. Through this we devalue what happens and cloud our vision of crime, perpetrators and victims.

Women with learning difficulties are 'sexually abused' whereas other women are raped. Men with learning difficulties are 'physically abused' whereas other men are assaulted. Steal something from someone with learning difficulties and it is 'financial abuse', not theft. Offenders against the general community are criminals but those who victimise people with learning difficulties are 'abusers'. Victims with learning difficulties are 'sufferers', and 'sufferers' do not report crimes to the police; they 'disclose abuse' to professionals.

To reduce the victimisation of people with learning difficulties we must see crimes as crimes, perpetrators as perpetrators and victims as victims. Only then can the invisible barriers within reporting routes and the justice system, which stand between people with learning difficulties and the achievement of equitable justice, be questioned.

References

Ashton, G. and Ward, A. (1992). *Mental Handicap and the Law*. Sweet and Maxwell, London.

Brindle, D. (1992). Staff sacked over patient tied to toilet. *The Guardian*, December 11.

Brown, H. and Craft, A. (1992). *Working with the 'unthinkable'*. Family Planning Association, London.

Gunn, M.J. (1990). The law and learning disability. *International Review of Psychiatry*, **2**, 13–22.

Hart, T. (1992). Make your own choices. *Disability Issues*, **9**, 3.

Hollins, S. (1992). *Jenny Speaks Out*. Division of Psychiatry of Disability, St Georges Hospital Medical School, London.

Hollins, S. (1992). *Bob Tells All*. Division of Psychiatry and Disability, St Georges Hospital Medical School, London.

Hollins, S. (1994). *Going to Court*. Division of Psychiatry of Disability, St Georges Hospital Medical School, London.

Independent (1994). Care home abuse inquiry. *The Independent*, 12 March.

NAPSAC/ARC (1993). *It Could Never Happen Here!* Department of Learning Disabilities, University of Nottingham.

NAPSAC (1993). *Who Can I Tell? Blowing the Whistle on Sexual Abuse*. Department of Learning Disabilities, University of Nottingham.

NAPSAC (1994). *Annotated Bibliography* (Sexual abuse). Department of Learning Disabilities, University of Nottingham.

National Society for the Prevention of Cruelty to Children (1993). *The Child Witness Pack*. NSPCC/Childline, London.

Williams, C. (1994). *Cracking Crime – A Learning Pack* (including video). Pavilion Publishers, Brighton.

Williams, C. (1995). *Invisible Victims: Crime and Abuse Against People with Learning Disabilities*. Jessica Kingsley, London.

Walsall Women's Group (1994). *Walsall Women's Group Safety Video – No means No*. The Women's Group, College of Continuing Education, Walsall.

Chapter 23

To have and have not: Addressing issues of poverty

Ann Davis, Ruth Eley, Margaret Flynn, Peter Flynn and Gwyneth Roberts

> Poverty is not only about shortage of money. It is about rights and relationships; about how people are treated and how they regard themselves; about powerlessness, exclusion and loss of dignity. Yet the lack of an adequate income is at its heart. (Archbishop of Canterbury's Commission, 1985).

Poverty characterises the lives of people with learning difficulties. It is etched into the services offered to them in the community and in segregated institutions. It is part of their everyday experience of managing on low incomes from the benefit system or work. Poverty cannot be ignored on any visionary agenda about changing services in the 1990s. Yet there is no tradition among service providers and policy makers of acknowledging the presence of poverty and the effects it has on the choices, opportunities and experiences of people using services (Sumpton, 1988). While poverty is central to the lives of service users it has been systematically ignored by those making decisions about allocating resources and by those striving to develop a new generation of high quality services.

We focus on issues of income as a core, but not an exclusive feature of poverty. This chapter has been written by a group of people with distinctly different insights into the poverty experienced by people with learning difficulties. We highlight, from our different perspectives, some of the key issues in this area and then go on to suggest ways in which services might address poverty in the future. We have found few examples of poverty-aware practice on which to draw for inspiration and argue that until professionals make a commitment to working with people on this issue, persistent poverty will continue to characterise their lives.

Peter Flynn: A personal story

'I can't remember how much pocket money I had when I was little. When I was 16 I went to the Adult Training Centre and I didn't get much money there. It used to be £2 a week – that's all for just putting things in boxes and other boring things. I kept the £2 and my mum used to make it up to £5. That was 27 years ago. I think I had more than my sisters because I was older. I spent it on going to clubs. I saved at the centre and went on holiday in Wales.

Living by myself, I get £62.45 a week and most of it goes on bills. I've saved £23 because I'm going abroad in 1995. I just put in £2 a week. Certain food I don't buy – they're too dear – like aubergines and things like that. So I buy things I can afford – for instance in the Arndale [a large Manchester shopping centre] they've got cheap shops and Kwik Save is cheap. Some weeks I've got money and some weeks I haven't. My sister, Margaret, buys my clothes and gives me money sometimes. I get some second hand ones myself sometimes. For birthdays and Christmas I prefer money.

My sister has an account because you can't declare it. What I'd really like is some money now. I'd like to buy a birthday present for a very good friend. When you're on benefits you can't afford too expensive presents. It's better sorting my own money out. I know what I'm doing. Margaret pays my phone bills. If I was in charge of the Benefits Agency I would give more money to people that need it. They don't know what it's like to live on £62. If I had £100 I'd go to Turkey. I've heard good reports of it. I know people who've been.

I can't afford to go on trains even though I like going places. Can't afford to go to the theatre and I'd like to see things like *Me and My Girl*. I like Irish tapes and I buy them in the market because there's a good Irish stall there and they're only £3.99. Sometimes people pester me for money and I don't give it them. I tell them "no."

I buy an evening newspaper – 30p. I like that. If I was stuck and had no money I would ask Margaret. Sometimes it's not easy asking. It's hard not having much money because of all the bills you've got to pay. There are things wrong with my flat and if I had enough money I'd get them repaired quickly. Instead I've got to wait for the housing and they take years.

Special schools aren't very good at learning you to manage your money. They should teach you more about it and so should everyone's parents.'

Margaret Flynn: A family perspective

When I think about my brother's financial circumstances a few things strike me:

- His learning difficulty has decided his economic fate.
- His net disposable income does not yield a satisfactory standard of living.
- He rarely has any surplus income.
- His income increases his dependency on subsidies from his family.
- Support in respect of his money has a history of inconsistency.
- Peter no longer dreams of being employed – having absorbed the preoccupation of "services" that he should not "lose" his benefits.
- Solicitors advise against leaving him more than a low fixed sum in wills.

Knowledge of such disadvantage leaves me bewildered by the government's populist card on the fraud and abuse of "welfare scroungers". This deflects attention from the squalid physical sur-roundings of the Department of Social Security (DSS) offices in which I have waited for hours with Peter; the inability of many DSS personnel to take the time to explain things simply; the highly discretionary manner in which his GP determined whether his "mental impairment" merited exception from the community charge (it did not); and the host of assumptions which surround most non-disabled people's decisions regarding Peter's ability to manage his income, most particularly, fears of vulnerability to exploitation and wasteful spending patterns.

A side effect of all of this is a rough and ready arrangement whereby Peter has holidays with his siblings. He goes out for meals with his siblings and friends and, as is his strong preference, he receives money for birthdays and Christmas. I have a deposit account from which when it was created I could draw money from for such outgoings as the replacement of his winter coat and occasional bills he could not pay. The increase in my financial well-being has meant that this "back-up" has not been drawn from in recent years.

When we meet we always spend some time talking about money. I have learned to be less punishing in my approach to Peter's need for cash. Our arrangement has become more satisfactory. On balance however, it is not a blueprint that either of us would commend. My uncontested position of control over subsidies to Peter's income results from the fragility of his capacity to budget; the remoteness of the administrative machinery which is available to assist disabled people in managing their money; and the knowledge that he is incredibly generous in many ways – a quality that, at times, I have found hard to value. I remain concerned that my control is not challenged – perhaps because this arrangement appears to work.

In contrast to the rest of his family, much of Peter's life displays material poverty. The array of financial services surrounding banking, investments, pensions, insurance, assurance and insolvency are all absent. There are no jostling offers to replace the services of welfare rights officers, benefits agencies, DSS personnel and social services personnel. The paper chases that characterise our dealings with the DSS and Benefit Agency personnel seem obstinately beyond the reach of improvement. Peter's letter to the Prime Minister for clarification about the implications of being a volunteer in a neighbourhood centre for his DSS benefits yielded some reassuring sentences, but for how long? The untender mercies of the community charge diminished his limited income and disadvantaged him further.

We continue in an unsought maze of discovery.

Ann Davis: Policy implications

The literature on this topic offers few signposts to Peter and Margaret in their journey of discovery. The policy agenda around community care in considering 'ordinary' living and 'normal' lives has consistently failed to acknowledge the way in which low incomes and poverty amongst people with learning difficulties shape their choices and opportunities (Davis et al., 1993). Professional and service agendas, though focussed on issues of challenging dependence and promoting independence through increasing valued opportunities, are strangely silent, too, on how this is to be achieved in the context of a benefit system which financially rewards people for trading on their incapacities in order to maximise their income from the complex packages of means-tested and disability benefits which are currently on offer. The preoccupation of policy makers and service providers and purchasers with 'effective' and 'cost-efficient packages of care' pays no heed to the way in which the personal income of those receiving services should be treated. It is as if it is no different from the other resources on which providers might draw without consultation with individual service users or their households.

In understanding why people with learning difficulties experience such different access to, and control over, their money than most other citizens we need to begin to gather systematic information about the way in which access and decision making in this area is taken on by others such as service providers and family members and why.

The subsistence levels of income made available to people with learning difficulties is a reflection of their low participation in the workforce and their consequent dependency on benefit incomes. Research has shown that benefit income alone is inadequate to maintain people's participation in the ordinary activities of their communities (Brown, 1985; Buckle, 1984; Flynn, 1989). Income inadequacy is sometimes a question of people failing to claim their full benefit entitlement (Wray and Wistow, 1987). For others it is the fact that full benefit entitlement covers daily survival but does not provide the means for participation (Davis et al., 1993). In addition, benefit income for disabled people is currently provided on declarations of 'incapacity' in relation to such activities as work, personal care and mobility. Such declarations serve to construct a devalued and power-less status for people with learning difficulties which reinforces their marginalisation as citizens.

The restructuring of the social security system which began in the mid-1980s has been promoted by government as having an explicit aim of targetting resources, more effectively, at those in most need. The targetting devices currently employed in the benefit system place financial disincentives in the paths of people with learning difficulties wishing to develop their capacities, pursue their interests and realise their work abilities. The combination of disability premiums in the means-tested benefits system with the extra financial rewards for establishing incapacity for personal care and mobility in Disability Living Allowance means that income loss is heavy for those people declaring themselves capable and available for work.

As Peter and Margaret's experiences suggest Benefit Agency staff who are making decisions about claims for benefits have little grasp of the facts that are relevant to the lives of people with learning difficulties. Their responses to the difficulties facing people are there-fore limited. The Benefits Agency has, so far, not set standards to develop work in this area. As the National Development Team's evidence to the House of Commons Select Committee argues:

> Performance standards in Benefit Agency offices should be developed in relation to, and in partnership with, people with learning disabilities. For example, quality assurance standards might outline how good individual face to face, adjudicative performance should be in order to be acceptable. (Davis *et al.*, 1993)

It is not, however, just a matter of the practice of central and local government benefit systems. Local authority, health and voluntary and private community-based accommodation and related service provision have been routinely devised on the basis of users maximising their income from the social security and local authority benefit systems. These services effectively lock individuals into patterns of daily life from which it is difficult to shift if change means a loss of benefit income (Davis *et al.*, 1993). The proliferation of charges for services in the mixed economy of current service provision is likely to intensify this impoverishing experience of service use. A similar pattern can be detected in those family households where people with learning difficulties are the highest benefit earners and household survival is dependent on that income being retained whatever the cost to individual autonomy, independence and choice.

The second issue of importance in this area is that of money management. In contrast to most adults in our society, people with learning difficulties produce little wealth and make little use of banks and building societies. Their experiences of education and training programmes are usually that little time and attention are paid to the knowledge and skills needed to manage personal finances. As a result, the management of personal income all too often becomes a matter of ad hoc informal and formal arrangements in which individuals may find themselves denied access to their income and its use. Experience suggests that the restrictions imposed on people's access and control of their income are unlikely to reflect the competence which they have or might learn to develop in this area. The ways in which institutions have arranged these matters in the past has received some consideration (Raynes *et al.*, 1987; Bradshaw and Davis, 1986). The routine practices of people being denied access to their DSS benefit books, given income in kind, offered substitute staff-controlled savings or bank arrangements, being enrolled in compulsory savings schemes and being subject to appointeeships have all been unquestioningly replicated in a number of the statutory and private community living arrangements which have been developed over the last 20 years. In addition, the way in which family households, relatives and paid carers have devised ways of managing individuals' money on an informal basis is a growing and complex area of activity which largely remains unaddressed by services and their personnel.

The scant evidence that is available on money management (Flynn, 1989; Davis *et al.*, 1993) suggests that the opportunities afforded most citizens to learn about managing personal income through experience, education, family and peer support and specialist advice is not generally experienced by people with learning difficulties. Nonetheless, there is evidence that many people with learning difficulties express a wish to take more responsibility for this area of their lives as well as being given opportunities to discuss the difficulties and dilemmas they may face in managing on limited incomes.

Ruth Eley: The role of social services departments

There are usually two reasons why social services departments intervene in the financial affairs of people with learning difficulties. Either they have difficulty managing their money and get into debt, or someone suspects they are being ripped off and sounds the alarm. In the former instance, it is often a combination of trying to live within an income which would test the business skills of the most able city finance manager with poor support and insufficient budgeting know-how. As Peter points out, the education system, particularly segregated special schooling, has not proved adept at teaching young people how to acquire and manage money. It is not just about basic numeracy, it involves enabling them to see the importance of money management, support for this and assisting them to make some fine judgements about spending priorities: do I pay the rent or buy shoes?

As far as exploitation is concerned, it is clear that those who have so little to start with do fall prey to the unscrupulous. Taking someone else's weekly benefit can double the income of someone dependent on Income Support. Also, there seems to operate an uncanny grapevine which is activated when people inherit money or property or receive a cash lump sum through retirement or compensation. The financial and legal institutions making the payments are often oblivious to the potential vulnerability of the recipients when a little preventive work would go a long way. Fortunately, there are bank clerks and building society managers who remain alert to such possibilities who do what they can to prevent disasters and refer the matter to us for attention. At the present time, the Court of Protection is the only recourse we have to intervene with legal authority. It is cumbersome and remote, and for people whose only assets are their weekly benefits or earnings, the Court is unwilling to act. Appointeeships (that is the appointment of a person to act on behalf of a claimant) apply only to benefits. Managing a bank or Post Office savings account on someone else's behalf is not possible without a Court of Protection order.

A hidden area of poverty arises for people who live with their families. The weekly benefits of people with learning difficulties are often subsumed into the family budget and some families do complain when requests are made, by day service staff, for example, for money to support activities such as going out for a drink. People living in residential units have a personal allowance of £13.35 (April 1995–April 1996 rates). This is not a lot to support the sorts of activities non-disabled people take for granted, such as the possibility of treating a friend to a drink or meal. It is relatively straightforward for staff working in residential units or supporting people in their own homes to assist or offer advice on money management. It is far more complex to intervene in family finances to try to untangle the weekly income of a daughter or son with learning difficulties. Furthermore, it is not a priority task for most social workers given other demands on their time.

There is no doubt that people with learning difficulties with whom social services are in contact experience a double disadvantage; not only do they depend on paid help to participate in the most basic of social activities, they also require subsidies. Depressed expectations which begin early, long-standing service provision and inadequate benefit incomes are all effective in closing off the possibility of employment and busy and interesting lives for too many people with learning difficulties.

Those people in touch with services, such as day centres or home support, should be able to expect basic advice and help on how to manage their money. Hard-pressed staff, though, may be tempted to adopt a controlling and directive approach rather than an educative and enabling one. If Peter did not have the active oversight and interest of Margaret and the rest of his family, it is not certain that it would be available from anywhere else, unless he got into difficulties.

Gwyneth Roberts: A new legal framework

The day-to-day lives of able people are based on a series of assumptions, so basic as to be almost unquestioned. One of the most fundamental is the assumption that they have a considerable degree of autonomy over the way they spend their money. For people with learning difficulties, what others perceive as a basic right, is too often treated, at best, as a grudging concession or an easily removed privilege, or, at worst, never even features in their lives. People with learning difficulties are entitled to a better deal than this. What we need is an appropriate legal framework which takes account of the particular needs of Peter and others. The rules should aim at safeguarding and promoting their right to 'take for themselves those decisions they are able to take', but

> . . . where it is necessary in their own interests or for the protection of others that someone else should take decisions on their behalf, the intervention should be as limited as possible and should be concerned to achieve what the person [her]/himself would have wanted; and . . . that proper safeguards should be provided against exploitation, neglect and physical, sexual or psychological abuse. (Law Commission, 1995).

Reform of the law on mentally incapacitated people and decision making which the Law Commission is currently engaged in, is long overdue, given the absence of a coherent legal framework and the evidence of abuse, including financial malpractice, which so many people with learning difficulties currently endure. What the Law Commission has so far proposed goes a considerable way towards achieving a better legal framework. The Commission proposes a general presumption of competence, but that where a person's incompetence is established, there should be a statutory framework for decision making based upon the best interest of the incapacitated person, taking into account his or her ascertainable past and present wishes and feelings; and recognising the need to encourage and permit that person to participate in any decision making to the full extent of which he or she is capable.

The Commission sees issues of substitute decision making and financial management as involving two separate interests: first, access to funds held by or due to the incapacitated person; and, second the authority of the carer or other person to use such resources on behalf of the incapacitated person. At present, there are few procedural safeguards in this field, and little opportunity in practice to monitor the performance of informal 'receivers'. The existing system of supervision through the Court of Protection is, as Ruth Eley says, widely perceived as remote, expensive and cumbersome to use. On the other hand, the current rules concerning appointees, although better framed (in that they allow individuals to confer responsibility on others even when they themselves are not incapacitated) are nevertheless flawed, since abuse of the system appears so widespread. Another problem arises from the fact that the DSS benefit income of those with learning difficulties who live with their families is frequently perceived as part of the family income. The Law Commission's final report No. 231 (1995) sets out proposals which aim to ensure that the current situation is tightened up in the future.

Key pointers to future service development

Over the last 20 years poverty has grown rapidly in the UK and the evidence suggests that this growth and its associated inequalities will continue in the 1990s (Oppenheim, 1993). Against this economic and social context, addressing the impact of poverty on the lives of people with learning difficulties becomes imperative in debates about service development.

Our experience suggests that the starting point for this work needs to be a systematic approach to establishing an understanding of how individuals and their households are managing poverty. Such an examination, undertaken in dialogue with individuals, is likely to reveal complex but recurring patterns of difficulties in managing on low weekly incomes, consequent exclusion from ordinary living and denial of the rights and choices which individuals with learning difficulties should have in respect of their access to, and use of, personal income. It is through such work that service purchasers, providers and professionals will be in a position to address the impact of poverty on the lives of people with learning difficulties. From this starting point, poverty needs to be placed on all personal and service agendas in a way which is consistent with service values and principles and which supports the delivery of creative, poverty-aware and rights-based practice.

In developing a properly aware approach, the following key pointers need to be considered:

- All service users are managing poverty in a variety of ways. These need to be identified, discussed and responded to as part of individual assessment, care planning and care management.

- Consequences of low income and the approaches to money management adopted by individuals, households and services need to be reviewed in the context of the stated values of good quality services.
- Implications for income and money management of any change in the situation of an individual needs to be identified and worked with by service personnel and independent advocates.
- Services for people with learning difficulties should identify the necessary resources and make arrangements for access to clear, relevant and independent information and advice about money and benefit rights for all service users.
- All service developments should be 'poverty-audited' in order to make explicit all the consequences of proposed service changes for the disposable incomes and income choices of people with learning difficulties.
- Charging policies and practice should be subject to poverty audits in order to consider their effects on the lives and options available to people with learning difficulties.
- Learning difficulty services should identify and make arrangements for the provision of clear, relevant and independent information and advice about the payment of service charges by users and their households.
- Independent advice should be available for service users and service providers about the consequences to personal income of choices people may wish to make in their lives (for example, with respect to work experience, changing accommodation, starting new relationships, pursuing new interests).
- Services should identify the education and support required by service users and their households in organising access to the shared management of money which will enhance personal autonomy and independence.
- Service contracts should make specific reference to the way in which access to and control of personal income should be managed in order to enhance individual autonomy, choice and independence.
- Services should make provision for an independent service to assist and negotiate the management of finance in the range of community, family and institutional settings in which people with learning difficulties may find themselves during their lives.
- Services should monitor and be responsive to the ways in which poverty shapes the quality of life experienced by service users.
- Services working with user groups should identify forums in which jointly they can seek to bring to the attention of government, local authorities and benefit agencies the impact which their policies and practice have on the lives of people with learning difficulties.
- Services should recognise the important contribution they have to make to the poverty campaigns which are currently addressing the problems facing the one in five citizens who are living on, or below, Income Support levels.

By using these key pointers to review current and future service development, we urge that a start is made in addressing an issue which has been too long ignored by most professionals, planners and providers in the learning difficulties field. This task, in our view, would be facilitated if it was supported by three further steps being taken. First, that the DSS, through the Benefits Agency, began to actively consider, in consultation, what service changes need to take place to improve the quality of its customer care to people with learning difficulties and their households. Second, that banks, building societies and those charged with the responsibility of issuing large sums of money to individuals work together to address vulnerability in relation to money matters. Third, that the Law Commission commends that procedural safeguards (with regard to people's finances) are put in place as a matter of urgency.

Poverty is an issue which people with learning difficulties have never been able to ignore, it confronts them each day. As Peter tells us 'It's hard not having much money'.

References

Archbishop of Canterbury's Commission (1985). *Faith in the City*. Church House, London.

Brown, R. (1985). *Money Matters for People with a Mental Handicap*. Disablement Income Group, London.

Bradshaw, M. and Davis, A. (1986). *Not a Penny to Call my Own – Poverty Amongst Residents in Mental Illness and Mental Handicap Hospitals*. King's Fund/Disability Alliance.

Buckle, J. (1984). *Mental Handicap Costs More*. Disablement Income Group, London.

Davis, A., Murray, J. and Flynn, M.C. (1993). *Normal Lives? The Financial Circumstances of People with Learning Disabilities*. National Development Team, Manchester.

Flynn, M.C. (1989). *Independent Living for Adults with Mental Handicap: A Place of my Own*. Cassell, London.

Law Commission (1995). *Mental Incapacity*, Report No. 231. HMSO, London.

Oppenheim, C. (1993). *Poverty: The Facts*. Child Poverty Action Group, London.

Raynes, N.V., Sumpton, R.C. and Flynn, M.C. (1987). *Homes for Mentally Handicapped People*. Tavistock, London.

Sumpton, R. (1988). Poverty, mental handicap and Social Work. In *Public Issues, Private Pain: Poverty, Social Work and Social Policy* (eds S. Becker and S. MacPherson). Insight, London.

Wray, K. and Wistow, G. (1987). Welfare initiative netted an extra £500,000. *Social Work Today*, 7th September.

Chapter 24

What the papers say: Media images of people with learning difficulties

Terry Philpot

In April 1991, Jo Ramsden, a 21-year-old woman with a learning difficulty, was abducted. She was found dead 11 months later. Apart from the initial news of her disappearance, there was little coverage of her story, even though the hunt for her included coastguards, local search parties and a police helicopter. Only one newspaper, *Today*, sent a reporter to her home town of Bridport, where she vanished; it then ran only a small photograph and a 250 word story. Even an arrangement to interrupt a Liverpool–Arsenal charity match (the missing woman was a Liverpool fan) failed to capture press interest. *The Sport*, seemingly conscious of its profession's failings, subsequently ran a two page spread: 'We haven't forgotten you, Jo!'

Almost at the same time as Jo Ramsden disappeared, so did Rachel McLean, a 19-year-old Oxford University student. But the story of the search for her (which included long features in some newspapers) was part of the daily fare for newspaper readers until she, too, was eventually found murdered. A letter from Lord (then Sir Brian) Rix, chairperson of MENCAP, contrasting the press treatment of the two cases, was refused by *The Times*. *The Independent* (5 May 1991), however, took up the story of the way the stories had been dealt with in a feature which had the effect of prompting greater media interest in Jo Ramsden.[1] Jo Ramsden's parents felt that greater publicity in the first weeks might have meant that she would have been discovered earlier.

---

[1] Interestingly, a later feature (21 December 1991) did not prevent *The Independent* from referring to her as 'part adult, part child'. And when the man believed to be Jo Ramsden's murderer was brought to trial for the abduction and rape of at least six women with

Jo Ramsden was a victim of a kind of treatment by the media which, by its nature, is difficult to detect; that the person with a learning difficulty is seen as a non-person. Yet what happened to her story was an example of the devaluing of people with learning difficulties which is more often expressed by negative stereotyping which attributes all manner of qualities, conjured up from some long-buried past. As Dowson (1991) writes: 'The theories [about the supposed characteristics of people with learning difficulties] have been largely forgotten, but the fears and fantasies which they expressed still live on in an assortment of stereotypes.' These stereotypes range from the 'eternal child' in need of constant, loving care and attention, to people with abnormal sexual appetites and low moral awareness. Stereotypes, historically, have often been more varied than is assumed. While some parts of the ancient world invested people with learning difficulties with magical properties and afforded them a kind of reverence, other parts of that world (as well as later ages and into our own) have portrayed them as dangerous or subhuman (Ryan and Thomas, 1988).

Wolfensberger (1972) says that people with learning difficulties (and other devalued groups) are typically represented in ways which devalue them as subhuman, menaces, objects of pity, holy innocents, diseased organisms, objects of ridicule and eternal children. One effect of this is that such descriptions prescribe the behaviour expected of people with learning difficulties. Whatever guise they are clothed in – from innocence to depravity – it is usually a negative one. The person with the learning difficulty is not seen as a person, but is invested with other qualities, is made 'special' in some way, which hides their essentially human qualities: 'Like other groups which are perceived to be different in some way, people with learning difficulties become a screen onto which public fears and uncertainties – the shadows of the collective unconscious – are projected.' (Dowson, 1991).

However, there is more ambivalence in public attitudes than this view implies. So far as community care policies are concerned, the public is very largely in favour of the *idea* of people with learning difficulties living ordinary lives in the community. Where their doubts arise (and, on occasion, their hostility is expressed) is when those lives are to be lived in the same streets and neighbourhoods as their own.

learning difficulties – it was ruled that there was insufficient evidence for him to stand trial for her kidnapping. *The Independent*'s crime reporter managed to refer to him (7 April 1993) as a 'retired psychiatric nurse' and a 'nursing assistant' who had worked with the 'mentally handicapped'.

Whatever devils may be lurking beneath 'the shadows of the collective unconscious' they need stoking up to survive; disablism, like sexism and racism, is socially learned, rather than innate. Barnes (1991) cites findings which showed that on the basis of looking at photographs, children were found not to react badly to 'abnormal' looks until they were at least 11 years of age, and thus 'discrimination against funny-looking people' is socially learned.

How far familiarity is a guard against stereotypes is arguable. But so far as people with learning difficulties are concerned, many still live separate lives. Despite the advances made in the closure of long-stay hospitals over the last decade, this form of 'care' is still home to 19 600 people with learning difficulties (Collins, 1993). Of the remainder, the great majority of children attend special schools which are segregated. From there they often go to segregated day centres and spent their time in segregated clubs. Yet it is much more common to see people with learning difficulties in a cafe, the street market, on a bus or in the local shop than was the case a couple of decades ago. McGill and Cummings (1990) opine that people are more likely to be influenced by negative images portrayed by the media where their contact with people with learning difficulties is limited.

If stereotypes and prejudice are socially learned, it is not unreasonable to speculate that our social attitudes are influenced by the media. As Troyna (1981) stated: 'For many people, the mass media represent a crucial source of beliefs and values from which they build up a picture of their social worlds.' Cohen and Young (1981) made the same point, somewhat more forcibly:

> In newspapers, books and magazines, on TV and in the cinema, on stage and through the airwaves, the media exert a uniquely powerful influence on how individuals come to understand the changing world around them. Whether one views any media form as a window of one's surroundings, the media's capacity to examine and communicate about people, places and ideas is unequalled.

Such influence is wider than just the print media. People with learning difficulties have long been the stock in trade of comedy (from traditional to alternative) and drama (from B movies and horror films to Shakespeare). Television, the most popular form of popular culture (Barnes, 1991), as well as children's comics, have a pervasive (and largely) negative influence in this respect. Advertising, whether run by disability charities or by commercial companies making use of disabled people (or, more commonly, not) can also shape public attitudes

(Wertheimer, 1988b; Scott-Parker, 1989; Morris, 1991; Hevey, 1992). This chapter though, is concerned with print media, and specifically, newspapers because they are probably the main source of *detailed* information for most people, and the coverage which they give to issues of disability and news as it affects people with learning difficulties is far greater than is found elsewhere.

What kind of images does the press portray? There have been a number of studies of media coverage of disability. Biklen and Bogdan (1977) identified ten commonly recurring stereotypes found in the treatment of disabled people by the mass media. Among these were the disabled person as laughable, as his or her worst enemy, as a burden, as asexual, and as being unable to participate in daily life. There are few significant differences in the way people with different sorts of disabilities are portrayed, with the possible exception of people with a mental illness (Glasgow Media Group, no date). While learning difficulties and mental illness are often confused in the media, where the latter is referred to correctly, notions of dangerousness are often attached. Keller *et al.* (1990) surveyed American newspaper coverage of people with disabilities to test the thesis that disability issues are not covered in the press, and where they are, the portrayal of the disabled person is a negative one. They found a substantial number of references to people with disabilities or their family members on a daily basis. These tended to be in features or 'soft' news, as opposed to 'hard' news, and to be about physically disabled people or people with learning difficulties identified generically as 'handicapped' or 'disabled'. When articles mentioned the impact of disability on an individual's life, it was often portrayed as negative; for example, if the articles considered the possibility for improvement in a person's condition, they frequently suggested that the condition could not be improved. Yoshida *et al.* (1990) describe several studies which show how disabled people are portrayed more negatively than positively. Their own study looked at the issues covered by big city newspapers regarding disability and found a lack of coverage on the topic of special education, as opposed to topics like policy, housing and treatment in institutions, sports, and medical advances. Special education's neglect could be accounted for by the fact that 47.9 per cent of the articles studied were about adults and 18.6 per cent featured children. The authors ascribed the dearth of coverage of the subject to the failure of those in the field to establish relationships with newspaper staff, and quote some staff as welcoming such contact.

The most recent and most extensive study of British newspapers' treatment of people with learning difficulties is by Wertheimer (1988a). News stories accounted for 81.8 per cent of her material, letters 9.4 per cent, comment (opinion pieces) 3.3 per cent, leaders 1.7 per cent and features 3.8 per cent. Despite some positive images, it was found that familiar negative stereotypes were perpetrated. The research was undertaken at the time of breaking of a story about relatives of the Queen Mother being found resident in a long-stay hospital (see later discussion). Two-thirds of the rest of the coverage was about fund raising and other aspects of charitable work. Like stories about services, these stories often reinforced notions of passivity and dependency. One of the most striking and revealing of Wertheimer's findings was that there was not a single example among 1489 cuttings of the direct reporting of an opinion of a person with learning difficulties. The language used was often negative: 'poor souls', 'born less than perfect', and 'a race apart'. The manager of an adult training centre who was featured as a bowls champion was described as 'a winner who looks after the losers in life'. When the Princess of Wales visited a day centre, which 'could have been distressing', she 'appeared unperturbed'.

While newspapers do shape people's attitudes and consciousness and can act as tools for change, that is not their primary purpose. They are a reflection of society. A good newspaper, according to the American playwright Arthur Miller is 'a nation talking to itself' (*Observer*, 26 November 1961). Anyone – from Cabinet ministers to a local residents' group – seeking to get their views across or pursue their own favoured changes may try to get the ear of a journalist. Thus, newspapers cannot always be blamed for reporting the statements or actions of others, which may reflect negatively on people with learning difficulties. But journalists are not unprejudiced and may be no more likely to have met or known someone with learning difficulties than the next person. They, like their informants, confuse mental illness with learning difficulties, and, more through ignorance than malice, perpetrate stereotypes and use highly charged, often inaccurate language. Take, for example, McGill and Cummings' study (1990) of *The Guardian* with its liberal reputation and social consciousness, and the role it played two decades ago in uncovering the 'scandals' at Ely and other long-stay hospitals. Their analysis of staff-written material and that written by outsiders suggested that the newspaper's own reporters were more likely to misrepresent people with learning difficulties than other writers. The articles included 11 letters, 23 features and one leading article. They depicted people with learning difficulties as sick and/or as children disproportionate to the degree of sickness found among people with learning difficulties or the numbers of them who were children. This was especially the case in articles written by the newspaper's own staff. Non-staff writers, while sometimes depicting people with learning difficulties as children, did not depict them as patients and used the term 'people' more frequently.

A more recent study of press coverage and disability generally by Smith and Jordan (1991) looked at 35 stories during eight weeks toward the end of 1990 and two weeks in February of the following year. The quality press ran four times as many disability stories as the tabloids; the most popular subjects were health, fund raising and charity, and personal interest stories. Community care, carers, mobility and council services were the least popular (this was, however, before the implementation of the NHS and Community Act which fuelled a lot of newspaper copy in its first years). The study concludes:

> The newspapers' choice of news does not correspond with the agenda priorities and expectations of disabled people, carers and disability organizations. So-called medical 'problems' of disabled people completely overshadow the political/social issues that relate to disability.

This latter ought not to be surprising. If society and, to an extent services, and charitable endeavour still harp more on the medical model of disability than social definitions, then the media is likely to reflect that. The study also found that words such as 'crippled', 'suffer', 'victim', and 'deformity' and 'defects' were commonly used and offered as a 'trigger mechanism' to sensationalise stories. Apart from some words which are peculiar to physical disability, these findings reflected those of earlier studies on the subject of learning difficulties.

Most negative stereotypes are attached to fairly run-of-the-mill stories (this is particularly so of the local press). Occasionally, stories break which allow the media (and not always the tabloid press) full vent to their penchant for the sensational and stereotyping. This was particularly so in the case of Dr Leonard Arthur, the physician, who, in 1981, was charged with (and acquitted of) murder for allowing a child with a learning difficulty to die by withholding treatment. This occasioned debates about the right to, and quality of life, and also brought out many suggestions that perhaps it was better for those born with a disability to be allowed to die. Negative coverage was evoked by two other cases. One was the case, also in 1981, of the 10-day-old baby

'Alexandra', whose parents refused to authorise fairly routine treatment for an intestinal blockage. The local authority, the London Borough of Hammersmith, successfully applied for the child to be made a ward of court so that it could, *in loco parentis*, authorise the operation. In the case of 'Jeanette', a young woman of 17 with a learning difficulty, her mother had a court application for her to be sterilised in 1987. She was a 'retarded youth', part of 'a breed apart', someone for whom 'childhood lasts a lifetime', who would undergo a 'sex op' and a 'spaying op'. Statements by judges in cases like that of Dr Arthur about whether some people have lives 'worth living' or are 'vegetables' not only have more to do with prejudice than legal argument, but also generate seemingly irresistible headlines that conjure up all the old myths and fears. Other stories have given a completely distorted view about learning difficulties. For example, in 1987, *The Sun* discovered that a niece of the Queen Mother had been living in a long-stay hospital for 46 years. Her sister had died the previous year but both sisters had been shown in *Debrett's* as dead. The newspaper's front page, four deck banner headline was: 'Queen's cousin locked in madhouse.' The fact that the *Daily Telegraph* a day later found three more royal relatives living at the hospital might suggest that the Dowson's 'shadows of the collective unconscious' fell across the Royal Family, or as *The Sun* put it, rather less elegantly, the relatives had been 'shunned and shut away' (Davies, 1987). There was much speculation about supposed hereditary 'insanity' and *The Guardian* leader, focussing almost wholly on mental illness, even managed to evoke Charlotte Brontë's Mrs Rochester (Wertheimer, 1988a).

Cases where the press actively harasses someone with a learning difficulty are rare. But when *The Sun* published a front page story about a small boy with behavioural problems under the heading 'The worst brat in Britain', the parents successfully sued.

If any influence is to be exerted on the media to try to make it more sensitive or better informed about certain issues, it needs to be done, as William Blake advised of doing good, in 'minute particulars'. The larger issues of the direction of the press seem lost somewhere in the labyrinth of multinational ownership and anonymous news rooms where it is difficult to speak to the same person twice. As Dowson says, the press is a very obvious medium to cultivate. But he rightly warns that its disadvantage is that it may not share the same concern to offer images which challenge negative stereotypes as does the person seeking to do so (Dowson, 1991).

So where to start? There is, in fact, a code of ethics by the National Union of Journalists, which states that journalists should not originate or process material which encourages discrimination on grounds of race, colour, creed, illegitimacy, disability, marital status (or the lack of it), gender or sexual orientation. The trouble with this (apart from the fact that few journalists will have seen it and fewer even read it) is that it is strong on good intentions but weak on interpretation. What does it mean not to 'process' material; to receive it from source, or to subedit it? And what about the borderline of free speech? Last year (1994), when successive Civil Rights Bills came before Parliament to outlaw discrimination against disabled people, some newspapers published articles and letters arguing that the Bill was well-intentioned but, for various reasons, mistaken. Should these not have been 'originated' or 'processed'? The code also states: 'A journalist shall at all times defend the principle of the freedom of the press and other media in relation to the collection of information and the expression of comment or criticism.' There are, arguably, points of conflict between these two parts of the code, if not an implicit inherent contradiction.

Newspapers have themselves agreed to a voluntary code of practice about fair reporting and 'fair representation'. This was drawn up in the face of increasing, but so far, empty threats about government regulation of newspapers. However, as the code has not stopped some spectacular invasions of privacy, it is unlikely to do much about the entirely ignored issues of how people with learning difficulties are represented. Newspapers have also instituted independent ombudspersons who deal with readers' complaints. While this is welcome for individuals, it deals with matters after the alleged offence has been committed and is, anyway, no substitute for more fundamental measures.

What is needed are both personal and structural approaches. The important thing is to cultivate the media, Dowson's caution notwithstanding, to establish a relationship between agency and newspaper. This is more likely to be successful at regional and local, rather than national newspaper levels. Press releases and letters to the editor are commonly employed, the latter having the virtue that while they may be cut, the emphasis which the writer wants is not likely to be changed. But publicity can be a double-edged sword. Too often disabled people make news in connection with fund-raising events and appeals. While this may gain publicity for the organisation, it can also have the effect of reinforcing the idea of the person with a learning difficulty being in need of 'care' and 'charity'. Again, news coverage about some achievement by a person with a learning difficulty can provoke some of the worst excesses of journalistic sentimentality and provoke thoughts of 'Aren't you wonderful!' As McConkey and McCormack (1983) advise, in a long list of practical approaches to the media:

> Fund-raising groups need to give careful thought to the way they portray disabled people, for unwittingly, they are very potent image-makers. The basis of their appeal to the public must shift from pity and poverty to participation and parity.

These authors also rightly emphasise that the problems which afflict people with learning difficulties, so far as the media are concerned, are often ones of omission:

> . . . in the absence of positive direction . . . media coverage merely reflects a condescending, outdated view of disabled people, which will at least partially undermine the best laid educational attempts. But given more positive direction, the media can become a powerful education tool, and while the final shape of the published material is in the hands of reporters, photographers and subeditors, they will generally take their cue from you, the 'expert'. (McConkey and McCormack, 1983).

Organisations of people with learning difficulties like People First have been increasingly assertive, and specialist media probably would not now consider running a major story on learning difficulties without a comment from them. This would probably not be so of the general media who may not even know of People First. Its first points of call would be the large voluntary agencies like MENCAP, which have highly skilled and sophisticated media departments. All the more important, then, that in such instances the large voluntaries should ensure that users themselves have a chance to express a view, either by making available user members of their organisations or by referring the inquirer to People First or other self-advocacy groups.

As to structural changes, these need to be both a matter of carrot and stick. Canada affords progressive examples of both. The Canadian Association for Community Living has put much energy in recent years into promoting positive success stories about community living. While the association has used whatever vehicle it could find, it first looked to what it had at its immediate disposal. This meant transforming its quarterly review, published by the associated Roehrer Institute, and now called *Entourage*, from a 'quasi-professional journal-cum-newsletter into a human interest magazine full of positive stories'. Other media were also used and developments were also publicised through workshops and conferences. The main news media were also cultivated and 'we made a commitment to always give priority to requests from the media since by spending time with them, educating them, and helping them to understand issues from a broad perspective, they then become our allies in conveying important information on a mass scale.' (Diane Richler, vice-president, CACL, personal communication, 3 January 1994). The association also instituted an awards scheme to reward positive journalism, with judging undertaken by well-known leaders in the communications field. Winners have numbered some of the most prestigious broadcasters and journalists in the country. With the help of a respected journalist who assists the association voluntarily, the association is now to launch an essay competition among community newspapers throughout the country. The Community Relations Commission in the UK has an awards competition for journalism about race relations, open to national, regional and local newspapers, as well as specialist magazines. Most media competitions in the UK tend to be either specialist in a broad sense (for example, farming, medicine and science) or general (that is, to award good journalism whatever the subject). One which rewarded local government journalism foundered a few years ago for lack of financial support, having failed to attract funding from the three local authority associations – the Associations of County Councils, District Councils and Metropolitan Authorities – whom, it might be thought, would have some interest in promoting good journalism in their field. This does not augur well for any British attempt to follow the Canadian example.

The Canadian stick is that there are strict guidelines for the representation of disabled people in the media. In Ontario, there are stringent regulations about the way television can portray disabled people. These say that disabled people should be part of the main-stream of programming and advertising, and not just used when a disabled character is required. There are always problems associated with the regulation of newspapers, as opposed to other media, due, perhaps, to the historical battles for freedom of expression which surrounded them when they and books were the only popular forms of communication. However, such considerations should not be allowed to stand in the way of examining the place of enforceable codes of practice and how those which exist for television could possibly be translated to newspapers. Such examination should be the more possible in that voluntary codes of conduct do exist. There is also the Press Complaints Commission, a Privacy Commissioner, and the continuing debate about whether, indeed, there should be statutory regulation of the press.

Some guidelines already exist. Those of the United Nations (UN, 1982), for example, suggest depicting people with a disability in the ordinary settings of work, home or at leisure; and that presenting stereotypes such as dependent, pitiful, saintly, asexual, dangerous or uniquely endowed with a special skill due to the disability should be avoided. The guidelines refer to presenting achievements and difficulties of the person with a disability in ways that do not overemphasise, exaggerate or 'emotionalise' the situation. Journalists are asked to consider carefully the words used to describe or characterise the disabled person and avoid demeaning terms such as 'mental defectives', 'high mod', 'subnormal', 'spastic', 'mongol' and 'holy innocent' (an unlikely media word, one would have thought). The disabled person should also be included as part of the general population in media presentations rather than in isolation or with other disabled people. He or she should be portrayed in the same 'multi-dimensional' way as others, and the curiosity and occasional awkwardness of the person who is not disabled should be acknowledged, and, where possible, positive examples should be provided of where curiosity is satisfied and awkwardness lessened (McCormack, 1991). The American National Easter Seal Society has even gone so far as adding to guidelines, broadly similar to those of the UN, a glossary of terminology and a detailed guidance on interviewing etiquette (National Easter Seal Society, no date).

There are alternative ways, other than by statutory enforcement, in which guidelines can be used and change implemented. Realistically, these are more realisable, certainly in the short- to medium-term. At a very basic level, all magazines and newspapers have style books, which list not only the publication's spelling and other conventions (for example, 'z' or 's' preferences, hyphenating, capitalising) but also terminology. *The Times* guide (Jenkins, 1992), for example, advises against 'gay' favouring 'homosexual' and has sections on the correct use of gender pronouns, and of 'girl', 'lady' and 'Ms'. It has no reference to 'handicap', or 'learning difficulties' but under 'disabled' states: 'beware of offensive metaphors. Also avoid the new and often patronising American euphemisms, such as "disadvantaged" and "physically challenged". But common usage changes here, so be sensitive.' The reader is then referred to 'medical' terms, where he or she finds the admonition: 'never use medical nomenclature metaphorically, as in geriatric, paralytic, schizophrenic, spastic.' The insertion of guidance about terminology in style books, as well as how people with learning difficulties should be written about, would be a step in the right direction.

Disabled people have themselves mapped out some changes they would like to see (Barnes, 1991). These include more disabled people working in, and being involved with, the media, with active policies to recruit or train them. At the moment, those few disabled people who are employed (largely in television and radio) often work on programmes for disabled people or about disability. However, while such employment policies would be helpful, journalists' training courses and media studies courses should put disability awareness on their curricula, too. The shortcoming of this approach however, is that journalists can enter their profession without having been on either type of course, and many do.

Another suggestion by disability groups on the subject of protecting privacy is one which would provoke the same objections that other proposals for statutory regulations have encountered. This is that representatives of disabled people should meet with representatives of the print, broadcasting and advertising industries to draw up 'an overriding policy framework or statement'. Existing bodies like the Press Complaints Commission, the Broadcasting Standards Commission and the Advertising Standards Authority would then monitor the effect of such a policy and have the power to impose sanctions on those who oppose 'agreed policy'. Leaving aside the media's almost instinctive objection to anything which smacks of sanctions, there is also the problem of who would consent to the 'agreed policy' in an industry like newspapers, which, like broadcasting, has constituent parts which have a habit of going their own way.

The answer to tackling media representation of people with learning difficulties is not an easy one. A mixture of exhortation, closer working with the media, more disabled people active in the mainstream media, changes in journalists' training, and more strictly enforced codes of practice along Canadian lines would go far. However, if the press reflects society, it will not change fundamentally until social attitudes toward people with learning difficulties and other disabled people change. Disabled people face disrimination in their everyday lives – in jobs, access, education, transport and leisure activities. If a comprehensive Civil Rights Bill became law, it would not only outlaw discrimination but express society's valuing of disabled people as fellow citizens. Newspapers, as a mirror of their times, would reflect that.

References

Barnes, C. (1991). *Disabled People in Britain and Discrimination. A Case for Anti-Discrimination Legislation*, Hurst and Company, London.

Biklen, D. and Bogdan, R. (1977). Media portrayal of disabled people: A study in stereotypes. In *Inter-Racial Children's Book Bulletin*, 8, 6 and 7.

Cohen, S. and Young, J. (1981). *The Manufacture of News: Deviancy, Social Problems and the Mass Media*. Sage, London.

Collins, J. (1993). *The Resettlement Game*. Values into Action, London.

Davies, P. (1987). Hounded by the press pack. *The Health Service Journal*, 23 April

Dowson, S. (1991). Promoting positive images of people with learning difficulties: problems and strategies. In *Social Work, The Media and Public Relations* (eds B. Franklin and N. Parton). Routledge, London.

Glasgow University Media Group (no date). *Media Representation and Mental Illness: Report for Health Education Board for Scotland*, Health Education Board for Scotland, Edinburgh.

Hevey, D. (1992). *The Creatures That Time Forgot. Photography and Disability Imagery*. Routledge, London.

Jenkins, S. (ed) (1992). *The Times Guide to English Style and Usage*. Times Books, London.

Keller, C., Hallahan, D.P., McShane, E.A., Crowley, E.P. and Blandford, B.J. (1990). The coverage of persons with disabilities in American newspapers. *The Journal of Special Education*, 24, 3.

McConkey, R. and McCormack, B. (1983). *Breaking Barriers. Educating People about Disability*. Souvenir Press, London.

McCormack, B. (1991). I don't think we've been introduced. *Frontline*, Winter.

McGill, P. and Cummings, R. (1990). An analysis of the representation of people with mental handicaps in a British newspaper. *Mental Handicap Research*, 3(1).

Morris, J. (1991). *Pride Against Prejudice. Transforming Attitudes to Disability*. Women's Press, London.

National Easter Seal Society (undated). *Portraying People with Learning Difficulties in the Media*. National Easter Seal Society, Chicago, Illinois.

Ryan, J. and Thomas, F. (1988). *The Politics of Mental Handicap* (revised edn). Free Association Books, London.

Scott-Parker, S. (1989). *They Are Not In The Brief*. King's Fund, London.

Smith, S. and Jordan, A. (1991). *What the Papers Say and Don't Say about Disability*. Spastics Society, London.

Troyna, B. (1981). *Public Awareness and the Media: A Study of Reporting on Race*, Community Relations Commission, London.

United Nations (1982). *Improving Communications about People with Disabilities*. United Nations, New York.

Wertheimer, A. (1988a). *According to the Papers: Press Reporting on People with Learning Difficulties*. Campaign for People with Mental Handicaps (now Values into Action), London.

Wertheimer, A. (1988b). *Images by Appointment. A Review of Advertising for Staff in Services for People with Learning Difficulties*. Campaign for People with Mental Handicaps (now Values into Action), London.

Wolfensberger, W. (1972). *The Principle of Normalization in Human Services*. National Institute on Mental Retardation, Toronto.

Yoshida, R.K., Wasilewski, L. and Friedman, D.L. (1990). Recent newspaper coverage about persons with disabilities. *Exceptional Children*, **56**, 5.

Part Four

Changing Strategies

Chapter 25

Building better communities: People with disabilities and their allies. Lessons from the USA

John O'Brien and Connie Lyle O'Brien

> The basis of people's lives with one another is twofold, and it is one – the wish of each person to be confirmed as what each person is, even as what that person can become; and the innate capacity in each person to confirm others in this way. That this capacity lies so immeasurably fallow constitutes the real weakness and questionableness of the human race; actual humanity exists only where this capacity unfolds. (Martin Buber, quoted in Friedman, 1960).

Three kinds of change, occuring at different scales, shape the opportunities for people with disabilities to participate in unfolding the capacity for mutual confirmation which Buber identifies at the foundation of humanity. Declarations of social policy, such as the Canadian Constitution's Charter of Rights and Freedoms and the Americans With Disabilities Act, reflect a new awareness of the rights (and political influence) of people with disabilities and their families by forbidding discrimination on the basis of disability. Services to people with substantial disabilities gradually shift away from congregating them together in large numbers in one place. So small but growing and visible numbers of people with disabilities live in ordinary housing, have support for ordinary employment, and attend ordinary schools. At the smallest scale are the efforts that concern this chapter. This kind of change involved people learning together how to build community across the imposed social barriers that separate people with substantial disabilities from other people.

Each of these changes serves as a platform for further change by revealing how much more must be done before people with disabilities take their rightful place as citizens. Even where they are in force, declarations of rights serve as much to expose contradictions with other policies, and conflicts with other political interests, as they do to stimulate habitual regard for the dignity of people with disabilities. The successes of people with disabilities in living, working, and learning in ordinary places increase dissatisfaction at the contrast between their situation and the far less satisfactory conditions still imposed on many people who remain segregated and controlled by the service programmes they rely on. These successes also yield disappointment because establishing people in typical settings seldom proves sufficient to support full and valued lives. More and more people who have worked hard for service reform nod a bit sadly when someone observes that people with disabilities are in communities without yet belonging to communities. Work to build community remains very small in scope, with many more people debating it than working to learn how to do it.

This chapter offers a perspective on efforts to build community. In general terms, we can define community building as the intentional creation of relationships and social structures, that extend the possibilities for shared identity and common action among people, outside usual patterns of economic and administrative interaction. We are especially interested when this work involves people with disabilities.

In particular, this chapter presents some of what we have learned by listening to the stories of people who have made important changes in their lives by working together. Our method for learning is simple: we locate people with disabilities who have been involved in an important change, ask involved people to tell us their stories of how the change happened, invite their reflections on what was most important in making the change, look for common images and themes across stories of change, reread the stories through different theoretical lenses, and, finally, retell the story and ask the original story tellers to correct or extend our account of the changes they have made. Clearly this method does not produce singular techniques or manuals of procedure for community building. Instead, it offers multiple ways to conceive action. (For complementary, but different, reading of the lessons in some of these same stories see Mount, 1991; O'Brien and Lyle-O'Brien, 1992; 1993).

The changes from which we have learned include establishing adequate support for family life; moving from an institution, medical hospital, nursing home, or group residence into one's own home; moving from one's family's home to a home of one's own; getting a job in an ordinary community workplace; and being in primary, secondary, or further education (from vocational and technical schools to community colleges to universities and adult education) as a member of ordinary classes. Because all of the people we learned from have disabilities, these changes have each required negotiating entry into new settings and new roles, usually as the first person with a disability to do so; arranging adequate systems of personal assistance; acquiring appropriate technical aids and devices; and finding adequate funding.

These important personal changes have additional significance because none of them resulted from the routine operation of welfare services available to the people involved. While people who work in services often play an important role in these stories of change, their contributions lie well outside their job descriptions and often challenge their employer's expectations. While money allocated for services usually contributes to making or sustaining the change, people have always had to work to change the established use of these funds, and sometimes have had to create new agencies, or even new policies and laws to make the change they seek.

Of course, these are not the only possible stories of community building. Some agencies, and a few authorities responsible for services, have invested in learning how to routinely offer assistance in ways that build community. But the changes we want to learn from here allocate resources elsewhere, around and with a particular person, and among people who discover new commitments and new ways to act through their shared effort. This context reshapes the usual functions and processes of services in ways which yield creative responses to common problems and important lessons for service reformers.

A brief sketch of a story of positive change provides a basis for a description of five types of person to person commitments, which people involved in community building have found useful in understanding and extending their efforts.

'There's a delicacy about her'

The phrase, 'There's a delicacy about her', captures an aspect of Lisa which was not apparent to the people who lived and worked with her during the years that she moved from one residential facility to another and another and another. In those settings, her inabilities, primarily her inability to use words, and her challenging behaviours defined her person and her life. She was moved from place to place as one agency after another concluded that she was too difficult to serve. Through these hard years, Lisa's mother, Gemma, remained a fierce advocate for appropriate services, providing Lisa with a firm anchor in a turbulent and threatening world. (This sketch of Lisa's story is drawn from Joyce, 1993.)

As Lisa faced yet another transfer to the behavioural ward of an institution, a setting which had proven dangerous to Lisa in the past, Gemma and Lisa found a committed assistant in John, an official in the regional bureaucracy that oversees services to people with disabilities. John decided that he wanted to respond to the political pressure about Lisa by developing individualised services for her. With Gemma's consent, John assigned Marilyn to design and develop services for Lisa. In the ensuing eight years Marilyn has proven herself as one of Lisa's strongest allies, though her job and family circumstances have changed several times.

Marilyn approached Lisa and Gemma with the image of a social structure in mind, an image transmitted from the experience of Judith Snow and her circle of friends as they developed individual supports for Judith (Pearpoint, 1990). She says: 'Once I would have asked, "*What* can I bring to Lisa?" But, instead, I asked, "*Who* can I bring to Lisa." . . . I introduced the idea to Gemma by saying that I thought we needed more people . . .'

Gemma consented, but she remembers: '[Marilyn] described a circle where Lisa would have people around her who'd care. I didn't think it would ever happen. I thought she was asking too much of herself and others. At first I was rather sceptical; I didn't think people would come through with their commitments. I didn't believe a support circle could happen – but it has!'

The support circle hasn't just happened. It developed initially from Marilyn's invitations to people she knew. Then, as action with and around Lisa grew, some people brought in others, like Elinore (the first person Marilyn invited) who involved her husband, Charlie, and then her daughter Lynne, who later became a key paid assistant to Lisa. As Marilyn continued to act outside Gemma's expectations of a paid worker, the circle grew stronger. Gemma says: '. . . I began to trust Marilyn because I saw her as a leader – she's determined and what she sets out to do she does. It's amazing to me that she brought in her friends' (Joyce, 1993).

Since its beginning, the circle has offered Lisa's brothers, Michael and Antosh, a specific focus for their desire to anchor their sister's future. The circle's early work was difficult, especially because no service providers were willing to offer individualised supports, even though Lisa had access to substantial amounts of funding. Michael says: 'The meetings were long, and there were lots of frustrations . . . A lot of the professionals were willing to listen and give advice, but few were willing to get their hands dirty or commit fully.' Antosh identifies the continuing concern of those closest to Lisa: 'I was afraid the circle would break down, that it would be too much of a burden.'

Dealing over time with the complexities of developing and maintaining good assistance for Lisa, as well as the challenge of understanding and clarifying Lisa's interests and capacities and finding opportunities for her, has been challenging. So, the circle's growth has not been smooth nor has its membership been stable. When an agency agreed to organise services for Lisa, many circle members assumed that the problem was solved and became less active. At one point, only three people were regularly involved.

However, as continuing problems clarified the fact that individualised services for Lisa posed too big a challenge to the culture of the only existing agency willing to serve her, the circle regenerated and enlarged. Members of Lisa's circle joined with several families whose dreams and desires outstripped the service system's capacity. They formed an association which has created a service agency called New Frontiers, whose job is to assist a small number of people with disabilities as they build their local community.

After eight years, 28 people identify themselves as members of Lisa's circle. Some were introduced to Lisa by other circle members. Some initially met Lisa when they were hired to work for her as assistants (though many of Lisa's assistants have not identified themselves as members of the circle). Some have come to her through the shared work of creating New Frontiers.

Circle members do much more than have planning meetings, and some members rarely attend the meetings that do occur. But each members identifies her or himself with Lisa and with the circle, each shares some mutually interesting activities with Lisa, and all have shown their willingness to act together to protect Lisa and promote a positive future for her. Lisa benefits from the many different ways in which people have come to know her, even though these differences have sometimes caused conflicts among circle members.

The circle benefits each of its members, though it holds Lisa at its centre. The circle demonstrates social concern to reshape its member's community; it is not an expression of pity for disability. All members can identify benefits from membership, including discovering new skills, making friends, overcoming stereotypes, joining in social activities, gaining confidence in ability to problem solve, finding opportunities to act vigorously on what seems right, finding support in personal hard times, and creating confirmation of hope that people can work together to make a real difference.

With the support of the circle and the assistance of New Frontiers, Lisa's life in her home is gradually becoming more stable overall, though some of her behavioural challenges persist, and she remains unable to use words to communicate. Lisa explores the places and activities available in her city. She regularly volunteers her time to meals on wheels and to a local community centre. She particularly enjoys many of the meals and parties that are part of the life of the circle. Through the shared work that builds and sustains the circle, she and her mother have gained many allies concerned for her future. One of them, Jennifer, says: 'It's one thing to think about how far Lisa has come – I think more about where Lisa can go.' (Joyce, 1993).

Herb, a psychologist who has visited Lisa and encouraged her circle, says: '. . . whenever I have been to Lisa's home or talked to the people who are in her circle, I have been struck by how much they love her and one another. Not in the everything-is-beautiful kind of way that has a hard time with conflict, but in the enduring, patient, and respectful way we all need, to get to the next and better version of ourselves.'

Five commitments that build community

As we have come to understand it, community building happens when people step outside the roles prescribed by the formal and informal administrative structures and assumptions that typically organise life for people with disabilities. Distinctions between staff and clients and family members and ordinary citizens dissolve as the familiar patterns of interaction that maintain them shift, and people discover new possibilities for shared action. This dissolution can be confusing and threatening, especially when people continue to fill administratively prescribed roles.

This confusion shows up in many ways, for example in debates about whether paid staff can be friends and advocates for people with disabilities. Many who believe they can seem to think that staff can presume that their clients will see them as friends and advocates, despite fundamental inequalities in power, and professional norms that dictate objectivity and detachment. Some, who have glimpsed the bureaucratic machinery beneath the mask of professionalised caring assert that paid people cannot be friends. Neither those who say yes nor those who say no seem to have adequate terms to describe the relationships that have developed between Lisa and Gemma and some paid staff people. Finding new terms outside the usual administrative vocabulary allows people to discuss some of the distinctions that emerge when people work together to make change. New words offer one way to help people make sense of this different way of acting.

Community building is an intentional move into a new space; if Marilyn had chosen to focus on what services to give Lisa rather than on who to bring into her life, the support circle would not exist. Far more an improvisation in response to changing circumstances than a carefully choreographed routine, community building needs ways of identifying the kinds of actions that can make positive differences to people's shared future. Invitation lies at the heart of community building and shapes the responses people offer. Searching for ways to communicate the different kinds of contributions that people can make to one another offers those who make invitations a vocabulary for considering their options.

As we have considered the differences between stories, like Lisa's, that include positive changes and stories that do not, as yet, include much change, we have labelled five different person-to-person commitments, which are identified on the figure below. In stories of change, we can usually identify people enacting these different commitments. In stories where no change has occurred, the absence of people making one or more of these commitments is notable. This does not mean that no change can happen without each commitment, only that significant change will require even more effort in the absence of one or more of them. When we describe these commitments to people who appear to display them, the people involved usually accept the description as more or less accurate for them, though they sometimes say that the words we have chosen seem a bit strange. So these descriptions have heuristic rather than predictive or technical value.

The notion of commitment involves accepting a particular kind of responsibility by acting on it. One person can share more than one commitment with a person with a substantial disability. Commitment

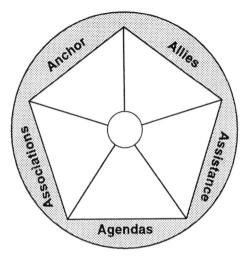

Fig. 25.1 Some person-to-person commitments

implies freedom; the roles assigned to people by administrative structures do not contain, nor can they compel, any of these commitments. Someone may be both a paid staff person and an ally, as Marilyn has been for Lisa. But John, as Marilyn's boss, cannot assign her to be Lisa's ally, though John could, as a person Marilyn respects because of his willingness to take personal risks on Lisa's behalf, invite and encourage her to consider alliance. Commitments are not disability specific; they seem necessary in any effort to build community. People with disabilities can, of course, undertake any of the commitments, just as people without disabilities can. These commitments are a matter of choice and desire, not of status.

People who commit to anchor another person love that person, are fundamental to them and their commitment is long-lasting. They share their life with the person and act as a source of continuity through the ups and downs of life; they have custody of important memories. They stand with the person in difficult times. They act vigorously to protect the person from harm. They seek ways to reconcile with the person when the person has offended them or when they have fallen out with the person. They want to continually grow in knowledge of the person, and especially of the person's gifts and capacities, even though this may be difficult when it challenges habitual patterns of expectation. They work to identify and create opportunities for the person. The other person figures in their decisions about their lives; when facing an important choice they will not need to be reminded of their importance to the person. They actively assist the person to expand relationships with others who may come to care.

People's family members may be anchors, as Gemma is for Lisa. But some family members can be overwhelmed by their own circumstances or by fear or by stereotyped thinking and be unable to anchor their son or daughter or brother or sister or spouse in making the kind of change that builds community. Unrelated people (including paid staff) can find themselves loving a person with a disability in this way, though this can be confusing and difficult for others to understand and can create significant conflicts for the staff person who is an anchor.

People who commit themselves to be allies share their time and resources for particular tasks with the person to make a jointly meaningful change. They offer practical help, assist with scheming and problem solving, lend experience and skills, and offer useful information. They make contacts for one another and bring others into the alliance. They usually enjoy the person's company in some mutual interest, and they often like to share food and drink. Because allies know the person in distinct ways, they come to have important knowledge of the person's interests and capacities. On the basis of this information, and their knowledge of community opportunities, they can join the person and the person's anchors to define a future worth working towards. Allies may be linked more closely to the person than they are to one another. If a shared project calls on them to work together, allies may have to deal with their differences with one another and be willing to negotiate conflicts instead of just walking away.

A person's allies may choose to consciously form a circle, as Lisa's have, or their relationship may be more like separate spokes related to the person, with no rim linking them together. Because many people with disabilities have been isolated and separated by prejudiced treatment, it may be necessary to purposely invite people to consider forming alliances with them around an important change, as Marilyn did when she formed a circle around developing individualised supports for Lisa.

Assistance provides the help a person requires to deal with the effects of disability so that they contribute their gifts to the change effort. Service managers offer assistance, as John did for Lisa, when they allocate funds with the flexibility to allow involved people to design and redesign a system of everyday personal assistance. Personal assistants provide necessary help with daily activities, from eating and dressing and housework to working and participating in community activities. Professional assistants offer specialised help to deal with difficulties in movement or communication, or learning, or problem solving, or dealing with problematic behaviours or feelings.

The particular commitment of assistance is to offer necessary help, in a respectful, creative, and flexible way, without taking over the person's life. The art is to assist without intruding between the person and other people or activities the person wants to be involved with. The gift of assistance is to resonate with and thus to amplify the person's bodily and mental contributions to the change effort.

Assistants can, of course, become deeply involved with the people they help: many of Lisa's allies have worked for her. But the commitment to the paradox of assisting without intruding or controlling remains a unique contribution, and it is important that assistants be clear when it is time for them to make it (Adler, 1993).

Some people with disabilities rely primarily on family members for the help they need, particularly their mothers and sisters. When publicly funded assistance fails to provide alternatives to care by family members, the person's relationship with caregivers can become deeply constraining for them all. When necessary assistance is only available in settings that segregate and control people, opportunities to make the kind of changes that build community are very limited.

Associations are the social structures groups of people create to further their interests. They may be structured formally or informally. They may be focussed on social change or on their members' protection or enjoyment or personal development or other political objectives. They may be organised around the particular interests of people with disabilities, as New Frontiers is, or they may be organised around other community purposes, as is the community centre where Lisa volunteers. People with disabilities have typically been excluded from the benefits and responsibilities of association membership, so a great deal of untapped energy can become available if a person's allies can facilitate their membership in associations that can share and shape the person's interests (Kretzmann and McKnight, 1993).

Agendas organise political action to ensure just and effective public policies and their proper implementation. People with disabilities and their families and allies have often joined political coalitions to work for such changes as personal assistance services and family support services under the control of users or people close to them; inclusive schooling; necessary assistance for individual employment; safe, accessible, and affordable housing; safe, convenient, and accessible transportation; access to adaptive technology and devices; and adequate cash income without stigma. The coalitions and actions that form around agendas multiply the influence of people and their circles.

People who share these five commitments and nurture them over time are likely to create new ways to build and be a community. Lisa and the support circle around her work slowly and modestly to increase the capacity of people in her city to deal creatively with diversity, to decide justly when prejudice threatens participation in the benefits and responsibilities of citizenship, and to make good use of the public funds allocated to the service of people with disabilities. Lisa and her allies have contributed direction and hard work to the creation of an innovative agency to assist them in defining and making their contribution to common life. They have claimed a new space for shared action, and thereby expanded possibilities for themselves and for other people with substantial disabilities.

Importance of community building

Community building matters significantly to people who claim the freedom to define and pursue a desirable future in a society whose economic sector threatens to colonise the whole of life. Community building matters particularly to people with disabilities because the modern economy typically assigns them either to be objects of professional work or to be on waiting lists to demonstrate the need for such work. Because this work is bureaucratically organised, people with disabilities are vulnerable to domination by state administrative mechanisms when they receive the services politically intended to relieve their kin from the unpaid work of caring for them.

When people with disabilities and their friends work together to build community, they can change the culture so that marginalised people can join people who are insiders to destroy delusions about disability and uncover shared meaning through joint projects. Within this new culture and revelation, people whose lives may be dominated by professional definitions of disability can find some relief, and even occasional liberation, from the burdens of full-time clienthood. Here, people can unfold the human capacity for confirmation of one another as each is, and as each can become.

Snow (1990), whose emancipation from a chronic care facility occurred through her shared life and work with a circle of support, reflected on the contribution outsiders can make to community building simply from the experience of being an outsider:

> The gift of surviving and growing through change belongs to the outcast . . . Living on the edge of chaos changes the people who survive it. You become very aware of the value of things ordinary citizens take for granted; things like having your opinion listened to, having a chance to make a mistake, to be forgiven and to have a chance to try again; things like having friends and family who celebrate holidays with you and who will tell their friends that you are looking for a job. Living on the margin either burns you out and kills you, or it turns you into a dreamer, someone who really knows what sort of change will help and who can just about taste it; someone who is prepared to do anything to bring about change. If these dreamers are liberated, if they are brought back into the arms of society, they become the architects of the new community; a community that has a new capacity to support everyone's needs and interactions. But how can this really be, especially since these dreamers still have the characteristics that marked them as outcasts in the first place? They will still lack good judgment, or find it hard to learn to read, or be disabled. Solving this problem is critical, for otherwise the outcasts and the ordinaries are very good at maintaining an invisible wall between their two worlds.

She goes on to say that this invisible wall can only be breached by long-term willingness to build new kinds of relationships between those who are reaching out and those who are reaching in. In the five commitments, we have tried to describe the terms of those new relationships.

Tensions in community building

A sort of discomfort surrounds these new relationships and some of the social structures that invite and support them. The very term 'community building' reflects the tensions that give rise to this discomfort and to some frank disagreements. For some people, community does not seem to be something that can be built: community is spontaneous, or it is not. To speak of building community violates what can, and should, only develop naturally and opens the door to a kind of clumsy, intrusive, and embarrassing social engineering, likely to be packaged in warm and fuzzy psycho-babble. For others, community is not worth building because it represents a failed structure for human development, incapable of dealing constructively with human diversity or addressing injustice. To speak of building community distracts from the necessity of living as successful individuals in a cosmopolitan and impersonal society. For still others, whether it is desirable or undesirable, the very possibility of community is gone. In their view, the turbulent forces that fragment our times replace community with cleverly marketed counterfeits, like community care, which masks impersonal rationing by joining two words with high appeal, emptying them of content, and filling the hollowed-out space with bureaucratic professional activity. To speak of building community is to be guilty of a kind of naive and dangerous flashback to the 1960s. It was in the latter period when a belief in the perfectability of people through social engineering sowed seeds which later led to effects to reverse disability.

Awareness of each of these disagreements and discomforts clarifies the work of community building. The economic and administrative forces that shape so much of modern life make it necessary to undertake conscious efforts to claim common spaces and to build within them. And conscious efforts can be and feel halting, tentative, uncertain, and uncomfortable. Recognising and honouring human diversity and enriching joint action with differing gifts presents so large a challenge that no one who sets out to build community will get far before encountering its threats and frustrations. Efforts to build community that overcome the invisible walls between those outside the social mainstream and 'ordinaries' (as Snow [1990] calls ordinary people) must be modest in scale and in expectation.

This kind of building is nothing like the massive imposition of individual will on masses of people through architectural technology which Rand characterises in *The Fountainhead*. It is much more like the kind of building celebrated by Rudofsky (1964) in *Architecture without Architects*. As Rudofsky beautifully illustrates, this kind of building is vernacular rather than formal; commonly practiced by inhabitants rather than sketched and controlled by professional experts who will not live within the results; rooted in a particular landscape rather than imposed upon it; purposely created for human comfort rather than scaled for mass consumption; and built in stages as use and resources expand rather than master planned and financed at high cost. He notes two inspiring qualities of successful vernacular builders: they work to make oases of public spaces, and, 'they do not hesitate to seek out the most complicated configurations in the landscape [often choosing] veritable eyries for their building sites . . .'

References

Adler, D. (1993). Perspectives of a support worker. In *Housing, Support, and Community: Choices and Strategies for Adults with Disabilities* (eds J. Racino, P. Walker, S. O'Connor and S. Taylor). Paul H. Brookes, Baltimore.

Friedman, M.S. (1960). *Martin Buber: The Life of Dialogue.* Harper Torchbooks, New York.

Joyce, S. (ed.) (1993). *Collages: Sketches of a Support Circle.* Realizations, Ontario.

Kretzmann, J. and McKnight, J. (1993). *Building Community from the Inside Out: A Path Toward Finding and Mobilising a Community's Assets.* Center for Urban Affairs and Policy Research, Northwestern University, Evanston, Illinois.

Mount, B. (1991). *Dare to Dream: An Analysis of the Conditions Leading to Personal Change for People with Disabilities.* Communitas Publications, Manchester, Connecticut.

O'Brien, J. and Lyle-O'Brien, C. (1992). Members of each other: perspectives on social support for people with severe disabilities. In *Natural Supports in Schools, at Work, and in the Community for People with Severe Disabilities* (ed. J. Nisbet). Paul H. Brookes, Baltimore.

O'Brien, J. and Lyle-O'Brien, C. (1993). Unlikely alliances: friendships and people with developmental disabilities. In *Friendships and Community Connections Between People With and Without Developmental Disabilities* (ed. A. Amado). Paul H. Brookes, Baltimore.

Pearpoint, J. (1990). *From Behind the Piano: The Building of Judith Snow's Unique Circle of Friends.* Inclusion Press, Toronto, Ontario.

Rand, A. (1952). *The Fountainhead.* NAL Dutton, New York.

Rudofsky, B. (1964). *Architecture without Architects: A short introduction to Non-pedigreed Architecture.* Doubleday, Garden City, New York.

Snow, J. (1990). Bradwin Address to the 89th Annual Meeting of Frontier College. Reprinted in Pearpoint, J. *From Behind the Piano: The Building of Judith Snow's Unique Circle of Friends.* Inclusion Press, Toronto.

Chapter 26
Count us in: Lessons from Canada on strategies for social change

Marcia Rioux and Diane Richler

Recent shifts in thinking about disability in general, and in learning difficulties in particular, have led to important changes in the struggle to improve the lives of disadvantaged people, and changes in where the 'deficit' is seen to be. These shifts also affect the definition of the goals sought by people in the disability movement. In Canada, the activities of the Canadian Association for Community Living have been profoundly influenced by changing perceptions of the source of problems facing persons who have a learning difficulty and their families.

Deficit as an individual responsibility

Until very recently – and the notion persists in some circles – the 'problem' of disability was perceived to reside in the individual. It was the individual who was out of step with the world. Once labelled with a learning difficulty, one did not fit into the labour market, one did not fit into the school system, one did not fit into recreation programmes, one did not fit generally into the community. The belief was that the individual had somehow to be changed to conform with the social, political and legal structures already in place. And, consequently, the professional community and service providers in the field tended to focus on ways to 'fix' the individual to reduce the deficit.

At first, the focus on 'fixing' the problem manifested itself as a strategy of prevention. In some cases, this even translated into 'preventing' life; whether through sterilisation or through withholding life supports or surgical procedures. Although these methods still occur, more recently prevention has meant therapy or habilitation to make the individual fit into an existing environment and social structure created to meet the needs of those without a disability.

Initially, intellectual disability was viewed as a medical problem. Specialists applied the medical model and sought medical solutions for what was accepted as an organic 'disease'. Doctors treated and diagnosed those with learning difficulties as patients and the latter assumed the role of 'invalids'. Much of the current literature still reflects this model with its emphasis on classification systems, diagnostic systems, criteria for evaluating disabilities, drugs administered and so on.

Over time, the medical model shifted to one of therapy. The individual was still seen as the locus of the problem, but the focus was not so much organic as therapeutic and educational. Specialists concentrated on teaching those in need the skills to adjust to their social milieu. In an overzealousness that surprises even the therapeutic community, every activity of people with learning difficulties became a form of therapy. Learning how to cook has become cooking therapy, caring for plants is horticultural therapy, having a pet is pet therapy and learning how to make friends has become social network therapy. The clinical nature of the medical model was carried over into the therapeutic model for addressing the needs of people with a learning difficulty.

Deficit as a service responsibility

With this shift to a therapeutic model came a focus on effective service design and delivery. Social workers, therapists and both government and not-for-profit organisations who provided services increasingly came to believe that the solution to the 'problem' of learning difficulties was to ensure good services to those with a learning difficulty – a need arising from services which did not properly support the targeted group of individuals – a deficit in services. This was to be rectified by close monitoring of services: Was the service actually benefiting the individual? Did the service reflect appropriate values? Did the service help or rehabilitate the individual? Did the service enable the individual to grow and learn? Did the service provide more than the basic needs of food and shelter? In other words, specialists placed a strong emphasis on services and delivery mechanisms rather than analysing the services in a larger social context. If the services were good enough, the 'problems' would be solved. In addition, services were evaluated by those who designed and delivered them rather than by service users.

We have now recognised that there are alternative ways to solve the 'problem' and evaluate how well we are doing – to decide where the deficit lies.

Deficit as a system responsibility

In Canada, recent events have shaped the way in which the issues and treatment of people with a learning difficulty are now being addressed. Over the past ten years, provincial and federal human rights laws have been amended to include individuals with mental and physical disabilities. The Canadian Charter of Rights and Freedoms, introduced in 1982, extends rights to, among other underprivileged groups, those with a learning difficulty. It goes so far as to recognise that affirmative action is necessary to redress discrimination against any Canadian. This has had, and continues to have, an important impact on people with a learning difficulty and on the discussions concerning their rights and citizenship as well as the place and structure of social services. It now seems outmoded, both legally and socially, to view people with a learning difficulty as social units in need of repair or rehabilitation before elevating them to the status of 'real' persons or citizens. Fitting in with the social structure has become much less important than changing the system to fit the individual. The locus of the problem— that is, the definition of the deficit and who is responsible for it—has shifted from the individual to the system. This has had repercussions on generic and specialist services and on the work of advocates, governments, families and individuals with a learning difficulty.

Promoting the social well-being of people with disabilities means the development of an overall disability framework. This involves interventions that seek to enable people with disabilities to live in ways that are personally satisfying and socially useful. People's self-determination, equality and participation as citizens are the goals sought by such policy. This is in contrast to many present policies which address disability through isolated interventions, usually treatments that include rehabilitation and training. These policies are made available or deemed desirable because it is believed they have the capacity to eliminate disability and social handicap.

The new concept of a disability framework is premised on the need to reorient or shift thinking about disability. It is not enough simply to add on new measures to deal with disability. This will neither meet the need that persists nor address the question of people's well-being. To address well-being we have to begin by recognising the connection between collective goals and what a society 'requires of, makes possible for, and even grants as a matter of right to its individual citizens' (Roeher Institute, 1993). Social policy, health policy and economic policy need to address explicitly how individuals will be involved in decision making and self-determination, that is, how they will achieve well-being. A new context for political debate about policy responsive to disability is critical. The alternative is to continue to tinker with the services and policies in place, with the overall impact of having a few more individuals, probably those with more socially acceptable (less disabling) disabilities participating but with no real recognition that society genuinely includes people with disabilities. In other words, tinkering will do little to change the basic message being conveyed about persons with disabilities: that they are peripheral members of the community who can participate when it is convenient or practical to fit them in. Although it may be helpful in the short run to have 'disability' services and policies, in the long run such policies are likely to further segregate and isolate people within a separate but unequal model. Instead, we need a policy framework progressive enough to recognise that those with disabilities are part of the population that any policy must be designed to meet.

In looking broadly at disability, we begin with the problem that most services and policies did not have the issues presented by disability in mind when they were conceived. Historically, they began from assumptions that people with disabilities would not be a part of the mainstream of society. Consequently, the structures established such as the education system, labour force, economic structure and so on, were not designed to deal with a population which included those with disabilities. This, as we are aware, has also been true for other disadvantaged groups. Assumptions about the role women would play in society have also made it very difficult to establish their place within the traditional structures. Now that people with disabilities are lobbying for a place within the mainstream institutions and structure of society, it is very difficult to accommodate them. There has been no major restructuring of the system which enables persons who have a disability to be a part of it.

Instead, there is a set of parallel services initially set up as charity but now, in fact, paid for out of the public budget. Therefore, we find segregated classes or schools paid for through the state school system, special transport in many cases operated by the municipal transportation systems and sheltered workshops or sheltered work paid for out of the social assistance and vocational rehabilitation budget and operated by not-for-profit organisations. With minor adaptations made so that some persons with disabilities can fit in, the existing social and economic structures are defended as acceptable.

Those with disabilities who are fortunate enough to be able to qualify for non-segregated services, and who have few needs beyond those of non-disabled people, may well be able to use generic resources to fit in. However, in most cases, because society and its mainstream services were designed without taking into account the needs of this group, it is particularly challenging for them to make it in that world.

Establishing parallel or add-on systems of transportation, education, employment, housing or recreation suggests that we are framing the question inappropriately. Rather than asking, as we should, what is wrong with existing policies that do not fully include those with disabilities, we ask how we can ensure that disabled people can have access to existing services in recreation, housing, education and so on. In other words, we misplace the responsibility for the deficit and then assume that we can tinker with the existing structures to meet the needs of those with disabilities. But this always leaves the person with a disability in a defensive position. If the basic structure is not changed the person with a disability will always be marginal, will always be, in some way, a lesser citizen and, so to speak, pleading to be taken seriously by the rest of society.

We need a critical shift in our thinking about disability and in how we structure our public policies and programmes. At present, eligibility for, and entitlement to, social benefits are treated as social privileges to be distributed on a discretionary basis to a select target population that can establish personal 'merit', rather than as matters of individual social right guaranteed on the basis of clearly defined conditions, or as an ethical imperative binding the state and community to the individual in need. The needs of individuals with disabilities should, however, not be thought of as special needs, any more than the needs of those without disabilities might have been seen as special had those with disabilities designed the world.

If the needs of one group are seen as special, they become pitted against the needs and rights of the rest of the population. Then, inevitably, those who argue for 'special' rights and needs must argue in a way that is quite distinct from how the issue would be addressed if the right were assumed. The discussion very often turns around the distribution of finite resources and how far one can go in denying this 'special' groups these 'special' requirements. But if the assumption is instead that these needs and rights are not, in fact, special, then the discussion is about the best and most expedient way to change the systems so that they take disability, a rather unexceptional human occurrence, into account. It puts the individual with a disability in the same position as any other citizen who requires that governments set up public programmes or policies that, by definition, take his needs or disabilities into account. In this kind of framework, if the government chooses not to implement a service or policy, the impact will be the same on those with and without disabilities.

The emergence of this new policy framework has both shaped and been shaped by the Canadian Association for Community Living (CACL). The goals and objectives of the community living movement have changed considerably since the first local associations of the federation were formed in the late 1940s. It is only within the last several years that people have begun to refer to a 'community living' movement. The changes in name of the national organisation – from Canadian Association for Retarded Children to the Canadian Association for the Mentally Retarded to the Canadian Association for Community Living – mirror the changes in the association's vision and preoccupations. These, in turn, were influenced by public policy discussions of the times.

Parents of sons and daughters who had a learning difficulty organised local associations spontaneously across Canada simultaneous with similar developments in other parts of the world. Before the Second World War, the preoccupation of families had been primarily on the medical aspects of learning difficulty. It was considered a medical problem and doctors were called on to help families deal with its consequences. The emergence of rehabilitation to cope with injuries from the Second World War inspired the families of people whose disabilities were intellectual rather than physical to turn to a rehabilitation model and to seek services which would help to overcome the challenges posed by the impairment. This was a major shift. The focus of the medical model has been solely 'treating' the individual; now there should also be a commitment to developing services which would help individuals develop to their fullest potential.

The rehabilitation model was the inspiration for the formation of local associations. They were preoccupied with the development and improvement of services. The emergence of the principle of normalisation in the late 1960s and 1970s reinforced this preoccupation. While the vision of parents, professionals and the association shifted to one which sought lifestyles for individuals with a learning difficulty which would be more like those of their non-disabled peers, the energy of the associations was clearly focussed on increasing the number and variety of services and on improving their quality.

The 1980s witnessed a dramatic shift in thinking. The emergence of the movement of physically disabled people advocating on their own behalf, the proclamation of the Canadian Charter of Rights and Freedoms and its prohibition of discrimination on the basis of mental or physical disability and the inclusion of individuals who had been labelled 'mentally handicapped' within the national association (then the Canadian Association for the Mentally Retarded) all led to the development of a new framework for thinking about learning difficulty – the community living framework. The shift in conceptual models has had a major impact on the activities of the national association.

While the conceptual model was primarily a medical one, the focus of the association was largely on educating the medical profession to 'treat' individuals with a learning difficulty. When the model shifted to a rehabilitation one, the focus of the association was largely on services. Since the most recent name change of the association in 1985, there has been another dramatic shift. In order to achieve the goal of community living for all individuals who have been labelled as having a learning difficulty, the focus is now on changing communities in order that they can and do include people with disabilities as full and participating members. This has meant a shift in focus away from services primarily for people who have a learning difficulty to a preoccupation with how people, regardless of degree of disability, can be accommodated in the mainstream of their communities. For this to become reality, major social changes must take place in how communities function so that individuals with a learning difficulty are not excluded. Therefore, the association has had to undergo a shift from agent for change in the quality and quantity of services to agent for broad social change.

This dramatic shift of goal has had major repercussions on the activities of the CACL. Helping communities to be inclusive requires dramatic changes in existing policies, laws, public attitudes and practice (behaviour). In other words, the association must achieve major social change in order to accomplish its goal. The association has attempted to understand the process of social change and to co-ordinate its activities for maximum effectiveness in achieving its goals.

The first step towards implementing its new vision of an inclusive society was to articulate the vision in a clear plan and agenda. Known as *Community Living 2000*, the plan sets out specific objectives and provides a framework for the association's activities until the end of the millennium. The objectives of the plan (CACL, 1987) are that by the year 2000:

- All children will have a meaningful family life.
- All children will go to school together in neighbourhood schools and be educated in ordinary classes.
- Everyone leaving secondary school will have the opportunity for meaningful work.
- Sheltered workshops will close and the people leaving them will become employed.
- Individuals will be supported to make their own decisions about the use of public money being spent on their behalf.
- No one will live in an institution.
- Individuals will be supported by a natural network of family and friends.

The vision articulated in the *Community Living 2000* plan was the result of a broad consultation process. The task force that drafted the plan sought opinions from all segments of the community living movement and informed itself about the challenges as perceived by different groups and individuals including individuals who had themselves been labelled as having a learning difficulty, parents, lay people and professionals at all levels of the association. The vision was then translated into a series of concrete goals and objectives that could be easily understood. Once the plan was in place, the association then embarked on a systematic examination of the barriers to its achievement.

In this process, the association has used two major strategies. One has been to focus the research capability of the Roeher Institute on disability as a public policy issue. (The Roeher Institute is Canada's national institute for the study of public policy affecting persons with a learning difficulty and other disabilities. It is sponsored by CACL.) This has meant a shift of the research efforts of the institute away from studying services for people who have a learning difficulty to looking at systems which exist for the general population and the barriers which exclude people who have been labelled from these systems. For example, rather than looking at how to change a system of sheltered workshops to one that employs people in the community, the institute is examining the barriers that exist in the workplace that make it difficult for people who have a learning difficulty to be employed (Roeher Institute, 1992). The research findings published in *Income Insecurity* (Roeher Institute, 1988) detailed how being relegated to a life of poverty excludes most people with disabilities from full participation in their communities. *Poor Places* (Roeher Institute, 1990) documents how existing services, particularly residential ones, do the same.

The second major way that the association has been able to examine existing barriers is to stay in touch with its membership base and with people who have been labelled and their families. Hearing the stories of their day-to-day challenges is an important factor in ensuring that the association's vision and agenda are consistent with the hopes and aspirations of those most affected by its work.

Once the barriers have been identified, a plan must be developed to erode them and finally to break them down. One approach has been for the Roeher Institute to develop policy options that can be reviewed, endorsed and promoted both by CACL and other disability advocacy organisations and equality-seeking groups. This strategy is essential for the most complex policy issues such as income and employment. Publishing research findings in straightforward language makes the information available to all of the association's constituency.

Other strategies involve participation in coalitions and public education, as well as more aggressive advocacy such as political lobbying and legal challenges. Each of these actions has been undertaken with careful consideration, recognising the limited resources available and the need for each single action to reinforce an overall strategy (Richler, 1993).

In order to break down the barriers to community living, many different target groups have been identified. These include politicians, key public officials, service planners, the media, business and trades unions, and the general public. For each of these target groups, a different strategy has been developed. In many cases, strategies overlap and are mutually reinforcing.

So, for example, in order to achieve integration in education, there must be strategies that will change policies, laws, public attitudes and practice. The first step of the CACL's strategy in this area was to identify problems in the existing segregated systems and to articulate the vision of what inclusion could mean. One critical step in the process was to bring together parents who favoured integration but who lacked the confidence and skills to make it a reality for their children. Providing them with training side-by-side with teaching professionals gave the parents the confidence to be more persistent in their demands and also encouraged a few professionals to take risks and try including disabled students in ordinary classes. Publicising the success stories helped to build the demand by other parents and also to break down the resistance of the school system. A delicate balance of supporting litigation by some families while working with school boards in other regions in order to develop better examples led to the creation of new training programmes (summer schools on integration are now being run at universities across the country). Work was done to have the media cover success stories as well as stories about unjust exclusion from ordinary schools and classes. This has helped to create public acceptance of integrated education (Porter and Richler, 1991).

Embarking on a mission to achieve social change means that all activities of the association must be planned within the context of the broad strategies. No decisions can be made in isolation. Whether planning a fund raising event or a presentation to a parliamentary committee, the overall objectives of the association must be considered and all opportunities for making advances seized. As a result, fund raising strategies include one component which encourages the business community to become employers of individuals who have a learning difficulty and another component providing broad public education about the benefits of community living for all.

Just as the new conceptual framework has identified that the only deficit is at the community level, so, too, the solutions offered by the association are presented as solutions that will solve the community's problems. Therefore, inclusion in education is not pursued as something good only for students who have a learning difficulty, but rather as an approach that can also be good for all students, teachers and administration. It has taken considerable work for the association to learn to present arguments that do not suggest that something must be given to persons with a learning difficulty and, therefore, *de facto* taken from others. Instead, changes are promoted as being good for the community at large and the association has learned about the problems perceived by the others involved. In this way it can propose solutions that can meet their needs while accomplishing the association's objectives.

Although CACL's agenda for social change was rooted in the personal hopes and aspirations of its members, the translation into strategies has often meant that CACL has had to invest its energies in activities that seem far from the daily realities of individuals who have a learning difficulty. For example, the achievement of fundamental changes to the poverty of people with a learning difficulty requires an understanding of the relationship between all the different levels of state and local services providing direct funds to these individuals. It also requires an understanding of how such services interconnect with other sectors such as employment. To that end, the Roeher Institute has done major research in this area. It will take years for this research to achieve the social change required, but the research provides the basic building blocks. Advocacy efforts by the association will move this part of the social change agenda forward.

Throughout this process of attempting to bring about social change there must be a realisation that, although theories and strategies make sense at the national level, members struggling at the grass roots of the association and coping with the reality of everyday problems often find them hard to relate to. Therefore, an additional component of the strategy must be to continually educate the membership about how the strategy connects to their daily realities and how they can capitalise on opportunities to help to move the agenda forward.

Challenges to a national organisation such as CACL are to maintain a consistent strategy for long enough to have a significant impact; to remain flexible enough to be able to capitalise on opportunities; to continue to build consensus within; and to continuously foster the emergence of new leadership. *Community Living 2000* provides the framework. Our joint efforts achieve the goal.

There are numerous examples of the strides made in Canada to advance social well-being and to include people with disabilities in the political agenda. These steps include the recently won right to vote for people residing in mental health and other specialist institutions and the precedent-setting right to integrated education for all children in the province of New Brunswick. The Canadian Supreme Court decision *Re Eve* has limited the power of the state and other third parties to perform intrusive medical and other procedures on non-consenting adults who have a learning difficulty. These developments, along with a federally supported policy of deinstitutionalisation, broad and continuing reviews of guardianship and competency, new employment equity measures and government establishment of special task forces on disability, are all indicators of progress.

Much remains to be done, however, to shift the power from service delivery mechanisms back to the people whose citizenship is in jeopardy. It is now recognised that a disability does not change a person's human value or his or her presumed right to citizenship, to health and well-being or to the other benefits of citizenship. Disability simply affects the nature of support a person requires. Legal and constitutional protection of those rights has become the centre of the advocacy movement for those with a learning difficulty.

It has taken a long time to achieve this fundamental shift in thinking about where the deficit lies; a shift to thinking about persons with a learning difficulty as equal members of our society. The mandate to accept and accommodate individual differences, no matter what colour, race, religion or disability, is a challenge that can no longer be ignored. Those concerned with disability will have to provide the leadership and the creativity to ensure it moves beyond the conceptual level. Justice demands no less than that the legal and social guarantees necessary for the protection of those rights be secured.

References

Canadian Association for Community Living (1987). *Community Living 2000*. CACL, Ontario.

Porter, G.L. and Richler, D. (eds) (1991). *Changing Canadian Schools: Perspectives on Disability and Inclusion*. Roeher Institute, North York, Ontario.

Richler, D. (1993). Organizing for social change: How to get what we want. *Entourage*, (special issue: Politics and Advocacy), 8(1).

Roeher Institute (1988). *Income Insecurity: The Disability Income System in Canada*. Roeher Institute, North York, Ontario.

Roeher Institute (1992). *On Target? Canada's Employment-Related Programs for Persons with Disabilities*. Roeher Institute, North York, Ontario.

Roeher Institute (1990). *Poor Places: Disability-Related Residential and Support Services*. Roeher Institute, North York, Ontario.

Roeher Institute (1993). *Social Well-being*. Roeher Institute, North York, Ontario.

Index

£16.99

Values and Visions

X

For our sons, Robert Philpot and Ollie Ward
and for Cyril Ward